Sleep-Disordered Breathing: Beyond Obstructive Sleep Apnea

Editor

CAROLYN M. D'AMBROSIO

CLINICS IN
CHEST MEDICINE

www.chestmed.theclinics.com

September 2014 • Volume 35 • Number 3

ELSEVIER

1600 John F. Kennedy Boulevard • Suite 1800 • Philadelphia, Pennsylvania, 19103-2899

http://www.theclinics.com

CLINICS IN CHEST MEDICINE Volume 35, Number 3
September 2014 ISSN 0272-5231, ISBN-13: 978-0-323-32317-8

Editor: Patrick Manley
Developmental Editor: Casey Jackson

Clinics in Chest Medicine (ISSN 0272-5231) is published quarterly by Elsevier Inc., 360 Park Avenue South, New York, NY 10010-1710. Months of issue are March, June, September, and December. Periodicals postage paid at New York, NY and additional mailing offices. Subscription prices are $345.00 per year (domestic individuals), $556.00 per year (domestic institutions), $165.00 per year (domestic students/residents), $380.00 per year (Canadian individuals), $690.00 per year (Canadian institutions), $470.00 per year (international individuals), $690.00 per year (international institutions), and $230.00 per year (international and Canadian students/residents). International air speed delivery is included in all Clinics subscription prices. All prices are subject to change without notice. **POSTMASTER:** Send address changes to Clinics in Chest Medicine, Elsevier Health Sciences Division, Subscription Customer Service, 3251 Riverport Lane, Maryland Heights, MO 63043. **Customer Service: Telephone: 1-800-654-2452** (U.S. and Canada); **1-314-447-8871** (outside U.S. and Canada). **Fax: 1-314-447-8029. E-mail: journalscustomerservice-usa@elsevier.com** (for print support); **journalsonlinesupport-usa@elsevier.com** (for online support).

Reprints. For copies of 100 or more of articles in this publication, please contact the Commercial Reprints Department, Elsevier Inc., 360 Park Avenue South, New York, NY 10010-1710. Tel.: 212-633-3874; Fax: 212-633-3820; E-mail: reprints@elsevier.com.

Clinics in Chest Medicine is covered in *MEDLINE/PubMed (Index Medicus), Current Contents/Clinical Medicine, EMBASE/ Excerpta Medica, Science Citation Index,* and *ISI/BIOMED.*

Contributors

EDITOR

CAROLYN M. D'AMBROSIO, MD, MS
Director, The Center for Sleep Medicine,
Tufts Medical Center; Associate Professor of
Medicine, Pulmonary, Critical Care, and Sleep
Medicine Division, Tufts University School of
Medicine, Boston, Massachusetts

AUTHORS

JASON AMATOURY, MBiomedE, PhD
Department of Respiratory and Sleep Medicine,
Neuroscience Research Australia, Randwick,
New South Wales, Australia; Ludwig Engel
Centre for Respiratory Research, Westmead
Millennium Institute, and Sydney Medical School,
University of Sydney at Westmead Hospital,
Westmead, New South Wales, Australia

GHADA BOURJEILY, MD
Associate Professor of Medicine, Department
of Medicine, The Miriam Hospital, The Warren
Alpert Medical School of Brown University,
Providence, Rhode Island

MICHAEL S. CARROLL, PhD
Computational Neuroscientist, Center for
Autonomic Medicine in Pediatrics (CAMP),
Ann & Robert H. Lurie Children's Hospital of
Chicago; Department of Pediatrics,
Northwestern University Feinberg School of
Medicine, Chicago, Illinois

CAROLYN M. D'AMBROSIO, MD, MS
Director, The Center for Sleep Medicine,
Tufts Medical Center; Associate Professor of
Medicine, Pulmonary, Critical Care, and Sleep
Medicine Division, Tufts University School of
Medicine, Boston, Massachusetts

MARYANN C. DEAK, MD
Division of Sleep and Circadian Disorders,
Departments of Neurology and Medicine,
Brigham and Women's Hospital; Instructor,
Department of Neurology, Harvard Medical
School, Boston, Massachusetts

BETH HOTT, BA
Women's Medicine Collaborative, The Miriam
Hospital, Providence, Rhode Island

ELIOT S. KATZ, MD
Division of Respiratory Diseases, Department
of Medicine, Boston Children's Hospital;
Assistant Professor of Pediatrics, Harvard
Medical School, Boston, Massachusetts

DAVID T. KENT, MD
Department of Otolaryngology, University of
Pittsburgh School of Medicine, UPMC,
Pittsburgh, Pennsylvania

WAJAHAT H. KHAN, MD
Assistant Professor of Medicine, Department
of Sleep Medicine, University of Pennsylvania,
Philadelphia, Pennsylvania

JASON P. KIRKNESS, PhD
Division of Pulmonary, Critical Care, and Sleep
Medicine, Department of Medicine, Johns
Hopkins University, Baltimore, Maryland

DOUGLAS B. KIRSCH, MD
Assistant Medical Director, Sleep Disorders
Service; Division of Sleep and Circadian
Disorders, Departments of Neurology and
Medicine, Brigham and Women's Hospital;
Instructor, Department of Neurology, Harvard
Medical School, Boston, Massachusetts

MEIR KRYGER, MD
Professor of Medicine, Section of Pulmonary,
Critical Care and Sleep Medicine, Yale
University School of Medicine, New Haven,
Connecticut

TEOFILO LEE-CHIONG, MD
Professor of Medicine, Division of Pulmonary, Critical Care and Sleep Medicine, National Jewish Health, University of Colorado, Denver, Colorado

MARIAM LOUIS, MD
Assistant Professor of Medicine, Department of Medicine, University of Florida, Jacksonville, Florida

VIPIN MALIK, MD
Assistant Professor of Medicine, National Jewish Health, University of Colorado, Denver, Colorado

MONIQUE MALOUF, FRACP
Lung Transplant Unit, St Vincents Hospital, Darlinghurst, Sydney, Australia

VAHID MOHSENIN, MD
Professor of Medicine, Department of Pulmonary and Critical Care Medicine, Yale Center for Sleep Disorders, Yale University School of Medicine, New Haven, Connecticut

KELLY NEWTON, MD
Fellow, Sleep Medicine Program, National Jewish Health, Denver, Colorado

DENNIS OYIENGO, MD
Pulmonary and Critical Care Fellowship Program, The Warren Alpert Medical School of Brown University, Providence, Rhode Island

SUSHEEL P. PATIL, MD, PhD
Division of Pulmonary, Critical Care, and Sleep Medicine, Department of Medicine, Johns Hopkins University, Baltimore, Maryland

PAOLA PIERUCCI, MD
Lung Transplant Unit, St Vincents Hospital, Darlinghurst, Sydney, Australia

CASEY M. RAND, BS
Research Director, Center for Autonomic Medicine in Pediatrics (CAMP), Ann & Robert H. Lurie Children's Hospital of Chicago, Chicago, Illinois

CAROL L. ROSEN, MD
Division of Pediatric Pulmonology and Sleep Medicine, Department of Pediatrics, Rainbow Babies and Children's Hospital, Case Western Reserve University School of Medicine, Cleveland, Ohio

DAVID ROSEN, MD
Fellow, Pulmonary Medicine, Montefiore Medical Center, Bronx, New York

KRISTIE R. ROSS, MD, MS
Division of Pediatric Pulmonology and Sleep Medicine, Department of Pediatrics, Rainbow Babies and Children's Hospital, Case Western Reserve University School of Medicine, Cleveland, Ohio

FRANCOISE JOELLE ROUX, MD, PhD
Connecticut Multispecialty Group, Division of Pulmonary, Critical Care and Sleep Medicine, Hartford, Connecticut

GILBERT SEDA, MD, PhD
Department of Pulmonary and Sleep Medicine, Naval Medical Center San Diego, San Diego, California

NEOMI SHAH, MD, MPH
Pulmonary Medicine, Montefiore Medical Center, Bronx, New York

RYAN J. SOOSE, MD
Director, Division of Sleep Surgery; Assistant Professor, Department of Otolaryngology, University of Pittsburgh School of Medicine, UPMC, Pittsburgh, Pennsylvania

MUDIAGA SOWHO, MD, MPH
Division of Pulmonary, Critical Care, and Sleep Medicine, Department of Medicine, Johns Hopkins University, Baltimore, Maryland

SHEILA TSAI, MD
Division of Pulmonary, Critical Care and Sleep Medicine, National Jewish Health, Denver, Colorado

DEBRA E. WEESE-MAYER, MD
Chief, Center for Autonomic Medicine in Pediatrics (CAMP), Ann & Robert H. Lurie Children's Hospital of Chicago, Professor of Pediatrics, Northwestern University Feinberg School of Medicine, Chicago, Illinois

CHRISTINE H.J. WON, MD, MS
Assistant Professor of Medicine, Section of Pulmonary, Critical Care and Sleep Medicine, Yale University School of Medicine, New Haven, Connecticut

Contents

Sleep and Breathing   451

Kelly Newton, Vipin Malik, and Teofilo Lee-Chiong

> The sleep state is associated with significant changes in respiratory physiology, including ventilatory responses to hypoxia and hypercapnia, upper airway and intercostal muscle tone, and tidal volume and minute ventilation. These changes are further magnified in certain disease states, such as chronic obstructive pulmonary disease, restrictive respiratory disorders, neuromuscular conditions, and cardiac diseases. This article discusses the regulation of breathing during sleep in health and associated comorbid conditions.

Sleep and Respiratory Physiology in Children   457

Kristie R. Ross and Carol L. Rosen

> Maturational changes of breathing during sleep contribute to the unique features of childhood sleep disorders. The clinician's ability to evaluate common disorders related to sleep in children relies on an understanding of normal patterns of breathing during sleep across the ages. This article reviews respiratory physiology during sleep throughout childhood. Specific topics include an overview of respiration during sleep, normal parameters through childhood including respiratory rate, oxygen saturation, and measures of carbon dioxide, normal patterns of apneas throughout childhood, and features of breathing during sleep seen in term and preterm infants.

Sleep and Respiratory Physiology in Adults   469

Mudiaga Sowho, Jason Amatoury, Jason P. Kirkness, and Susheel P. Patil

> Respiration during sleep is determined by metabolic demand; respiratory drive is determined by a central respiratory generator. Changes in pharyngeal dilator muscle tone resulting in increased upper airway resistance and collapsibility contribute to hypoventilation. Relative hypotonia of respiratory muscles, body posture changes, and altered ventilatory control result in additional physiologic changes contributing to hypoventilation. This article reviews mechanisms of central control of respiration and normal upper and lower airway physiology. Understanding sleep-related changes in respiratory physiology will help in developing new therapies to prevent hypoventilation in susceptible populations.

Sleep in Asthma   483

Wajahat H. Khan, Vahid Mohsenin, and Carolyn M. D'Ambrosio

> Many patients with asthma experience worsening of symptoms at night. Understanding the mechanism of nocturnal asthma and the factors that exacerbate asthma during sleep would lead to better management of the condition.

Sleep disturbances are frequently observed in cystic fibrosis (CF). The resultant sleep fragmentation, short sleep duration, and gas-exchange abnormalities are postulated to contribute to the neurocognitive, cardiovascular, and metabolic abnormalities associated with CF. There are no outcomes data to establish the optimal procedure for screening and treating CF patients for sleep-related respiratory abnormalities. Therapy with supplemental oxygen and bilevel ventilation are widely considered to be effective in the short term, but there are few evidence-based data to support long-term improvements in morbidity and mortality.

Restrictive lung disease leads to ventilatory defects and diffusion impairments. These changes may contribute to abnormal nocturnal pathophysiology, including sleep architecture disruption and impaired ventilation and oxygenation. Patients with restrictive lung disease may suffer significant daytime fatigue and dysfunction. Hypercarbia and hypoxemia during sleep may impact progression of lung disease and related symptoms. Little is known about the impact of treatment of sleep disruption on sleep quality and overall prognosis in restrictive lung disease. This review discusses the pathophysiology of sleep and comorbid sleep disorders in restrictive lung diseases including interstitial lung disease, neuromuscular disease, and obesity hypoventilation syndrome.

During the past 20 years, lung transplantation (LTX) has evolved and it is now accepted as a mainstream modality for care of patients with severe life-threatening respiratory diseases that are refractory to maximal conventional therapies. Improvements in surgical techniques and in antirejection medications have resulted in prolonged survival in these patients. Several studies have explored quality of life after LTX and its improvement has been noted especially in the early period between 3 and 6 months. This article discusses the salient features of the physiology of breathing and sleep disturbances before and after LTX and its alterations during sleep.

Heart failure (HF) is one of the most prevalent and costly diseases in the United States. Sleep apnea is now recognized as a common, yet underdiagnosed, comorbidity of HF. This article discusses the unique qualities that sleep apnea has when it occurs in HF and explains the underlying pathophysiology that illuminates why sleep apnea and HF frequently occur together. The authors provide an overview of the treatment options for sleep apnea in HF and discuss the relative efficacies of these treatments.

Congenital central hypoventilation syndrome (CCHS), a rare neurocristopathy with disordered respiratory control, is characterized by alveolar hypoventilation and diffuse autonomic nervous system (ANS) dysregulation. Mutations in the paired-like homeobox 2B (*PHOX2B*) are causative, leading to physiologic ANS dysregulation and pathologic abnormalities. Presentation is typically during the newborn period with alveolar hypoventilation during sleep, or in more severely affected individuals, during sleep and wakefulness. Breathing complications occur despite the lungs and airways being normal. Disordered respiratory control demonstrated by absent or severely attenuated ventilatory, behavioral, and arousal responses to both endogenous and exogenous hypoxemia and hypercarbia results in severe physiologic compromise.

Sleep-related breathing disorder or sleep-disordered breathing (SDB) encompasses central sleep apnea (CSA), obstructive sleep apnea (OSA), and sleep-related hypoventilation or hypoxemic syndromes. SDB is common in neurologic conditions that affect the central and/or peripheral nervous systems. Patients with neurologic conditions are at risk for SDB due to a combination of factors such as muscular weakness, damage to areas of the brain that control respiration, use of sedating medications, and weight gain from limited physical activity. This article discusses recognition and treatment of SDB as important aspects of treating patients with neurologic disease.

Sleep respiration is regulated by circadian, endocrine, mechanical and chemical factors, and characterized by diminished ventilatory drive and changes in Pa_{O_2} and Pa_{CO_2} thresholds. Hypoxemia and hypercapnia are more pronounced during rapid eye movement. Breathing is influenced by sleep stage and airway muscle tone. Patient factors include medical comorbidities and body habitus. Medications partially improve obstructive sleep apnea and stabilize periodic breathing at altitude. Potential adverse consequences of medications include precipitation or worsening of disorders. Risk factors for adverse medication effects include aging, medical disorders, and use of multiple medications that affect respiration.

Sleep disturbances are common in pregnancy and may be influenced by a multitude of factors. Pregnancy physiology may predispose to sleep disruption but may also result in worsening of some underlying sleep disorders, and the de novo development of others. Apart from sleep disordered breathing, the impact of sleep disorders on pregnancy, fetal, and neonatal outcomes is poorly understood. In this article, we review the literature and discuss available data pertaining to the most common sleep disorders in perinatal women. These include restless legs syndrome, insomnia, circadian pattern disturbances, narcolepsy, and sleep-disordered breathing.

Allergic rhinitis and associated symptomatic nasal obstruction negatively affect sleep through a variety of mechanisms and may contribute to persistent symptoms and poor adherence with medical device therapy for sleep apnea. A history of sino-nasal symptoms, particularly those that occur at night or in the supine position, is the cornerstone of the medical evaluation. Further research into the relationship between allergic rhinitis and sleep disturbance would benefit from improved anatomic and pathophysiologic phenotyping as well as more advanced outcome measures such as spectral electroencephalogram analysis or other polysomnography variables beyond the apnea-hypopnea index.

PROGRAM OBJECTIVE

The goal of the *Clinics in Chest Medicine* is to provide provide practitioners with state-of-the-art information that is clinically useful, concise, well referenced, and comprehensive.

TARGET AUDIENCE

All practicing physicians and healthcare professionals who provide patient care utilizing findings from *Chest Medicine Clinics of North America*.

LEARNING OBJECTIVES

Upon completion of this activity, participants will be able to:
1. Review sleep disorders in pregnancy.
2. Discuss sleep and respiratory physiology in adults and children.
3. Recognize sleep disordered breathing in asthma, cystic fibrosis, lung disease, congestive heart failure, and neurological disorders.

ACCREDITATION

The Elsevier Office of Continuing Medical Education (EOCME) is accredited by the Accreditation Council for Continuing Medical Education (ACCME) to provide continuing medical education for physicians.

The EOCME designates this enduring material for a maximum of 15 *AMA PRA Category 1 Credit*(s)™. Physicians should claim only the credit commensurate with the extent of their participation in the activity.

All other health care professionals requesting continuing education credit for this enduring material will be issued a certificate of participation.

DISCLOSURE OF CONFLICTS OF INTEREST

The EOCME assesses conflict of interest with its instructors, faculty, planners, and other individuals who are in a position to control the content of CME activities. All relevant conflicts of interest that are identified are thoroughly vetted by EOCME for fair balance, scientific objectivity, and patient care recommendations. EOCME is committed to providing its learners with CME activities that promote improvements or quality in healthcare and not a specific proprietary business or a commercial interest.

The planning committee, staff, authors and editors listed below have identified no financial relationships or relationships to products or devices they or their spouse/life partner have with commercial interest related to the content of this CME activity:

Jason Amatoury, MBiomedE, PhD; Ghada Bourjeily, MD; Michael S. Carroll, PhD; Carolyn M. D'Ambrosio, MS, MD; Maryann C. Deak, MD; Kristen Helm; Beth Hott, BA; Brynne Hunter; Casey Jackson; Eliot S. Katz, MD; David T. Kent, MD; Wajahat H. Khan, MD; Jason P. Kirkness, PhD; Douglas B. Kirsch, MD; Meir Kryger, MD; Sandy Lavery; Mariam Louis, MD; Vipin Malik, MD; Monique Malouf, FRACP; Patrick Manley; Jill McNair; Vahid Mohsenin, MD; Palani Murugesan; Kelly Newton, MD; Dennis Oyiengo, MD; Susheel P. Patil, MD, PhD; Paola Pierucci, MD; Casey M. Rand, BS; Carol L. Rosen, MD; David Rosen, MD; Kristie R. Ross, MD, MS; Francoise Joelle Roux, MD, PhD; Gilbert Seda, MD, PhD; Neomi Shah, MD, MPH; Mudiaga Sowho, MD, MPH; Sheila Tsai, MD; Debra E. Weese-Mayer, MD; Christine H.J. Won, MD, MS.

The planning committee, staff, authors and editors listed below have identified financial relationships or relationships to products or devices they or their spouse/life partner have with commercial interest related to the content of this CME activity:

Teofilo Lee-Chiong, MD has stock ownership, research grant and an employment affiliation with Philips Respironics; is a consultant/advisor for Elsevier and CareCore National; and has royalties/patents with Elsevier, Wiley, Oxford University Press and Lippincott.
Ryan J. Soose, MD is a consultant/advisor for Inspire Medical Systems, Inc. and Philips Respironics; has research grant from Inspire Medical Systems, Inc.

UNAPPROVED/OFF-LABEL USE DISCLOSURE

The EOCME requires CME faculty to disclose to the participants:
1. When products or procedures being discussed are off-label, unlabelled, experimental, and/or investigational (not US Food and Drug Administration (FDA) approved); and
2. Any limitations on the information presented, such as data that are preliminary or that represent ongoing research, interim analyses, and/or unsupported opinions. Faculty may discuss information about pharmaceutical agents that is outside of FDA-approved labelling. This information is intended solely for CME and is not intended to promote off-label use of these medications. If you have any questions, contact the medical affairs department of the manufacturer for the most recent prescribing information.

TO ENROLL

To enroll in the *Chest Medicine Clinics* Continuing Medical Education program, call customer service at 1-800-654-2452 or sign up online at http://www.theclinics.com/home/cme. The CME program is available to subscribers for an additional annual fee of USD $345.

METHOD OF PARTICIPATION

In order to claim credit, participants must complete the following:

1. Complete enrolment as indicated above.
2. Read the activity.
3. Complete the CME Test and Evaluation. Participants must achieve a score of 70% on the test. All CME Tests and Evaluations must be completed online.

CME INQUIRIES/SPECIAL NEEDS

For all CME inquiries or special needs, please contact elsevierCME@elsevier.com.

CLINICS IN CHEST MEDICINE

FORTHCOMING ISSUES

December 2014
Acute Respiratory Distress Syndrome (ARDS)
Lorraine B. Ware, Julie A. Bastarache, and
Carolyn Calfee, *Editors*

March 2015
Non-Tuberculosis Mycobacteria
Gwen A. Huitt and Charles Daley, *Editors*

June 2015
Chest Imaging
David Lynch and Jonathan Chung, *Editors*

RECENT ISSUES

June 2014
**Pulmonary Rehabilitation: Role and
Advances**
Linda Nici and Richard L. ZuWallack, *Editors*

March 2014
Chronic Obstructive Pulmonary Disease
Peter J. Barnes, *Editor*

December 2013
Pulmonary Arterial Hypertension
Terence K. Trow, *Editor*

RELATED INTEREST

Sleep Medicine Clinics, Vol. 3, No. 4 (December 2008)
Respiratory Disorders and Sleep
U.J. Magalang, *Editor*

Preface

The Multifaceted Origins of Sleep-Disordered Breathing

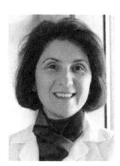

Carolyn M. D'Ambrosio, MD, MS
Editor

Sleep and breathing are intimately related. Pathologic conditions of one can adversely affect the other. The connection between sleep and breathing starts during fetal maturation and is influenced by many factors throughout life. Sleep is a very vulnerable time for patients with respiratory illness: the brainstem centers are blunted to both hypoxia and hypercapnea, and respiratory mechanics are affected by sleep. Patients with lung disease can have both significant breathing abnormalities due to the physiology of sleep and sleep disruption from the lung disease. Several previous issues of the *Clinics in Chest Medicine* were devoted to Sleep Medicine. This issue is different, because it focuses solely on Sleep-Disordered Breathing.

This issue contains 13 articles by 32 authors from institutions across the globe. To introduce this topic, Drs Newton, Malik, and Lee-Chiong review briefly the neurologic mechanisms involved in the control of breathing and highlight a few conditions, such as Obstructive Sleep Apnea and Central Sleep Apnea, that are not mentioned in depth elsewhere. Following this introduction of the topic, the first section is on Sleep and Respiratory Physiology. Drs Ross and Rosen discuss maturational changes of breathing during sleep from fetal development through infancy and childhood as well as normal respiratory physiology in these age groups. The next article, by Drs Sowho, Amatoury, Kirkness, and Patil, builds on this and reviews in great detail the interconnection of sleep and respiratory control at the neurologic level and the physiologic processes.

After introducing the normal physiology of sleep and breathing, the second section of this issue focuses on sleep in patients with respiratory conditions. Drs Khan, Mohsenin, and D'Ambrosio provide an update on the effects of sleep in patients with asthma. This article builds on an original article for the 1998 *Clinics in Chest Medicine* on Sleep and presents new data and recommendations for these patients. Dr Katz discusses the sleep-related breathing abnormalities that affect patients with cystic fibrosis and emphasizes the need to treat the sleep-related breathing difficulties as part of comprehensive care. The next article, by Drs Won and Kryger, focuses on the sleep-related breathing abnormalities of patients with restrictive lung disease. This article highlights that, although changes in breathing during sleep and changes in sleep patterns occur in patients with restrictive lung disease, little is known about how treating the breathing and sleep abnormalities might benefit these patients. To complete this section, Drs Pierucci and Malouf discuss sleep and breathing difficulties in patients undergoing lung transplantation. Although the neural circuits that control breathing by receiving and sending information from the lung are interrupted during transplant, little is actually known about sleep and breathing in this population.

Primary respiratory diseases are not the only conditions that can adversely affect sleep and breathing. The third section in this issue is dedicated to discussing sleep in patients with conditions that adversely affect the respiratory system

Clin Chest Med 35 (2014) xiii–xiv
http://dx.doi.org/10.1016/j.ccm.2014.07.001

and control of breathing. The respiratory system and the central nervous system are intertwined in regulating breathing. Many disorders that affect the central nervous system can have significant ramifications on breathing, especially during sleep. Drs Rosen, Shah, and Roux review the pathophysiology of how congestive heart failure plays a critical role in the development of sleep-disordered breathing. Environmental factors such as allergies can have a role in worsening breathing during sleep. One of those conditions, central congenital hypoventilation syndrome, is reviewed in great detail by Drs Rand, Carroll, and Weese-Mayer. With this inherited syndrome, patients are born with an inability to breathe properly when sleeping. Other neurologic conditions that affect sleep and breathing are discussed in another article by Drs Deak and Kirsch.

Many medications affect breathing during sleep. Drs. Seda, Tsai and Lee-Chiong provide an extensive review of common medications and the role each may have in sleep-disordered breathing. Congestive Heart Failure is well known to contribute to Cheynes-Stokes Respiration and other breathing abnormalities during sleep.

A non-pathologic condition that affects sleep and breathing is pregnancy. Complaints of disrupted sleep if quite common in pregnancy but it is important to know when a sleep disorder or sleep disordered breathing is the cause as treatment can be quite beneficial. Drs. Oyiengo, Louis and Bourjeilly with Ms. Hatt review the literature on sleep and pregnancy and make important diagnostic and treatment recommendations.

Finally, in this last article, Dr. Soose provides an extensive discussion of how environmental allergies affect the respiratory system and thus breathing during sleep.

I am deeply grateful to all of the contributors to this edition, to Patrick Manley and Casey Jackson at Elsevier for their invaluable guidance in this endeavor, and finally, to all the patients I have encountered with difficulty breathing especially during sleep as they are the inspiration for this work.

Carolyn M. D'Ambrosio, MD, MS
The Center for Sleep Medicine
Tufts Medical Center
Pulmonary, Critical Care, and
Sleep Medicine Division
Tufts University School of Medicine
800 Washington Street, #4
Boston, MA 02111, USA

E-mail address:
cdambrosio@tuftsmedicalcenter.org

Sleep and Breathing

 CrossMark

Kelly Newton, MD[a],*, Vipin Malik, MD[a,b], Teofilo Lee-Chiong, MD[a,b]

KEYWORDS

- Sleep • Breathing • Respiratory physiology • Sleep-disordered breathing

KEY POINTS

- Complex interaction between neurophysiological controllers and mechanical effectors regulate ventilation.
- Upper-airway narrowing and excess weight along with sleep related positional changes affect the mechanics of breathing and gas exchange.
- These changes are further magnified in certain disease states, such as COPD, restrictive respiratory disorders, neuromuscular conditions, and cardiac diseases.

INTRODUCTION

Control of breathing during sleep involves a complicated physiologic process that differs from that during wakefulness. Complex neurologic and respiratory mechanisms are impacted by host disease states, including specific sleep-related anatomic considerations (eg, upper airway, intercostal, and diaphragm muscles). Derangements in any of these factors can give rise to abnormalities of gas exchange, such as hypoxemia and hypercapnia, or sleep-disordered breathing, including snoring, obstructive and central sleep apneas, Cheyne-Stokes respiration, Biot breathing, and the various hypoventilation syndromes. This article introduces the basic physiology and concepts that are discussed in greater detail in the ensuing articles.

This article discusses the regulation of breathing during sleep as well as screening, diagnostic approaches, and current treatment modalities for sleep-disordered breathing.

NEURAL CONTROL OF BREATHING DURING SLEEP

Medullary respiratory neurons, including the dorsal respiratory group (DRG), ventral respiratory group (VRG), and cranial motor neurons innervating the pharyngeal and laryngeal muscles, receive efferent fibers from the pontine respiratory group.[1] The dorsomedial medulla in the ventrolateral nucleus of the solitary tract contains inspiratory neurons, whereas the VRG contains the nucleus ambiguous, expiratory neurons (Bötzinger complex and caudal retroambigualis), and inspiratory neurons (pre-Bötzinger complex and rostral retroambigualis).[2,3] Pre-Bötzinger complex neurons are thought to possess pacemakerlike properties that generate the basic respiratory rhythm.[4,5]

Afferent neurons (vagal from the lung, carotid/aortic chemoreceptors and baroreceptors) project to the dorsal respiratory group and assorted subnuclei of the medullary solitary tract. Information regarding Pa_{CO_2}, Pa_{O_2}, acid-base balance (pH), and blood pressure are integrated via this mechanism. Inspiratory and expiratory neurons are also present in the ventral respiratory group.[2,3] Motor neurons innervating the pharyngeal and laryngeal muscles are located in subregions of the nucleus ambiguus and extend rostrocaudally.[1] Cranial nerves (hypoglossal, trigeminal, and facial motor nuclei) innervate the upper airway muscles to maintain the latter's patency.[6] Finally, the DRG and VRG neurons project to spinal motor neurons that, in turn, innervate their respective respiratory muscles.[2,3]

[a] Sleep Medicine Program, National Jewish Health, 1400 Jackson Street, Denver, CO 80206, USA; [b] National Jewish Health, University of Colorado, 1400 Jackson Street, Denver, CO 80206, USA
* Corresponding author.
E-mail address: newtonk@NJHealth.org

Clin Chest Med 35 (2014) 451–456
http://dx.doi.org/10.1016/j.ccm.2014.06.001

The respiratory propriobulbar, premotor neuron and motor neurons are responsible for generating the respiratory rhythm and the central respiratory drive. There are several models regarding the generation of the respiratory rhythm, namely, the pacemaker, network, and hybrid models.[1,2,5] During inspiration, central neurons (DRG and VRG) innervate the phrenic and intercostal motor neurons. Expiratory neurons inhibit the inspiratory neurons allowing exhalation to occur.[2]

Mechanisms that control the activity of the pharyngeal motor neurons differ from those that control the spinal respiratory muscles.[2] Inspiratory drive to the hypoglossal motoneurons arises predominately from the reticular formation, which provides tonic drive to the respiratory system; it is significantly affected during sleep.[1,2] Activity of muscles with respiratory and nonrespiratory (postural/behavioral) functions, such as intercostal and pharyngeal muscles, is suppressed during sleep.[7]

RESPIRATORY PHYSIOLOGY DURING SLEEP

Muscles of respiration do not possess an intrinsic pacemaker and have to be controlled centrally. The respiratory center responds to chemical information (Pao_2 and $Paco_2$) via the carotid/aortic chemoreceptors and baroreceptors; mechanical information from vagal afferent neurons (stretch, deflation, congestion of lungs); and behavioral data (wakefulness stimulus).[8]

HYPOXIA

Ventilatory response to hypoxia is blunted during sleep.[9–12] A sex difference in hypoxic drive has been described. Hypoxic ventilatory response during wakefulness is much higher in men than women.[12] In addition, although hypoxic ventilatory response is lower during non–rapid eye movement (NREM) sleep than wakefulness among men, it is similar during NREM sleep and waking in women.[9,10] Whether this contributes to the decreased prevalence of sleep-disordered breathing among premenopausal women is unclear.[11–14] The hypoxic ventilatory response declines further during REM sleep.[9–12] Isocapnic hypoxia is not a major stimulus for arousal in normal adults, who can remain asleep even if arterial saturation decreases to as low as 70%.[9–11]

HYPERCAPNIA

The hypercapnic ventilatory response is also reduced during sleep and is most blunted during REM sleep.[15] As in the case with hypoxia, the ventilatory drive to hypercapnia does not change significantly from wakefulness to NREM sleep in women, who have higher ventilatory responses during sleep compared with men.[16,17]

Hypercapnia produces arousals from sleep, generally when end-tidal carbon dioxide levels reach 15 mm Hg more than baseline values.[11,15,18,19] Concurrent hypoxia increases the sensitivity to hypercapnic arousal.[20]

AIRWAY RESISTANCE

Increases in airway resistance, including the addition of inspiratory resistance or occlusion during inspiration, also lead to arousals.[21,22] Arousal frequency increases during NREM stages 2 and 3 sleep and REM sleep when inspiratory resistance is added.[23] The frequency of arousals from additional inspiratory resistance is lowest during slow wave sleep.[24,25] In contrast, airway occlusion produces more arousals during REM sleep.[26,27]

Upper airway resistance is increased during sleep, as a reduction in upper airway muscle tone causes anatomic structures to become more prone to collapse. This effect is compounded by positional changes during sleep or increased vascular congestion.

Regularity of Breathing During Sleep

Irregular breathing patterns can develop during sleep, especially during stages NREM 1 and 2 sleep. Periodic breathing, including episodic central apneas, can arise when carbon dioxide sensitivity and threshold changes from wakefulness (lower) to sleep (higher) levels.[19,28] Experimental hypocapnia with and without hypoxia has been demonstrated to induce irregular breathing patterns during NREM sleep.[29] The apnea threshold is higher in premenopausal women than in both men and postmenopausal women.[30] Hypocapnia in conjunction with increased airway resistance may lead to occlusive apneas.[31]

Respiratory Muscle Function During Sleep

Respiratory functional residual capacity is reduced in the supine, compared with the upright, position because of the relative inability of chest wall expansion to counter an increased abdominal pressure. During REM, sleep-associated atonia of the intercostal muscles results in decreased chest wall compliance and leaves the diaphragm as the sole musculature of respiration. Respiratory muscle atonia along with decreased hypercapnic and hypoxic chemosensitivity, can lead to hypoventilation during REM sleep.

Other important changes in respiratory physiology occur during sleep: (1) reduced ventilatory response to elastic loading, (2) decreased minute ventilation, and (3) increased upper airway resistance. The decreased minute ventilation is primarily caused by lower tidal volumes, with less marked changes in the respiratory rate and no significant change in the inspiratory time ratio.

CLINICAL IMPLICATIONS

Sleep-related impairments in ventilatory drive, blunted responses to hypercapnia, and increased upper airway resistance contribute to the development of sleep-disordered breathing. Obstructive sleep apnea (OSA) results from a combination of several factors, including upper airway collapsibility, genioglossus hyporesponsiveness, and low arousal threshold.[32–42]

OSA

The prevalence of OSA is currently estimated at 5% to 10% of the general population.[43,44] Balance between collapsing and dilating forces determines the patency of the upper airways. Collapse of the upper airway occurs at a critical closing pressure (Pcrit). Retrognathia, enlarged tonsils/adenoids, and nocturnal rostral fluid shift during sleep can increase Pcrit,[45–55] thereby increasing the likelihood of obstructive apnea-hypopneas occurring.

The activity of the upper airway dilator muscles, including the genioglossus, is controlled by respiratory pattern-generating neurons in the medulla, the wakefulness stimulus mediated by wake-promoting neurons, and mechanoreceptors located in the larynx. Central respiratory input to the pharyngeal muscles is reduced during sleep, as are reflex dilatory activity and tonicity of the genioglossus and tensor palatini. Tension on the airway walls is also reduced during sleep and in the supine position because of the loss of caudal traction. Collectively, these events increase upper airway collapsibility and cause airflow obstruction. To compensate for this greater airflow resistance, the work of breathing increases; this, in turn, results in higher $Paco_2$ levels.

Positive airway pressure therapy for OSA can, itself, give rise to sleep disruption because of pressure intolerance or mask discomfort. It can also result in the emergence of central apneas (discussed in the next section).

CENTRAL SLEEP APNEA

The concept of loop gain can explain several pathophysiologic mechanisms affecting chemoregulatory control of breathing during sleep. In simple terms, a given disturbance in any system usually elicits a specific response. A response is appropriate when it results in movement of the disturbance in a desired direction and to a desired extent, consequently reestablishing system stability. On the other hand, instability in a system can be caused by a delay in response or a markedly exaggerated response to a given disturbance.

Both controller and plant gain affect loop gain. Controller gain refers to chemoresponsiveness, whereas plant gain is ventilatory efficiency in eliminating carbon dioxide. With high controller gain, a smaller change in $Paco_2$ is required to reach the apneic threshold (ie, brisk hypercapnic responsiveness). With high plant gain, a small change in ventilation will result in exaggerated carbon dioxide clearance. Sleep results in reduced functional residual capacity, metabolic rate, and cardiac output as well as higher $Paco_2$, all of which increases plant gain. These mechanisms lead to significant respiratory instability and can predispose to central apneas in susceptible individuals.

The term *complex sleep apnea* refers to the emergence, persistence, or worsening of central apneas during PAP titration or treatment, oral appliance therapy, or upper airway surgery in a patient with predominantly obstructive or mixed apnea-hypopneas during a baseline diagnostic sleep study. The probability of complex sleep apnea developing is greater if there is a narrow difference between baseline $Paco_2$ and the apneic threshold (carbon dioxide reserve) or if respiratory sensitivity to $Paco_2$ is increased (controller gain).

OBSTRUCTIVE LUNG DISEASE

Sleep can significantly affect gas exchange and worsen both hypoxemia and hypercapnia in patients with chronic obstructive pulmonary disease (COPD) caused by sleep-related reductions in airflow, decreased response to increments in work of breathing, ventilatory hyporesponsiveness, and ventilation perfusion mismatch. Changes in blood gas values are particularly prominent during REM sleep.

Patients with COPD present with sleep maintenance/initiation insomnia, frequent nighttime awakenings, and reduced sleep efficiency.[56] In emphysema, intrinsic positive end-expiratory pressure, hyperinflation, and reduced resistive loading can stimulate pulmonary mechanoreceptors and, consequently, increase arousals. Nocturnal coughing and wheezing (reported in up to 53% patients) can also disrupt sleep continuity.[57] The coexistence of COPD and OSA, known as the *overlap syndrome*, also results in sleep fragmentation.[58]

Sleep disturbance in COPD is predictive of exacerbations, respiratory-related emergency utilization, and all-cause mortality.[59,60]

RESTRICTIVE LUNG DISEASE

Significant sleep disturbance can complicate chronic interstitial lung disease. Nocturnal dyspnea and cough, increased work of breathing, and abnormal gas exchange can negatively impact sleep quality. Nonrestorative sleep can, in turn, worsen daytime fatigue and diminish activity levels.[61–66]

Noninvasive ventilation can improve oxygen saturation and sleep quality in patients with chronic respiratory failure caused by thoracic restrictive disorders.[67,68]

SUMMARY

The sleep state is associated with significant changes in respiratory physiology, including ventilatory responses to hypoxia and hypercapnia, upper airway and intercostal muscle tone, and tidal volume and minute ventilation. These changes are further magnified in certain disease states, such as COPD, restrictive respiratory disorders, neuromuscular conditions, and cardiac diseases.

REFERENCES

1. Orem J, Kubin L. Respiratory physiology: central neural control. In: Kryger MH, Roth T, Dement WC, editors. Principles and practice of sleep medicine. 3rd edition. Philadelphia: Saunders; 2000. p. 205–20.
2. Duffin J. Functional organization of respiratory neurons: a brief review of current questions and speculations. Exp Physiol 2004;89:517–29.
3. Rekling JC, Feldman JL. Pre-Botzinger complex and pacemaker neurons: hypothesized site and kernel for respiratory rhythm generation. Annu Rev Physiol 1998;60:385–405.
4. Smith JC, Ellenberger HH, Ballanyi K, et al. Pre-Botzinger complex: a brainstem region that may generate respiratory rhythm in mammals. Science 1991;254:726–9.
5. Feldman JL, Del Negro CA. Looking for inspiration: new perspective on respiratory rhythm. Nat Rev Neurosci 2006;7:232–41.
6. Horner RL. Motor control of the pharyngeal musculature and implications for the pathogenesis of obstructive sleep apnea. Sleep 1996;19:827–53.
7. Worsnop C, Kay A, Pierce R, et al. Activity of respiratory pump and upper airway muscles during sleep onset. J Appl Physiol 1998;85:908–20.
8. Kryger MH, Roth T, Dement WC. Principles and practice of sleep medicine. 5th edition.
9. Douglas NJ, White DP, Weil JV, et al. Hypoxic ventilatory response decreases during sleep in normal men. Am Rev Respir Dis 1982;125:286–9.
10. Berthon-Jones M, Sullivan CE. Ventilatory and arousal responses to hypoxia in sleeping humans. Am Rev Respir Dis 1982;125:632–9.
11. Hedemark LL, Kronenberg RS. Ventilatory and heart rate responses to hypoxia and hypercapnea during sleep in adults. J Appl Physiol 1982;53:307–12.
12. White DP, Douglas NJ, Pickett CK, et al. Hypoxic ventilatory response during sleep in normal women. Am Rev Respir Dis 1982;126:530–3.
13. Gothe B, Goldman MD, Cherniak NS, et al. Effect of progressive hypoxia on breathing during sleep. Am Rev Respir Dis 1982;126:97–102.
14. Tarbichi AG, Rowley JA, Shkoukani MA, et al. Lack of gender difference in ventilatory chemoresponsiveness and post-hypoxic ventilatory decline. Respir Physiol Neurobiol 2003;137:41–50.
15. Douglas NJ, White DP, Weil JV, et al. Hypercapnic ventilatory response in sleeping adults. Am Rev Respir Dis 1982;126:758–62.
16. Berthon-Jones M, Sullivan CE. Ventilation and arousal responses to hypercapnia in normal sleeping adults. J Appl Physiol 1984;57:59–67.
17. Davis JN, Loh L, Nodal J, et al. Effects of sleeping on the pattern of CO2 stimulated breathing in males and females. Adv Exp Med Biol 1978;99:79–83.
18. Birchfield RI, Sicker HO, Heyman A. Alterations in respiratory function during natural sleep. J Lab Clin Med 1959;54:216–22.
19. Bulow K. Respiration and wakefulness in man. Acta Physiol Scand 1963;59(Suppl 209):1–110.
20. Sullivan CE, Issa FG. Pathophysiological mechanisms in obstructive sleep apnea. Sleep 1980;3:235–46.
21. Iber C, Berssenbrugge A, Skatrud JB, et al. Ventilatory adaptations to resistive loading during wakefulness and non-REM sleep. J Appl Physiol 1982;52:607–14.
22. Gothe B, Cherniak NS, Williams L. Effect of hypoxia on ventilatory and arousal responses to CO2 during non-REM sleep with and without flurazepam in young adults. Sleep 1986;9:24–37.
23. Gugger M, Molloy J, Gould GA, et al. Ventilatory and arousal responses to added inspiratory resistance during sleep. Am Rev Respir Dis 1989;140:1301–7.
24. Santiago TV, Sinha AK, Edelman NH. Respiratory flow-resistive load compensation during sleep. Am Rev Respir Dis 1981;123:382–7.
25. Netick A, Dugger WJ, Symmons RA. Ventilatory response to hypercapnia during sleep and wakefulness in cats. J Appl Physiol 1984;56:1347–54.
26. Issa FG, Sullivan CE. Arousal and breathing responses to airway occlusion in healthy sleeping adults. J Appl Physiol 1983;55:1113–9.
27. Gugger M, Bogershausen S, Schaffler L. Arousal response to added inspiratory resistance during

REM and non-REM sleep in normal subjects. Thorax 1993;48:125–9.

28. Douglas NJ, White DP, Pickett CK, et al. Respiration during sleep in normal man. Thorax 1982;37: 840–4.

29. Skatrud JB, Dempsey JA. Interaction of sleep state and chemical stimuli in sustaining rhythmic ventilation. J Appl Physiol 1983;55:813–22.

30. Rowley JA, Zhou XS, Diamond MP, et al. The determinants of the apnea threshold during NREM sleep in normal subjects. Sleep 2006;29:95–103.

31. Onal F, Burrows DL, Hart RH, et al. Induction of periodic breathing during sleeping causes upper airway obstruction in humans. J Appl Physiol 1986;61:1438–43.

32. Eckert D, White D, Jordan A, et al. Defining phenotypic causes of obstructive sleep apnea. Am J Respir Crit Care Med 2013;188:996–1004.

33. Gleadhill IC, Schwartz AR, Schubert N, et al. Upper airway collapsibility in snorers and in patients with obstructive hypopnea and apnea. Am Rev Respir Dis 1991;143:1300–3.

34. Jordan AS, Wellman A, Heinzer RC, et al. Mechanisms used to restore ventilation after partial airway collapse during sleep in humans. Thorax 2007;62: 861–7.

35. Loewen AH, Ostrowski M, Laprairie J, et al. Response of genioglossus muscle to increasing chemical drive in sleeping obstructive sleep apnea patients. Sleep 2011;34:1061–73.

36. Eckert DJ, Owens RL, Kehlmann GB, et al. Eszopiclone increases the respiratory arousal threshold and lowers the apnoea/hypopnoea index in obstructive sleep apnoea patients with a low arousal threshold. Clin Sci (Lond) 2011;120:505–14.

37. Younes M. Role of arousals in the pathogenesis of obstructive sleep apnea. Am J Respir Crit Care Med 2004;169:623–33.

38. Younes M, Ostrowski M, Atkar R, et al. Mechanisms of breathing instability in patients with obstructive sleep apnea. J Appl Physiol 2007;103:1929–41.

39. Longobardo GS, Evangelisti CJ, Cherniack NS. Analysis of the interplay between neurochemical control of respiration and upper airway mechanics producing upper airway obstruction during sleep in humans. Exp Physiol 2008;93:271–87.

40. Younes M. Role of respiratory control mechanisms in the pathogenesis of obstructive sleep disorders. J Appl Physiol 2008;105:1389–405.

41. Younes M, Ostrowski M, Thompson W, et al. Chemical control stability in patients with obstructive sleep apnea. Am J Respir Crit Care Med 2001; 163:1181–90.

42. Wellman A, Jordan AS, Malhotra A, et al. Ventilatory control and airway anatomy in obstructive sleep apnea. Am J Respir Crit Care Med 2004;170: 1225–32.

43. Tishler PV, Larkin EK, Schluchter MD, et al. Incidence of sleep-disordered breathing in an urban adult population; the relative importance of risk factors in the development of sleep-disordered breathing. JAMA 2003;289:2230–7.

44. Young T, Peppard PE, Gottlieb DJ. Epidemiology of obstructive sleep apnea; a population health perspective. Am J Respir Crit Care Med 2002; 165:1217–39.

45. Yumino D, Redolfi S, Ruttanaumpawan P, et al. Nocturnal rostral fluid shift: a unifying concept for the pathogenesis of obstructive and central sleep apnea in men with heart failure. Circulation 2010; 121(14):1598–605.

46. Dempsey J. Crossing the apnoeic threshold: causes and consequences. Exp Physiol 2004;90: 13–24.

47. White DP. Pathogenesis of obstructive and central sleep apnea. Am J Respir Crit Care Med 2005; 172:1363–70.

48. Sawicka EH, Branthwaite MA. Respiration during sleep in kyphoscoliosis. Thorax 1987;42:801–8.

49. McNicholas WT, Fitzgerald MX. Nocturnal death among patients with chronic bronchitis and emphysema. BMJ 1984;289:878.

50. McNicholas WT, Carter JL, Rutherford R, et al. Beneficial effects of oxygen in primary alveolar hypoventilation with central sleep apnea. Am Rev Respir Dis 1982;125:773–5.

51. Labanowski M, Schmidt-Nowara W, Guilleminault C. Sleep and neuromuscular disease: frequency of sleep-disordered breathing in a neuromuscular disease clinic population. Neurology 1996;47:1173–80.

52. Johnson MW, Remmers JE. Accessory muscle activity during sleep in chronic obstructive pulmonary disease. J Appl Physiol 1984;57:1011–7.

53. Jackson M, Smith I, King M, et al. Long-term non-invasive domiciliary assisted ventilation for respiratory failure following thoracoplasty. Thorax 1994;49: 915–9.

54. Hudgel DW, Martin RJ, Johnson BJ, et al. Mechanics of the respiratory system and breathing pattern during sleep in normal humans. J Appl Physiol Respir Environ Exerc Physiol 1984;56: 133–7.

55. Hetzel MR, Clark TJ. Comparison of normal and asthmatic circadian rhythms in peak flow rate. Thorax 1980;35:732–8, 24.

56. McSharry DG, Ryan S, Calverley P, et al. Sleep quality in chronic obstructive pulmonary disease. Respirology 2012;17:1119–24.

57. Klink M, Quan SF. Prevalence of reported sleep disturbances in a general adult population and their relationship to obstructive airways diseases. Chest 1987;91:540–6.

58. Krachman SL, Chatila W, Martin UJ, et al. Effects of lung volume reduction surgery on sleep quality and

nocturnal gas exchange in patients with severe emphysema. Chest 2005;128:3221–8.

59. Zhang L, Samet J, Caffo B, et al. Power spectral analysis of EEG activity during sleep in cigarette smokers. Chest 2008;133:427–32.

60. Omachi TA, Blanc PD, Claman DM, et al. Disturbed sleep among COPD patients is longitudinally associated with mortality and adverse COPD outcomes. Sleep Med 2012;13:476–83.

61. Perez-Padilla R, West P, Lertzman M, et al. Breathing during sleep in patients with interstitial lung disease. Am Rev Respir Dis 1985;132: 224–9.

62. American Thoracic Society. Statement on home care for patients with respiratory disorders. Am J Respir Crit Care Med 2005;171:1443–64.

63. Nugent AM, Smith IE, Shneerson JM. Domiciliary-assisted ventilation in patients with myotonic dystrophy. Chest 2002;121:459–64.

64. Swigris JJ, Kuschner WG, Jacobs SS, et al. Health-related quality of life in patients with idiopathic pulmonary fibrosis: a systematic review. Thorax 2005; 60:588–94.

65. Swigris J, Stewart A, Gould M, et al. Patients' perspectives on how idiopathic pulmonary fibrosis affects the quality of their lives. Health Qual Life Outcomes 2005;3:61.

66. Vries JD, Kessels BLJ, Drent M. Quality of life of idiopathic pulmonary fibrosis patients. Eur Respir J 2001;17:954–61.

67. Schönhofer B, Köhler D. Effect of non-invasive mechanical ventilation on sleep and nocturnal ventilation in patients with chronic respiratory failure. Thorax 2000;55(4):308–13.

68. Contal O, Janssens JP, Dury M, et al. Sleep in ventilatory failure in restrictive thoracic disorders. Effects of treatment with non invasive ventilation. Sleep Med 2011;12:373–7.

Sleep and Respiratory Physiology in Children

Kristie R. Ross, MD, MS*, Carol L. Rosen, MD

KEYWORDS

- Respiration • Reference values • Oxygen saturation • Carbon dioxide • Sleep/physiology • Child
- Infant • Adolescent

KEY POINTS

- The maturation of respiratory physiology during sleep contributes to the unique features of childhood sleep disorders.
- Ventilation decreases during sleep in children as it does in adults, with variability related to sleep state.
- Knowledge of the range of normal values of respiratory parameters during sleep, including respiratory rates, oxygen saturation, measures of carbon dioxide, and number and patterns of apneas, is crucial for the physician to evaluate common sleep disorders in children.

INTRODUCTION

Sleep is a critical determinant of health. As a child develops from infancy through adolescence, important changes in respiratory physiology occur. Maturational changes of breathing during sleep contribute to the unique features of childhood sleep disorders. The clinician's ability to evaluate common disorders related to sleep in children, including apnea of prematurity, sudden infant death syndrome (SIDS), apparent life threatening events (ALTE), obstructive sleep apnea syndrome, and other forms of sleep-disordered breathing relies on an understanding of normal patterns of breathing during sleep across the ages. The purpose of this article is to review respiratory physiology during sleep throughout childhood.

OVERVIEW OF NORMAL RESPIRATION DURING SLEEP

Breathing during sleep is controlled by voluntary and behavioral factors in addition to metabolic and mechanical factors.[1] Chemical information is relayed through peripheral chemoreceptors in the carotid and aortic bodies. The carotid chemoreceptors, although small, have a uniquely high blood supply, and sense the arterial concentration of O_2 and relay the information to the medulla. The carotid body chemoreceptors are responsible for about 90% of the ventilatory response to hypoxemia. Chemosensory function in the carotid bodies is immature at birth and increases with age. Carbon dioxide (CO_2) is also sensed in the carotid body, accounting for 20% to 50% of the response to arterial hypercapnia. The remaining response to hypercapnia comes from central brainstem receptors in the medulla. The central chemoreceptors respond primarily to changes in pH, mediated by CO_2 tension, in the cerebrospinal fluid. Laryngeal chemoreflexes (LCR) located in the epithelium that surrounds the airway respond to acidic solutions with reflexes that include startle, swallowing, laryngeal constriction, apnea, and bradycardia. Mechanical information sensed through receptors in the lung and chest wall are also relayed to the

Disclosure: The authors have no disclosures relevant to this article.
Division of Pediatric Pulmonology and Sleep Medicine, Department of Pediatrics, Rainbow Babies and Children's Hospital, Case Western Reserve University School of Medicine, 11100 Euclid Avenue, RBC 3001, Cleveland, OH 44106, USA
* Corresponding author.
E-mail address: Kristie.ross@uhhospitals.org

Clin Chest Med 35 (2014) 457–467
http://dx.doi.org/10.1016/j.ccm.2014.06.003

medulla via the vagal nerve. Higher central nervous system centers can override the respiratory centers to control nonbreathing functions such as speaking and laughing. These voluntary and behavioral controls are affected by sleep state. Clinical problems associated with disorders of respiratory control are listed in **Box 1**.

In general, ventilation decreases during sleep compared with wakefulness, but varies with sleep state. During non–rapid eye movement (NREM) sleep, breathing is regulated primarily by carbon dioxide and is characterized by the absence of behavioral controls. Breathing is regular with reduced tidal volume and respiratory rate compared with wakefulness, resulting in decreased minute ventilation. This decline, in combination with the supine position and decrease in intercostal muscle tone, results in a decrease in functional residual capacity. Upper airway tone and lung volume also decrease during sleep, resulting in increased upper airway resistance. Compared with the regular breathing seen during NREM sleep, breathing during rapid eye movement (REM) sleep is irregular in terms of both respiratory rate and tidal volume. Short central respiratory pauses are common during REM sleep in children. Inhibition of tonic activity of the intercostal muscles during REM results in a further decline in functional residual capacity. At the same time, activity of the diaphragm remains stable, and this incoordination between the intercostal muscles and diaphragm results in paradoxic chest and abdominal movement during REM sleep that usually resolves by the age of 3 years. A relative decrease in upper airway muscle tone when diaphragmatic contractions remain unchanged can predispose to obstructive apnea, especially when the airway is already small or narrow. Finally, hypoxic and hypercapnic ventilatory drives decrease during sleep. Therefore, normal children experience a small increase in the partial pressure of CO_2 and a small decrease in arterial oxyhemoglobin saturation (Spo_2) during sleep. The magnitude of these changes has not been systematically studied in large pediatric samples of healthy children, but is believed to average 2% for Spo_2 and 4 to 6 mm Hg for CO_2.[2] These sleep-related changes in ventilation, upper airway stability, and gas exchange can be exaggerated in children with underlying pulmonary, upper airway, and neuromuscular problems, resulting in increased vulnerability to sleep-disordered breathing. Differences between newborn and adult respiratory systems that make the infant more vulnerable to ventilatory failure are summarized in **Box 2**.

DEVELOPMENTAL CHANGES IN RESPIRATORY CONTROLLERS

Postnatally there is an increase in the hypoxic sensitivity (resetting) of both carotid and aortic chemoreceptors, and a diminishing influence of descending inhibitory effects on breathing in hypoxia.[3] Compared with the adult, peripheral chemoreceptors assume a greater role in the newborn. Although not essential for initiation of fetal respiratory movements, animal studies show that peripheral chemoreceptor denervation in the newborn period results in severe respiratory impairment and a high probability of sudden death. In the newborn, steady-state hypoxia produces a transient increase in ventilation followed by a decrease back to or below baseline level. With maturation, this biphasic response to hypoxia changes to a sustained ventilatory response. By contrast, a steady-state response to CO_2 is present at all ages from birth and increases with advancing postnatal age. There are only limited data on ventilatory responses in different sleep states in infants, but the directionality is similar to the findings in adults, with responses to hypoxia and hypercapnia that are reduced in REM compared with NREM sleep. In the newborn, hypercapnia and hypoxic ventilatory responses interact to augment respiratory responses. With increasing age, peripheral chemoreceptors undergo progressive decrement in their relative sensitivity.[4] LCR responses are significantly more active in the immediate postnatal period compared with later in life, and the pattern of the response also changes with maturation. The predominant LCR response in the newborn includes swallowing and apnea, and differs from the LCR responses seen in the older infant or adult (cough and the expiration reflex).[5,6]

VENTILATION, RESPIRATORY PATTERNS, AND APNEAS

Normative data on tidal volume and minute ventilation in children are not readily available, as most studies have focused on describing respiratory rates and patterns, gas exchange, and the frequency and type of apneas seen in healthy children of various ages. More data are available for preterm and full-term infants in the first months of life than for children and adolescents, but several new reports of normative sleep and breathing data in these age groups have been published.[7–9]

Respiratory Frequency

As would be predicted from knowledge about the inverse relationship between respiratory rate and body size in other mammals,[10] respiratory rates

Box 1
Clinical problems associated with disorders of respiratory control in children

Psychogenic
Hyperventilation
Habitual cough
Vocal cord dysfunction

Reflexive
Breath-holding spell
Expiratory apnea

Neurometabolic or Genetic Disorders
Central congenital hypoventilation syndrome
Central hypoventilation associated with hypothalamic or endocrine dysfunction
Rett syndrome
Leigh disease
Prader-Willi syndrome

Conditions Associated with Brainstem Malformation or Brainstem Lesions
Arnold-Chiari malformation
Dandy-Walker malformation
Möbius syndrome
Hypoxic-ischemic encephalopathy
Tumors
Vascular abnormality, infarction, or hemorrhage

Other Central Nervous System Disorders
Spinal muscular atrophy
Polio
Familial dysautonomia

Peripheral Nervous System Disorders
Myasthenia gravis
Guillain-Barré syndrome
Muscular dystrophy
Myotonic dystrophy

Thoracic Cage, Lung, or Airway Disease
Kyphoscoliosis
Asphyxiating thoracic dystrophy (Jeune disease)
Interstitial lung disease
Asthma

Conditions that Affect Multiple Respiratory Systems
Sudden infant death syndrome
Obstructive sleep apnea syndrome
Apnea of prematurity

Cerebral palsy
Depressant drugs
Craniofacial syndromes
Obesity hypoventilation syndrome
Trisomy 21

are highest in newborns and decrease until they reach normal adult values in middle childhood.[11,12] The changes in respiratory frequency with maturation are shown in **Table 1**. Infants have higher respiratory rates per unit body weight than older children, and this relationship is not proportional to body size.[13] During both sleep and waking states, respiratory rates decrease during the first 3 years of life with increasing body weight, but this decrease is not directly proportional to body size. Boys have a higher respiratory rate for a given body weight than girls.[13] The mean difference between the waking and sleep respiratory rate is greatest in infants, and decreases to 1 to 2 breaths per minute in adolescents. Respiratory rate varies with sleep state in infants, children, and adolescents, with changes being most prominent and clinically relevant in infants. In general, the respiratory frequency is higher during REM than during NREM sleep in newborns and infants.[14] In a small sample of healthy children aged 9 to 13 years, respiratory rates during sleep were variable but were highest during waking and light N1 sleep, and lowest during stage 2 sleep later in the night. Rates

Box 2
Characteristics of the respiratory system in infants that increase vulnerability to respiratory failure

Difficulty transitioning to mouth breathing during nasal obstruction, particularly during rapid eye movement (REM) sleep

Laryngeal reflexes trigger more profound cardiorespiratory depression

Increased chest-wall compliance

Barrel-shaped chest wall with more horizontal position of the ribs

Increased REM sleep time with loss of stabilizing intercostal muscle tone

Loss of expiratory braking in REM sleep

Lower specific lung compliance

Higher metabolic demand

Immaturity of chemoreceptors

Table 1
Respiratory rates during sleep from birth through adolescence

	Newborn	Infant	Preschool	School Age	Adolescent
Mean (SD)		29 (6)[77] 32.3 (4.9)[48]			15.3 (1.6) NREM[16] 16.4 (1.5) REM[16]
Median (IQR)	40 (34–52)[80]	29[81]	20 (18–21)[82]	18 (17–19)[82]	18 (17–18)[82]
Range		21–62[81]	14–26[82]	15–25[82]	15–22[82]

Abbreviations: IQR, interquartile range; NREM, non–rapid eye movement sleep; REM, rapid eye movement sleep; SD, standard deviation.

were slightly higher in boys than in girls in all stages of sleep.[15] In a small sample of healthy adolescents, respiratory rate and minute ventilation decreased by 8% from wakefulness to NREM sleep, and increased by 4% from NREM to REM sleep.[16]

Tidal Volume and Minute Ventilation

Minute ventilation is the product of respiratory rate and tidal volume, and is related to metabolic rate. To respond to increased metabolic demand, minute ventilation can be increased by increasing the respiratory rate, increasing the tidal volume, or both. In the newborn and young child, increasing the respiratory rate (rather than tidal volume) is the most energy-efficient strategy to cope with higher ventilatory needs.[13,17] This strategy of changing respiratory frequency rather than tidal volume is consistent with data in resting humans showing that both tidal volume and dead space per body weight remains essentially unchanged from birth to adulthood (about 6 mL/kg for tidal volume and 2.2 mL/kg for dead space).[18] There are limited data on normal tidal volume and minute ventilation in healthy children from newborn and adolescent age groups.[14,16] In general, minute ventilation is slightly higher in REM than in NREM sleep, consistent with the higher respiratory rates in REM. As expected, minute ventilation decreases with age (from 250 mL/kg/min in newborns to 100 mL/kg/min in adolescents), and parallels the maturational changes in respiratory frequency and metabolic needs.

Apnea Type, Duration, and Frequency

Numerous studies have investigated the frequency and duration of apnea in newborns and infants in the first year of life, with fewer studies in older children and adolescents.[7–9,19–23] Comparisons among the different studies are difficult for a variety of reasons. Definitions of respiratory events are not standardized, in terms of both length of event and how they are classified. Measurement conditions and methodology vary from study to study. Some studies have included children with snoring while others have not. Findings by age groups are discussed in this section.

Apnea in full-term infants

Central apneas are respiratory events defined by the absence of both airflow and respiratory effort. Apnea in infants is most commonly defined as a pause in breathing for at least 20 seconds, or a shorter pause that is associated with bradycardia or oxygen desaturation.[7] Although the term "prolonged" is often used to describe central apneas with a duration of at least 20 seconds, clinicians should be aware that apnea durations of 20 seconds or longer occur occasionally, and those of 30 seconds or longer rarely, in healthy term infants. Shorter (<20 seconds) central pauses are commonly seen in REM sleep, after a sigh breath or a body movement, and during transition from wakefulness to sleep. Determining normative values for central apneas across different age groups can be challenging because studies have used different technologies, time frames, and respiratory event definitions, and there is some debate about the evidence base for the currently accepted definition.[24]

Nevertheless, in full-term infants central respiratory pauses are common, occur frequently after body movements, and are more frequent during active sleep and REM sleep.[25] Most events meeting the aforementioned criteria for apnea in term infants are central in nature,[26] with substantial evidence that obstructive and mixed apneas are rare in healthy infants.[26–28] In the first 6 months of life, central apneas are very frequent with median apnea indices of approximately 5 per hour and the highest values in the first 5 weeks of life, 8/h. In the second 6 months of life, the median central apnea indices of 6.4/h in REM and 1.7/h in NREM sleep are reported. The frequency of central apneas declines after the first year of life. When recorded, obstructive apneas occur mainly during REM sleep.[29] Mechanisms for the greater respiratory instability in infants during REM compared with NREM sleep include immaturity of central respiratory control and phasic inhibitory-excitatory mechanisms inherent to REM sleep.[30] The sleeping position (prone or supine) does not alter the incidence, duration, or type of apnea in healthy infants.[28] The incidence of both central and obstructive apneas decreases with increasing postmenstrual age.[26,31] Although apnea was at one time hypothesized to be the pathophysiologic precursor to SIDS, extensive research has failed to support this concept.[32–35]

Apnea in preterm infants

Apnea of prematurity usually refers to the sudden cessation of breathing that lasts for at least 20 seconds or, if of shorter duration, is accompanied by bradycardia or oxygen desaturation in an infant younger than 37 weeks gestational age.[36] Apnea of prematurity generally resolves when the child reaches term, but may persist for several additional weeks in the most premature infants.[37–39] Extreme episodes lasting at least 30 seconds usually cease at approximately 43 weeks postmenstrual age.[40] In contrast to term infants in whom obstructive events are rare, apnea of prematurity is characterized by a combination of obstructive, central, and mixed apneas,[41] although there is little consensus regarding the frequency of these events. The difficulty of distinguishing central apneas (no effort, no airflow) from obstructive apneas (effort, no airflow) is technically challenging in these fragile infants.[42] Continuous positive airway pressure has been shown to reduce apnea in preterm infants, suggesting that upper airway obstruction is an important contributor to apnea of prematurity.[43] Obstructive apnea decreases with increasing postmenstrual age,[31] which may be related to the improvement in extrathoracic airway stability with maturation.[44] In addition, the degree to which laryngeal chemoreflexes trigger cardiorespiratory depression seems to be increased in prematurity.[6] Chronic hypoxemia related to immature lungs appears to enhance the ventilatory response of the peripheral chemoreceptors to hypoxemia, which may also explain the increased frequency of apnea in prematurity.[45] In healthy preterm infants, apnea triggered by desaturation decreases over time because of developmental improvements in chest-wall stability[46] and ventilation-perfusion matching.[47]

Periodic breathing

Periodic breathing, a common respiratory pattern in infants, is defined as 3 or more episodes of apnea lasting 3 or more seconds, separated by continued respiration of 20 seconds or less. Periodic breathing is more frequent in preterm infants, varies across studies in full-term infants, and decreases during the first 2 years of life. Episodes of periodic breathing can be seen in 80% to 100% of 1-week-old term infants. In term infants, the upper limits for sleep time spent in periodic breathing are 5% to 10% at 1 month of age, decreasing to 2% at 3 months of age. In preterm infants, the upper limits are higher: 15% to 20% at 1 month of age and 5% to 10% at 3 months of age.[48–50] In otherwise asymptomatic preterm infants with long episodes of periodic breathing that result in reduced saturation values, administration of supplemental O_2 is associated with decrease in time spent in periodic breathing.[51] The pathophysiology of periodic breathing is thought to be due to increased sensitivity of the peripheral chemoreceptors.[45] This hypothesis is supported by work in animal models, and findings that periodic breathing does not occur in the first 48 hours of life when the hypoxic response of peripheral chemoreceptors is suppressed.[52] In addition, compared with older children and adults, infants breathe very close to their CO_2 apneic threshold. The average threshold of eupneic partial pressure of CO_2 (P_{CO_2}) in neonates (1.1 ± 0.2 mm Hg above the apneic threshold) is much lower than the adult threshold (3.4 ± 0.4 mm Hg). This closeness of the eupneic and apneic CO_2 thresholds creates greater vulnerability in the respiratory control system for infants such that minor oscillations in breathing may bring eupneic P_{CO_2} values below threshold, causing apnea. Lower lung volumes and faster desaturation rates also contribute to this instability.[53] Older studies suggesting that increased periodic breathing was a marker for increased risk of SIDS have been challenged.[50,52,54]

CARDIORESPIRATORY EVENTS IN INFANCY

Bradycardia, apnea, and hypoxemia are closely related in preterm infants.[2] Heart rate varies with sleep state. In a cohort of healthy term infants aged 1 to 4 months, a decrease in heart rate was more likely to be associated with NREM sleep than with REM sleep.[55] The precise mechanisms underlying these relationships, and the thresholds that define abnormal heart rate and Spo_2 in this population, remain controversial. In preterm infants, 83% of bradycardic episodes were associated with apnea and 86% were associated with desaturation.[56] To test the hypothesis that cardiorespiratory events including apnea and bradycardia are more common in infants at increased risk for SIDS, researchers in 5 cities conducted a 6-month longitudinal cohort study of in-home cardiorespiratory event recording in a total of 1079 infants. The sample included healthy term infants and infants considered to be at increased risk for SIDS for a variety of reasons, including a history of ALTE, having a sibling who had died of SIDS, or prematurity (<34 weeks' gestation with birth weight <1750 g).[40] Surprisingly, apneas using conventional criteria of an event lasting 20 or more seconds, or of shorter duration but associated with bradycardia, were common even in the healthy term infants. Forty-three percent of healthy term infants had at least 1 event that met criteria for a "conventional" apnea. There was no difference in the frequency of these conventional apneas in the healthy term infants and the term infants at increased risk for SIDS. Only preterm children had an increased risk of conventional apneas. The investigators also examined the occurrence of "extreme" apneas, defines as apnea longer than 30 seconds or an age-adjusted bradycardia threshold of a specific duration. Only 2% of the healthy term infants experienced 1 or more extreme apneas. Similar to the conventional apneas, only preterm children had a significant increase in the risk of experiencing extreme apneas. This increased risk persisted until about 43 weeks postmenstrual age. Of concern, a follow-up study of developmental outcomes in this same cohort in the second year of life showed that 5 or more cardiorespiratory events per hour was associated with lower adjusted mean differences in the mental development index of the Bayley Scales of Development in both term and preterm infants.[57]

RESPIRATORY EVENTS DURING SLEEP BEYOND THE FIRST YEAR OF LIFE

The first study to establish normal values for respiratory events using polysomnography during sleep in children was published in 1978, and included 22 children aged 9 to 13 years.[15] Short respiratory pauses, more frequent during stage 1 and REM sleep, were reported. No obstructive events were described. In 1992, Marcus and colleagues[20] published a more comprehensive study of 50 children aged 1 to 17 years. A limitation to this study was the lack of neurophysiologic confirmation of sleep. Obstructive apneas were found to be rare in children, occurring in only 18%, with an average index of 0.1 ± 0.5 per hour (range 0–3.1) and no obstructive apneas longer than 10 seconds. Central apneas were more common, with 30% of children in this study having a central apnea longer than 10 seconds. Subsequent studies have confirmed that short central pauses (generally 10 seconds or less) are part of the normal pattern of breathing during sleep in children and adolescents,[21,58] and occur more often in REM than in NREM sleep.[59] The frequency of respiratory pauses, summarized

in **Table 2**, decreases from infancy through adolescence.[58] Obstructive apneas of any length are rare in both normal full-term infants and children.[7–9,20,22,26,58] Obstructive apneas occur mainly in REM and lighter NREM sleep. Despite the variation in measurement techniques, respiratory event definitions, scoring approach, and sample population, these studies are remarkably similar in their findings: (1) obstructive apneas are extremely rare; and (2) central pauses are seen frequently in healthy infants, including pauses that last up to 30 seconds, and decrease in frequency but are still present throughout childhood.

GAS EXCHANGE

There are several changes in gas exchange during sleep in normal adults. The partial pressure of CO_2 increases 3 to 7 mm Hg the partial pressure of arterial O_2 (PaO_2) decreases 3 to 9 mm Hg, and the SpO_2 decreases 2% in comparison with wakefulness.[1] Similar changes are seen in children. As in adults, these changes can be exaggerated in children with lung disease or upper airway obstruction. Most information about gas exchange during sleep in children comes from the use of noninvasive monitoring techniques including pulse oximetry measurements of SpO_2, transcutaneous measurement of CO_2 ($tcCO_2$), and end-tidal CO_2 ($EtCO_2$) measurement. Normal values from infancy to adolescence are summarized in **Table 3**.

OXYGEN

The ventilatory response to changes in PaO_2 is exponential. There is little increase in ventilation until PaO_2 falls below 60 mm Hg. The response to hypoxemia is augmented by hypercapnia, and decreases with age and training. Normative data for noninvasive measures of oxygenation (SpO_2 by pulse oximetry) from infancy through adolescence are summarized in **Table 3**. Data from the Collaborative Home Infant Monitoring Evaluation study published in 1999 provides the most comprehensive study of SpO_2 during infancy.[60] Their report of longitudinal data of SpO_2 during the first 25 postnatal weeks in 64 healthy term infants provided valuable information not addressed in earlier studies, which were generally limited to 1 to 2 nights of monitoring, or brief recording periods during respiratory events spread out over weeks.[61–63] The median baseline SpO_2 in these healthy infants was 97.9% (10th percentile SpO_2 95.2%) and did not change with age or sleep position. Most infants in this study had at least one 3-minute epoch with SpO_2 lower than 90%, and

Table 2
Central apnea indices in healthy children from infancy through adolescence

	1.4 y (1.1–1.9)	3 y (2.2–3.5)	5 y (4.3–5.8)	8 y (6.3–10.1) Tanner I	11.5 y (9.7–13.2) Tanner II	12.5 y (11.4–17.2) Tanner III	15.2 y (13.4–17.2) Tanner IV	16.9 y (15.8–17.9) Tanner V
Central apnea index (episodes per hour of total sleep time)	2.8 (1.0–4.3)	1.5 (0.7–6.9)	1.1 (0.5–3.2)	0.9 (0.3–2.7)	0.4 (0.0–1.2)	0.5 (0.1–1.8)	0.1 (0.0–0.8)	0.1 (0.0–1.3)
Maximum apnea duration (s)	11.7 (10.1–14.5)	13 (9.7–18.8)	14.1 (10.1–17.4)	15.5 (9.7–20.1)	13.3 (9.0–18.2)	13.0 (9.9–16.3)	12.5 (10.9–20.3)	11.2 (8.8–24.0)
Spo$_2$ nadir (%)	92.0 (87.6–95.0)	92.0 (88.8–95.0)	94.0 (83.6–96.0)	93.5 (87.0–96.0)	94.0 (91.4–96.0)	93.5 (90.5–96.0)	93.5 (91.0–96.0)	94.0 (91.5–96.0)

Data are presented as median (10th–90th percentile). These indices are based on central apneas that are scored without requiring an associated desaturation or arousal.
Data from Scholle S, Wiater A, Scholle HC. Normative values of polysomnographic parameters in childhood and adolescence: cardiorespiratory parameters. Sleep Med 2011;12(10):988–96.

Table 3
Oxygen saturation and carbon dioxide normal values in infancy through adolescence

	Infant	Preschool	School Age	Adolescent
Spo_2 mean or median	97–99[60,67,77]	99[8,9,82]	96–99[8,9,71,72,82]	97–99[16,68,82]
Spo_2 lower limit of normal (5th percentile or 2 SD below mean)	94–95[58,64,74]	95[8,9,82]	95[8,9,71,72,82]	95[12,55,65]
Desaturation index (≥4)		0.3[9]	0.5–1.2[9,71,72]	
Decreases in Spo_2 to less than 90% (per hour)				
Median (IQR)		0.0 (0.0–0.2)[82]	0.0 (0.0–0.3)[82]	0.0 (0.0)[82]
Range		0.0–2.7	0.0–0.6	0.0–0.3
$tcco_2$ mean or median	40–41[49,77,80]	42		
Interquartile range	37–44[49,80]	40–46		
$Etco_2$ mean (SD)		40.6 (4.6)[9]	40.7 (4.5)[9]	40.7 (4.5)[9]
Percent sleep time with $Etco_2$ >45 mm Hg, mean (SD)		20.4 (28)[9]	1.6 (3.8)[7] 6.9 (19.1)[20] 21.6 (29)[9]	1.6 (3.8)[7] 6.9 (19.1)[20]

acute decreases in Spo_2 occurred in most infants. These transient acute decreases improved with age and reduced the frequency of periodic breathing pattern, and based on this and earlier work the investigators concluded that they are part of the normal breathing and oxygenation behavior in infants.[60,61]

Gestational age and sleep state influence the development of stability in arterial oxygenation. Although healthy preterm infants have baseline Spo_2 values in the same range as full-term infants, the variability about the baseline is greater in preterm infants. The frequency of transient desaturation episodes to 80% or less varies considerably with age and between individual patients, with rates being highest in preterm infants, lower in term infants,[60,61,64–67] and lowest in older children and adolescents. During the regular breathing of quiet or NREM sleep, most infants do not have episodes of desaturation, or when episodes do occur they are brief. By contrast, during active or REM sleep, the brief apneic pauses are more likely to be associated with desaturation.

In healthy children 2 to 16 years of age, using a desaturation criterion of 90% or less, most children do not show any episodes of desaturation.[7–9,16,20,21,68–72] This increased stability in oxygenation may be partially explained by developmental changes in the relationship between lung volume and oxygen consumption. Infants have a highly compliant chest wall, resulting in a functional residual capacity that is significantly lower than that of adults when compared on the basis of metabolism.[73] Lung volume in infants decreases even further during apneic pauses[74] and during REM sleep.[75] Because lung volume at the onset of breath-holding is a major determinant of

the severity of resulting hypoxemia, the increase in the stability of oxygenation with age is likely due to increased and more stable lung volumes relative to oxygen consumption in the older child.

CARBON DIOXIDE

Arterial CO_2 is maintained with relatively little variation. Ventilation increases linearly in response to increasing CO_2 production in wakefulness and sleep. This response is augmented by hypoxia; the slope of the increase in ventilation in response to a given pressure of arterial CO_2 ($Paco_2$) is increased in the presence of a lower Pao_2. Although most healthy children maintain a resting $Paco_2$ near 40 mm Hg, there is substantial variation in the set point and sensitivity. Under normal conditions during NREM sleep, changes in $Paco_2$ of 2 mm Hg or less are promptly recognized by chemoreceptors. The rapid negative feedback system between the brain and lungs maintains $Paco_2$ within a small range between the eupnea and apnea thresholds.

Arterial CO_2 can be estimated noninvasively using transcutaneous $tcco_2$ and $Etco_2$; each method has advantages and disadvantages.[76] Normative data using these noninvasive measurements are summarized in **Table 3**. In a sample of healthy term infants during the first 9 months of life, $tcco_2$ values averaged 40.5 ± 2.25 mm Hg, with no differences between active and quiet sleep.[77] $tcco_2$ values during sleep change little with postnatal age during the first 2 years of life.[77–79] Normal children show an increase in $Etco_2$ values of 4 to 10 mm Hg during sleep, spending an average of 6.9 +/− 19.1% of sleep time with $Etco_2$ values above 45 mm Hg.[20] In a sample of 50 healthy children and adolescents, children had $Etco_2$ values above 45 mm Hg for an average of 6.9% ± 19.1% of sleep time. In this same population, peak $Etco_2$ values ranged from 38 to 53 mm Hg, with a mean of 46 ± 4 mm Hg.[20] CO_2 values are statistically lower in REM than in NREM sleep, but the difference (1–2 mm Hg) is clinically trivial. The limited normative data for CO_2 values measured during polysomnography from infancy to childhood are summarized in **Table 3**. A recent study[9] describes much higher values during sleep in children than previously reported.[7,20]

SUMMARY

Sleep-related changes in respiratory physiology in children vary with age, but generally include a reduction in respiratory rate and minute ventilation, mild reductions in Spo_2, mild increases in Pco_2, the presence of short central respiratory pauses, and rare obstructive respiratory events. Knowledge of the maturation of breathing patterns from infancy through adolescence is crucial to the ability of the physician to evaluate children for common disorders of sleep.

REFERENCES

1. Kreiger J. Breathing during sleep in normal subjects. In: Kryger M, Roth T, editors. Principles and practices of sleep medicine. Philadelphia: Elsevier Saunders; 2005. p. 232–44.
2. Rosen CL. Maturation of breathing during sleep. In: Marcus CL, Carroll JL, Donnelly DF, et al, editors. Sleep and breathing in children, second edition, developmental changes in breathing during sleep. New York: Informa Healthcare USA, Inc; 2008. p. 117–30.
3. Carroll JL, Donnelly DF. Postnatal development of carotid chemoreceptor function. In: Marcus CL, Carroll JL, Donnelly DF, et al, editors. Sleep and breathing in children, second edition, developmental changes in breathing during sleep. New York: Informa Healthcare USA, Inc; 2008. p. 47–73.
4. Marcus CL, Glomb WB, Basinski DJ, et al. Developmental pattern of hypercapnic and hypoxic ventilatory responses from childhood to adulthood. J Appl Physiol (1985) 1994;76(1):314–20.
5. Thach BT. Maturation and transformation of reflexes that protect the laryngeal airway from liquid aspiration from fetal to adult life. Am J Med 2001; 111(Suppl 8A):69S–77S.
6. Praud JP, Samson N. Laryngeal function and neonatal respiration. In: Marcus CL, Carroll JL, Donnelly DF, et al, editors. Sleep and breathing in children, second edition, developmental changes in breathing during sleep. New York: Informa Healthcare USA, Inc; 2008. p. 19–46.
7. Uliel S, Tauman R, Greenfeld M, et al. Normal polysomnographic respiratory values in children and adolescents. Chest 2004;125(3):872–8.
8. Traeger N, Schultz B, Pollock AN, et al. Polysomnographic values in children 2-9 years old: additional data and review of the literature. Pediatr Pulmonol 2005;40(1):22–30.
9. Montgomery-Downs HE, O'Brien LM, Gulliver TE, et al. Polysomnographic characteristics in normal preschool and early school-aged children. Pediatrics 2006;117(3):741–53.
10. Crosfill ML, Widdicombe JG. Physical characteristics of the chest and lungs and the work of breathing in different mammalian species. J Physiol 1961; 158:1–14.
11. Iliff A, Lee VA. Pulse rate, respiratory rate, and body temperature of children between two months and eighteen years of age. Child Dev 1952;23(4): 237–45.
12. Bardella IJ. Pediatric advanced life support: a review of the AHA recommendations. American Heart Association. Am Fam Physician 1999;60(6):1743–50.
13. Gagliardi L, Rusconi F. Respiratory rate and body mass in the first three years of life. The working party on respiratory rate. Arch Dis Child 1997; 76(2):151–4.
14. Gaultier C. Respiratory adaptation during sleep from the neonatal period to adolescence. In: Guilleminault C, editor. Sleep and its disorders in children. New York: Raven Press; 1987. p. 67–98.
15. Carskadon MA, Harvey K, Dement WC, et al. Respiration during sleep in children. West J Med 1978;128(6):477–81.
16. Tabachnik E, Muller NL, Bryan AC, et al. Changes in ventilation and chest wall mechanics during sleep in normal adolescents. J Appl Physiol Respir Environ Exerc Physiol 1981;51(3):557–64.
17. Mortola JP. Some functional mechanical implications of the structural design of the respiratory system in newborn mammals. Am Rev Respir Dis 1983;128(2 Pt 2):S69–72.
18. Polgar G, Weng TR. The functional development of the respiratory system from the period of gestation to adulthood. Am Rev Respir Dis 1979;120(3): 625–95.
19. Acebo C, Millman RP, Rosenberg C, et al. Sleep, breathing, and cephalometrics in older children and young adults. Part I – normative values. Chest 1996;109(3):664–72.
20. Marcus CL, Omlin KJ, Basinki DJ, et al. Normal polysomnographic values for children and adolescents. Am Rev Respir Dis 1992;146(5 Pt 1):1235–9.
21. Tang J, Rosen CL, Larkin EK, et al. Identification of sleep-disordered breathing in children: variation with event definition. Sleep 2002;25(1):72–9.

22. Verhulst SL, Schrauwen N, Haentjens D, et al. Reference values for sleep-related respiratory variables in asymptomatic European children and adolescents. Pediatr Pulmonol 2007;42(2):159–67.

23. Witmans MB, Keens TG, Ward SL, et al. Obstructive hypopneas in children and adolescents. Am J Respir Crit Care Med 2003;168(12):1540.

24. Elder DE, Campbell AJ, Galletly D. Current definitions for neonatal apnoea: are they evidence based? J Paediatr Child Health 2013;49(9):E388–96.

25. Ellingson RJ, Peters JF, Nelson B. Respiratory pauses and apnea during daytime sleep in normal infants during the first year of life: longitudinal observations. Electroencephalogr Clin Neurophysiol 1982;53(1):48–59.

26. Guilleminault C, Ariagno R, Korobkin R, et al. Mixed and obstructive sleep apnea and near miss for sudden infant death syndrome: 2. Comparison of near miss and normal control infants by age. Pediatrics 1979;64(6):882–91.

27. Flores-Guevara R, Plouin P, Curzi-Dascalova L, et al. Sleep apneas in normal neonates and infants during the first 3 months of life. Neuropediatrics 1982;13(Suppl):21–8.

28. Kahn A, Groswasser J, Sottiaux M, et al. Clinical symptoms associated with brief obstructive sleep apnea in normal infants. Sleep 1993;16(5):409–13.

29. Kahn A, Groswasser J, Rebuffat E, et al. Sleep and cardiorespiratory characteristics of infant victims of sudden death: a prospective case-control study. Sleep 1992;15(4):287–92.

30. Haddad GG, Epstein RA, Epstein MA, et al. Maturation of ventilation and ventilatory pattern in normal sleeping infants. J Appl Physiol Respir Environ Exerc Physiol 1979;46(5):998–1002.

31. Hoppenbrouwers T, Hodgman JE, Cabal L. Obstructive apnea, associated patterns of movement, heart rate, and oxygenation in infants at low and increased risk for SIDS. Pediatr Pulmonol 1993;15(1):1–12.

32. Franks CI, Watson JB, Brown BH, et al. Respiratory patterns and risk of sudden unexpected death in infancy. Arch Dis Child 1980;55(8):595–9.

33. Southall DP, Richards JM, Rhoden KJ, et al. Prolonged apnea and cardiac arrhythmias in infants discharged from neonatal intensive care units: failure to predict an increased risk for sudden infant death syndrome. Pediatrics 1982;70(6):844–51.

34. Southall DP, Richards JM, Stebbens V, et al. Cardiorespiratory function in 16 full-term infants with sudden infant death syndrome. Pediatrics 1986;78(5):787–96.

35. Gordon D, Southall DP, Kelly DH, et al. Analysis of heart rate and respiratory patterns in sudden infant death syndrome victims and control infants. Pediatr Res 1986;20(7):680–4.

36. Committee on Fetus and Newborn. American Academy of Pediatrics. Apnea, sudden infant death syndrome, and home monitoring. Pediatrics 2003;111(4 Pt 1):914–7.

37. Henderson-Smart DJ. The effect of gestational age on the incidence and duration of recurrent apnoea in newborn babies. Aust Paediatr J 1981;17(4):273–6.

38. Eichenwald EC, Aina A, Stark AR. Apnea frequently persists beyond term gestation in infants delivered at 24 to 28 weeks. Pediatrics 1997;100(3 Pt 1):354–9.

39. Darnall RA, Kattwinkel J, Nattie C, et al. Margin of safety for discharge after apnea in preterm infants. Pediatrics 1997;100(5):795–801.

40. Ramanathan R, Corwin MJ, Hunt CE, et al. Cardiorespiratory events recorded on home monitors: comparison of healthy infants with those at increased risk for SIDS. JAMA 2001;285(17):2199–207.

41. Albani M, Bentele KH, Budde C, et al. Infant sleep apnea profile: preterm vs. term infants. Eur J Pediatr 1985;143(4):261–8.

42. Upton CJ, Milner AD, Stokes GM. Upper airway patency during apnoea of prematurity. Arch Dis Child 1992;67(Spec No 4):419–24.

43. Miller MJ, Carlo WA, Martin RJ. Continuous positive airway pressure selectively reduces obstructive apnea in preterm infants. J Pediatr 1985;106(1):91–4.

44. Duara S, Silva Neto G, Claure N, et al. Effect of maturation on the extrathoracic airway stability of infants. J Appl Physiol (1985) 1992;73(6):2368–72.

45. Gauda EB, McLemore GL, Tolosa J, et al. Maturation of peripheral arterial chemoreceptors in relation to neonatal apnoea. Semin Neonatol 2004;9(3):181–94.

46. Heldt GP. Development of stability of the respiratory system in preterm infants. J Appl Physiol (1985) 1988;65(1):441–4.

47. Woodrum DE, Oliver TK Jr, Hodson WA. The effect of prematurity and hyaline membrane disease on oxygen exchange in the lung. Pediatrics 1972;50(3):380–6.

48. Kelly DH, Riordan L, Smith MJ. Apnea and periodic breathing in healthy full-term infants, 12-18 months of age. Pediatr Pulmonol 1992;13(3):169–71.

49. Schluter B, Buschatz D, Trowitzsch E. Polysomnographic reference curves in the first and second year of life. Somnologie 2001;5:3–16.

50. Glotzbach SF, Baldwin RB, Lederer NE, et al. Periodic breathing in preterm infants: incidence and characteristics. Pediatrics 1989;84(5):785–92.

51. Simakajornboon N, Beckerman RC, Mack C, et al. Effect of supplemental oxygen on sleep architecture and cardiorespiratory events in preterm infants. Pediatrics 2002;110(5):884–8.

52. Barrington KJ, Finer NN. Periodic breathing and apnea in preterm infants. Pediatr Res 1990;27(2):118–21.

53. Khan A, Qurashi M, Kwiatkowski K, et al. Measurement of the CO_2 apneic threshold in newborn infants: possible relevance for periodic breathing and apnea. J Appl Physiol (1985) 2005;98(4):1171–6.

54. Finer NN, Barrington KJ, Hayes B. Prolonged periodic breathing: significance in sleep studies. Pediatrics 1992;89(3):450–3.

55. Haddad GG, Bazzy AR, Chang SL, et al. Heart rate pattern during respiratory pauses in normal infants during sleep. J Dev Physiol 1984;6(4):329–37.

56. Upton CJ, Milner AD, Stokes GM. Apnoea, bradycardia, and oxygen saturation in preterm infants. Arch Dis Child 1991;66(Spec No 4):381–5.

57. Hunt CE, Corwin MJ, Baird T, et al. Cardiorespiratory events detected by home memory monitoring and one-year neurodevelopmental outcome. J Pediatr 2004;145(4):465–71.

58. Scholle S, Wiater A, Scholle HC. Normative values of polysomnographic parameters in childhood and adolescence: cardiorespiratory parameters. Sleep Med 2011;12(10):988–96.

59. Gaultier C. Apnea and sleep state in newborns and infants. Biol Neonate 1994;65(3–4):231–4.

60. Hunt CE, Corwin MJ, Lister G, et al. Longitudinal assessment of hemoglobin oxygen saturation in healthy infants during the first 6 months of age. Collaborative Home Infant Monitoring Evaluation (CHIME) Study Group. J Pediatr 1999;135(5):580–6.

61. Stebbens VA, Poets CF, Alexander JR, et al. Oxygen saturation and breathing patterns in infancy. 1: full term infants in the second month of life. Arch Dis Child 1991;66(5):569–73.

62. Levene S, McKenzie SA. Transcutaneous oxygen saturation in sleeping infants: prone and supine. Arch Dis Child 1990;65(5):524–6.

63. Hunt CE, Hufford DR, Bourguignon C, et al. Home documented monitoring of cardiorespiratory pattern and oxygen saturation in healthy infants. Pediatr Res 1996;39(2):216–22.

64. Poets CF, Stebbens VA, Alexander JR, et al. Oxygen saturation and breathing patterns in infancy. 2: preterm infants at discharge from special care. Arch Dis Child 1991;66(5):574–8.

65. Poets CF, Stebbens VA, Alexander JR, et al. Arterial oxygen saturation in preterm infants at discharge from the hospital and six weeks later. J Pediatr 1992;120(3):447–54.

66. Richard D, Poets CF, Neale S, et al. Arterial oxygen saturation in preterm neonates without respiratory failure. J Pediatr 1993;123(6):963–8.

67. Poets CF, Stebbens VA, Lang JA, et al. Arterial oxygen saturation in healthy term neonates. Eur J Pediatr 1996;155(3):219–23.

68. Chipps BE, Mak H, Schuberth KC, et al. Nocturnal oxygen saturation in normal and asthmatic children. Pediatrics 1980;65(6):1157–60.

69. Owen G, Canter R. Analysis of pulse oximetry data in normal sleeping children. Clin Otolaryngol Allied Sci 1997;22(1):13–22.

70. Rosen CL, Larkin EK, Kirchner HL, et al. Prevalence and risk factors for sleep-disordered breathing in 8- to 11-year-old children: association with race and prematurity. J Pediatr 2003;142(4):383–9.

71. Urschitz MS, Wolff J, Von Einem V, et al. Reference values for nocturnal home pulse oximetry during sleep in primary school children. Chest 2003;123(1):96–101.

72. Moss D, Urschitz MS, von Bodman A, et al. Reference values for nocturnal home polysomnography in primary schoolchildren. Pediatr Res 2005;58(5):958–65.

73. Cook CD, Cherry RB, O'Brien D, et al. Studies of respiratory physiology in the newborn infant. I. Observations on normal premature and full-term infants. J Clin Invest 1955;34(7 Pt 1):975–82.

74. Olinsky A, Bryan MH, Bryan AC. Influence of lung inflation on respiratory control in neonates. J Appl Physiol (1985) 1974;36(4):426–9.

75. Henderson-Smart DJ, Read DJ. Reduced lung volume during behavioral active sleep in the newborn. J Appl Physiol Respir Environ Exerc Physiol 1979;46(6):1081–5.

76. Morielli A, Desjardins D, Brouillette RT. Transcutaneous and end-tidal carbon dioxide pressures should be measured during pediatric polysomnography. Am Rev Respir Dis 1993;148(6 Pt 1):1599–604.

77. Horemuzova E, Katz-Salamon M, Milerad J. Breathing patterns, oxygen and carbon dioxide levels in sleeping healthy infants during the first nine months after birth. Acta Paediatr 2000;89(11):1284–9.

78. Hoppenbrouwers T, Hodgman JE, Arakawa K, et al. Transcutaneous oxygen and carbon dioxide during the first half year of life in premature and normal term infants. Pediatr Res 1992;31(1):73–9.

79. Schafer H, Koehler U, Ewig S, et al. Obstructive sleep apnea as a risk marker in coronary artery disease. Cardiology 1999;92(2):79–84.

80. Schafer T, Schafer D, Schlafke ME. Breathing, transcutaneous blood gases, and CO_2 response in SIDS siblings and control infants during sleep. J Appl Physiol (1985) 1993;74(1):88–102.

81. Poets CF, Stebbens VA, Southall DP. Arterial oxygen saturation and breathing movements during the first year of life. J Dev Physiol 1991;15(6):341–5.

82. Poets CF, Stebbens VA, Samuels MP, et al. Oxygen saturation and breathing patterns in children. Pediatrics 1993;92(5):686–90.

Sleep and Respiratory Physiology in Adults

Mudiaga Sowho, MD, MPH[a], Jason Amatoury, MBiomedE, PhD[b,c], Jason P. Kirkness, PhD[a], Susheel P. Patil, MD, PhD[a,*]

KEYWORDS

- Respiratory physiology • Control of breathing • Sleep effects • Hypoventilation • Upper airway
- Lower airway

KEY POINTS

- Sleep is a potentially vulnerable state for the respiratory system.
- Respiratory drive is determined by a central respiratory generator located within the brainstem.
- Withdrawal of wakefulness stimuli and the initiation of active sleep processes results in ventilation being determined primarily by metabolic demand.
- The respiratory system is regulated by central and peripheral chemoreceptors and mechanoreceptors that provide negative feedback to maintain ventilation.
- Sleep onset results in alterations in upper and lower airway physiology to maintain eucapnia.

The respiratory system is a complex interplay between the central nervous system, respiratory-related motor neurons, and the muscles of respiration. During wakefulness, both volitional and metabolic pathways are active in determining the minute ventilation necessary to maintain eucapnia (the CO_2 level during stable breathing). With sleep onset, wakefulness stimuli are withdrawn as active central processes for sleep are initiated, leaving metabolic demand as the primary determinant of minute ventilation. Individuals with respiratory abnormalities such as an anatomically small upper airway, restrictive lung disease, obstructive lung disease, or neuromuscular weakness, may depend on the wakefulness stimuli through recruitment of accessory muscles to maintain ventilation. Sleep onset results in a marked reduction of compensatory mechanisms, which can promote hypoventilation and the development of sleep-related breathing disorders. Thus, sleep represents a potentially vulnerable state for the respiratory system.

BASIC RESPIRATORY NEUROBIOLOGY
Respiratory Anatomy and Neuromotor Control

From classical transection experiments, the medulla and pons have been identified as the primary central nervous system location responsible for determining respiratory drive.[1] Medullary respiratory neurons vital to breathing include 2 groups of neurons referred to as the dorsal respiratory group (DRG) and the ventral respiratory group (VRG; **Fig. 1**).[2] The DRG contains predominantly inspiratory neurons and is located in the nucleus tractus solatarius, an area responsible for central sensory integration of vagal afferents coming from the lungs, central chemoreceptors (pH),

Disclosure: The authors have nothing to disclose.
[a] Division of Pulmonary, Critical Care, and Sleep Medicine, Department of Medicine, Johns Hopkins University, 5501 Hopkins Bayview Circle, Baltimore, MD 21224, USA; [b] Neuroscience Research Australia, Barker Street, Randwick, New South Wales 2031, Australia; [c] Ludwig Engel Centre for Respiratory Research, Westmead Millennium Institute, and Sydney Medical School, University of Sydney at Westmead Hospital, Hawkesbury Road, Westmead, New South Wales 2145, Australia
* Corresponding author.
E-mail address: spatil@jhmi.edu

Clin Chest Med 35 (2014) 469–481
http://dx.doi.org/10.1016/j.ccm.2014.06.002
0272-5231/14/$ – see front matter © 2014 Elsevier Inc. All rights reserved.

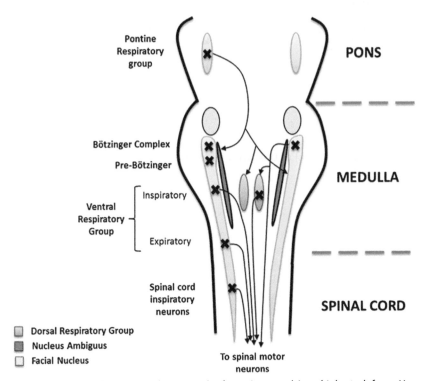

Fig. 1. Brainstem centers contributing to the control of respiratory drive. (*Adapted from* Horner RL. Sleep Research Society basics of sleep guide: control of ventilation. In: Amlaner CJ, Buxton O, editors. Sleep and respiratory physiology in adults. Darien (IL): Sleep Research Society; 2008; with permission.)

carotid and aortic chemoreceptors (CO_2 and O_2), and baroreceptors (blood pressure). The VRG contains both inspiratory and expiratory neurons and includes several important nuclei, or neuronal groups, including the nucleus ambiguus, the Botzinger complex (expiratory neurons), the pre-Botzinger complex (inspiratory neurons), the rostral retroambigualis neurons (inspiratory neurons), and the caudal retroambigualis neurons (expiratory neurons).[2] Bulbospinal neurons from the VRG and DRG then project to spinal motor neurons that innervate the respiratory pump muscles. In close proximity to the VRG are important cranial motor neurons (nucleus ambiguous, contributes to the glossopharyngeal nerve; trigeminal, facial, and hypoglossal nuclei) that innervate muscles of the larynx and pharynx, but are driven by different premotor neurons than those that drive the pump muscles, presumably because the laryngeal and pharyngeal muscles contribute to other functions, such as swallowing and phonation. Above the VRG, in close proximity to the Botzinger complex, is the pre-Botzinger complex, which has pacemakerlike properties that generate an underlying respiratory rhythm.[3] This complex of neurons contains mu-opioid receptors and neurokinin receptors, which has important clinical implications. The mu-opioid receptors when stimulated slow

the pacemaker, whereas the neurokinin receptors speed the pacemaker.[4] Neuroactive medications, such as opiates, used in the treatment of pain can, therefore, significantly impact ventilation. The pons also plays an important role in modulating respiratory activity, receiving input from the pontine respiratory group (Kolliker fuse and parabrachial nuclei).[5]

The connections and interactions between respiratory propriobulbar neurons, premotor neurons, and motor neurons, referred to as a central respiratory generator (CRG), are ultimately responsible for producing an underlying respiratory drive (tonic activity) and respiratory rhythm (phasic activity) to the respiratory pump muscles (**Fig. 2**).[2] The level of tonic drive generated by the CRG is based on input from peripheral and central chemoreceptors.[6] During inspiration, the CRG generates phasic activity, through inspiratory premotor neurons from the VRG and DRG that synapse with phrenic and intercostal motor neurons. Inspiratory activity is terminated by inhibitory projections from expiratory neurons in the Botzinger complex to the brainstem and spinal cord. In contrast with the phrenic and intercostal motor neurons, control of respiratory drive to pharyngeal muscle motor neurons, such as the hypoglossal nerve, is not actively inhibited with expiration. Instead, tonic activity to

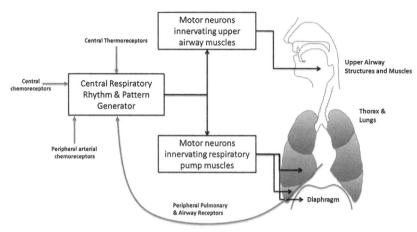

Fig. 2. Overview of central respiratory generators and feedback systems in determining respiratory drive. (*Adapted from* Horner RL. Sleep Research Society basics of sleep guide: control of ventilation. In: Amlaner CJ, Buxton O, editors. Sleep and respiratory physiology in adults. Darien (IL): Sleep Research Society; 2008; with permission.)

these motor neurons is determined by inputs from the reticular formation rather than the VRG and DRG.[7] The brief periods of inspiratory activity from some pharyngeal muscle-related motor neurons are owing to an underlying respiratory-related activity within the motor neuron. At sleep onset, reticular formation activity is withdrawn and leads to a reduction in tonic drive to muscles of the upper airway, making the airway vulnerable to collapse.[2]

Effects of Sleep on Central Neural and Neuromotor Control

Multiple neuronal networks between the brainstem and cortex (ascending arousal system) are important for both arousal and wakefulness (**Table 1**).[8,9] These systems include serotonergic neurons (dorsal raphe nucleus), noradrenergic neurons (locus

coeruleus), histaminergic neurons (tuberomammilary nucleus), dopaminergic neurons (ventral periacqueductal gray), cholingeric neurons (basal forebrain), and orexin (perifornical region of the hypothalamus). These systems affect respiration through projections to the medulla, pons, and spinal cord.

Non-rapid eye movement (NREM) sleep is a dynamic process generated by activity from the ventrolateral preoptic area, the hypothalamus, and basal forebrain (see **Table 1**).[2] A circadian-mediated decline in body temperature activates the ventrolateral preoptic area. Ascending inhibitory cortical projects to the cortical arousal systems and descending inhibitory projections to brainstem arousal neurons assist to promote sleep via the neurotransmitters GABA and galanin.[10] The prominence of GABA helps to explain the sedative

Table 1		
Central nervous system (CNS) centers and neurotransmitters associated with states of wakefulness and sleep		
State	**CNS Centers**	**Neurotransmitters**
Wakefulness	Dorsal raphe nucleus	Serotonin
	Locus coeruleus	Norepinephrine
	Tuberomammillary nucleus	Histamine
	Ventral periacqueductal gray	Dopamine
	Basal forebrain	Acetylcholine
	Hypothalamus–perifornical region	Orexin
Non-rapid eye movement	Ventrolateral preoptic area	γ-Aminobutyric acid
	Hypothalamus	Galanin
	Basal forebrain	
Rapid eye movement	Pedunculopontine tegmentum	Serotonin
	Laterodorsal tegmentum	Norepinephrine
	Pontine reticular formation	Acetylcholine
	Medullary reticular formation relay neurons	Glycine

properties of medications, such as benzodiazepines, imidazopyridines, and barbiturates.[11] The diffuse projections of sleep-state–related neurons ultimately can act to influence respiratory neurons and motor neurons, and lead to a reduction in the tonic drive to the respiratory system.[2]

REM sleep is characterized by a decrease in serotonin and noradrenergic neuron activity that results in a loss of inhibition to the pedunculopontine tegmental and laterodorsal tegmental nuclei (see **Table 1**).[2,9] This leads to acetylcholine release in the pontine reticular formation promoting REM sleep. The motor suppression observed during REM sleep occurs through activation of the medullary reticular formation relay neurons, which inhibit spinal motor neurons via glycine release. Pontine neurons may also inhibit spinal motor neurons through glutamine-mediated activation of motor neurons of the ventral horn of the spinal cord, activating glycine interneurons that inhibit the spinal motor neurons.

CONTROL OF VENTILATION

The primary purpose of the ventilatory control system is to regulate the exchange of respiratory and blood gases, particularly arterial CO_2 ($Paco_2$), within a relatively narrow range (**Table 2**). $Paco_2$ is determined by a hyperbolic relationship between metabolic CO_2 production and alveolar ventilation (V_A). Assuming a constant CO_2 production and dead space, a 50% decrease in V_A would result in a doubling of the $Paco_2$.[12] The consequence of homeostatic regulation of $Paco_2$ is that the Pao_2 depends relative atmospheric pressure (P_{us}), the $Paco_2$, and the respiratory quotient. Several processes are responsible for

regulating ventilation during wakefulness and include metabolic control, behavioral control, and the wakefulness stimulus.[13] With the onset of sleep, behavioral control and wakefulness stimuli recede and metabolic control becomes the primary stimulus for ventilation. Ventilatory control mechanisms respond to changes in both chemical and mechanical information (**Table 3**) that arise from metabolic demand. The primary sensors for chemical stimuli include the central (ventral medulla) and peripheral chemoreceptors (carotid body; see **Table 3**). With increasing hypoxemia, the carotid body sends afferent impulses to the nucleus tractus solatarius via the glossopharyngeal and vagus nerves to increase ventilation, particularly as the Pao_2 falls below 60 mm Hg.[14] Similarly, with hypercapnia or hypocapnia, linear changes in ventilation occur in response to central and peripheral chemoreceptors stimuli. Mechanical information from the thoracic cage and lungs is also received by the nucleus tractus solatarius via vagal afferent pathways responding to intrapulmonary stretch receptors, irritant receptors, and unmyelinated C fibers (see **Table 3**). Stimulation of these receptors typically results in the development of a rapid, shallow breathing pattern and provides a negative feedback to limit overinflation of the lungs (Herring-Breuer reflex).[14]

Ventilatory Control Stability (Respiratory Loop Gain Concept)

Control of ventilation is tightly organized as a negative feedback system to maintain the $Paco_2$ at approximately 40 mm Hg during wakefulness. The concept of respiratory loop gain is used to characterize the negative feedback response.[13]

Table 2
Normative arterial blood gas values

Blood Gas Analyte	Normal Ranges	Value Meaning and Interpretation
Arterial carbon dioxide partial pressure ($Paco_2$)	35–45 mm Hg	An indicator of metabolic production of CO_2. Hypercapnia refers to an elevated $Paco_2$ owing to hypoventilation. Hypocapnia refers to a reduced $Paco_2$ owing to hyperventilation.
Arterial oxygen partial pressure (Pao_2)	75–100 mm Hg	Intermittent or sustained reductions in Pao_2 indicate poor oxygenation or hypoxemia.
pH	7.34–7.44	Hydrogen ion concentration [H^+]. Increased levels result in alkalemia (pH>7.45). Decreased levels result in acidemia (pH<7.35).
H^+	35–45 nmol/L	H^+ >45: acidemic or H^+ <35: Alkalemic.
HCO_3^-	22–26 mEq/L	Bicarbonate ion (HCO_3^-) is a blood CO_2-buffering electrolyte. Low HCO_3^- results in metabolic acidosis. High HCO_3^- results in metabolic alkalosis.

Table 3
Chemoreceptors and mechanoreceptors of the respiratory system

	Sensor Type	Location	Action
Chemoreceptors			
Central	pH-sensitive membrane bound proteins	Ventrolateral medulla	Signal respiratory efferent neurons for control of eupneic breathing; contribute to ~75% of the ventilatory response to small change in $Paco_2$
Peripheral	Glomus cells sensitive to Pao_2, pH, and $Paco_2$ sensitive	Carotid body, aortic body	Combined ~25% of the chemical control of ventilation; afferent signal of glossopharyngeal and vagus nerves
Lung and airway mechanoreceptors			
Stretch	Myelinated afferent fibers sensitive to pressure	Airway smooth muscle and extrapulmonary airway	Increased firing by elevated bronchial transmural pressure; afferent transmission via vagus nerve
Irritant	Myelinated afferent fibers stimulated chemically by nitrogen dioxide, sulfur dioxide, ammonia, inhaled antigens	Airway epithelial cells	Cough, bronchoconstriction, apnea and glottal closure
Unmyelinated C fibers	Unmyelinated afferent fibers and local receptors stimulated by chemical irritants	Lung interstitium and alveolar walls	Vagal afferent signal causing irritation, burning and choking sensations; localized vasodilation and mucosal swelling
Chest wall mechanoreceptors			
Joint	Receptors responding to deep pressure, stress or change in position	Joint capsules and associated ligaments	Proprioception of rib movement during inspiration and expiration
Muscle spindle	Stretch-sensitive nerve fibers imbedded in muscles	Muscle fibers of intercostal and abdominal wall muscles	Spindle afferent fibers project to the cerebral cortex; posture and rib cage stabilization response to increases in airway resistance or by decreases in lung compliance
Tendon organs	Branched nerve endings respond to stretch	Tendons	Response proportion to stimulus; causes relaxation of the attached muscle

The 3 major components of the ventilatory control system include a plant, a circulatory delay, and a controller (**Fig. 3**). The respiratory plant is represented by the CO_2 that is present in the lungs, body tissue, and blood. The plant gain is represented by the change in $Paco_2$ for a given change in ventilation ($\Delta Paco_2/\Delta V_A$). A circulatory delay exists owing to the transit time from the pulmonary

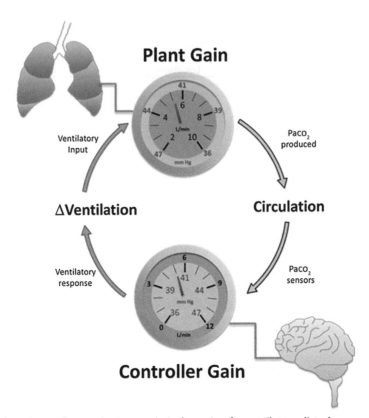

Fig. 3. Principle of respiratory loop gain. Loop gain is the ratio of a ventilatory disturbance and the consequent ventilatory response. When a disturbance such as an apnea or hypopnea occurs (ie, a ventilatory disturbance), hypoventilation occurs resulting in a rise in $Paco_2$. After a circulatory delay, the relative hypercapnia is sensed by chemoreceptors and results in increased ventilation (ie, a ventilatory response) returning the system to eucapnic levels. High respiratory loop gains are associated with an unstable ventilatory system.

capillaries to reach the central and peripheral chemoreceptors. Central respiratory controllers subsequently respond to the change in $Paco_2$ through negative feedback that to appropriately change V_A. The controller gain is represented by a change in V_A for a given change in $Paco_2$ ($\Delta V_A/\Delta Paco_2$).[12]

Respiratory loop gain is thus a ratio of a ventilatory response for a given ventilatory disturbance, and is considered a measure of ventilatory stability.[13] For example, a transient reduction in ventilatory drive as seen with an apnea or hypopnea (ie, a ventilatory disturbance) results in an increase in $Paco_2$, which, after a circulatory delay, translates into a transient increase in ventilatory drive (ie, a ventilatory response) and consequent reduction in $Paco_2$ and eventual return to a steady-state $Paco_2$ level. A high loop gain indicates an inherently unstable system prone to frequent oscillation and an inability to achieve a steady state. In contrast, a low loop gain is characteristic of a stable respiratory system.[15,16]

Hypoxic and Hypercapnic Ventilatory Responses

The hypoxic and hypercapnic ventilatory responses represent the important elements of the controller gain in the respiratory loop gain model. Increases in ventilation occur in response to a given rise in $Paco_2$ (ie, hypercapnic ventilatory response [HCVR]) and to reductions in Pao_2 (ie, hypoxic ventilatory response [HOVR]) to maintain chemical homeostasis.[14] The slope of the HCVR and HOVR is a measure of the sensitivity of the chemoreceptors to hypercapnia and hypoxia, respectively, and can be diminished owing to heritable or acquired factors (eg, neuromuscular diseases, pulmonary disorders, obesity, or central nervous system depressants).[17]

The combined effects of hypercapnic hypoxemia (eg, asphyxia) create a greater ventilatory stimulus than either in isolation.[18] In general, both the HCVR and HOVR seem to decline during NREM sleep and decline further with REM sleep.[19,20] The etiology of the decline of chemoreceptor responsiveness with NREM sleep remains controversial; some studies suggest a sleep-related decline in chemoresponsiveness and others suggest diminished load compensation (eg, increased upper airway resistance).

HCVR

The HCVR is composed of a slope and a ventilatory set point. The HCVR slope is reduced during NREM sleep (~50% from wakefulness) and reduced further during REM sleep (~28% from NREM; **Fig. 4**).[21] The resting ventilatory set point (the point at which further increases in $Paco_2$ result in increased ventilation) during NREM sleep shifts rightward owing to changes in the eupneic CO_2 set point with sleep (see apnea threshold discussion). Gender differences in HCVR may be present; women demonstrate a preserved HCVR with NREM sleep.[22] During REM sleep, however, the decline in HCVR is much more evident and may be associated with leptin-mediated pathways.[23]

HOVR

The slope of the HOVR is not constant, but can be linearized if expressed as ventilation versus SaO_2.[24] The HOVR also seems to be reduced during NREM sleep and is reduced further during REM sleep (see **Fig. 3**).[14] However, the decline in HOVR during NREM sleep is noted only in studies where men predominate, suggesting that women may have an intact HOVR during NREM sleep.[25,26] During REM sleep, however, the decline in HOVR is much more evident and consistent in both men and women.

Apnea Threshold/CO₂ Reserve and Changes with Sleep Onset

All healthy humans hypoventilate at sleep onset with eupneic CO_2 levels (the CO_2 level during stable breathing), typically 2 to 8 mm Hg above wakefulness levels. This transient state unmasks a highly sensitive, hypocapnia-induced apneic threshold, whereby apnea is initiated by small, transient reductions in arterial CO_2 pressure ($Paco_2$) by 3 to 6 mm Hg below eupnea and respiratory rhythm is not restored until $Paco_2$ has returned to eupnoeic levels during sleep. The absolute CO_2 level at which apnea occurs during sleep, however, is about 1 to 2 mm Hg lower than the waking CO_2 level, suggesting that waking eupneic CO_2 levels are inadequate to maintain eupneic breathing during sleep.[27,28] Ventilatory oscillations then continue until steady-state sleep and the eupneic CO_2 level during sleep is obtained, unless an inherent ventilatory instability is present, in which case persistent cyclical ventilatory overshoots may persist. Another measure of this ventilatory stability is the CO_2 reserve represented by the difference in eupneic CO_2 and the apnea threshold during sleep. Increases in plant gain resulting in higher $Paco_2$ levels (which may occur with chronic pulmonary, neuromuscular, and neurologic disorders) or an high HCVR (eg, seen with congestive heart failure or patients with idiopathic central sleep apnea) results in a narrow CO_2 reserve and promote ventilatory instability, particularly during NREM sleep.[12,28]

Arousal Responses and Ventilation

Although arousals from sleep may seem undesirable, they represent an important protective

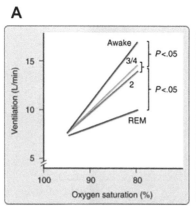
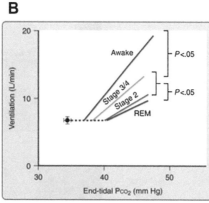

Fig. 4. (*A*) Hypoxic ventilatory response across sleep stages. (*B*) Hypercapnic ventilatory responses across sleep stages. (*From* Douglas NJ. Respiratory physiology: understanding the control of ventilation. In: Kryger M, Roth T, Dement WC, editors. Principles and practice of sleep medicine. 5th edition. Philadelphia: Elsevier Saunders; 2011; with permission.)

response during periods of compromised ventilation or airway obstruction.[29] Conversely, ventilatory overshoot during arousal can contribute to instability and promote disordered breathing. Specifically, individuals that have a low arousal threshold are at risk for ventilatory instability.[30]

Several factors, including hypoxia, hypercapnia, and increased airway resistance, can influence arousal responses during sleep. Hypoxia is considered a poor stimulus for arousal induction with somewhat variable responses. Studies have demonstrated that individuals can remain asleep even with oxygen saturation as low as 70% during REM and NREM sleep.[31,32] Hypercapnia is a more consistent stimulus for arousals within 15 mm Hg of eupneic wakefulness values.[33] Hypercapnic hypoxia has a synergistic effect in reducing the arousal threshold,[34] because hypercapnia increases the sensitivity of the carotid and aortic bodies to hypoxia. Added inspiratory resistance or airway occlusion increases arousal frequencies during NREM and REM sleep, but is lowest during stage N3 sleep.[35] A common pathway for these stimuli contributing to increased arousal frequency is increasing respiratory drive, where a particular threshold of respiratory drive is associated with arousal and is generally reproducible within a given individual.[36]

SLEEP EFFECTS ON UPPER AND LOWER AIRWAY PHYSIOLOGY

The purpose of respiration is to allow for gas exchange, by delivering oxygen to the pulmonary and systemic circulation and eliminating carbon dioxide from the lungs. In this section, the contribution of the mechanics of the upper and lower airway in maintaining normal gas exchange is briefly reviewed along with the effects of sleep on upper and lower airway mechanics.

Upper Airway Anatomy and Physiology

The upper airway extends from the external entrance of the nares and oral cavity to the glottis, at the entrance of the larynx (**Fig. 5**).[37] The upper airway is traditionally divided into 4 anatomic regions (see **Fig. 5**): (i) The nasopharynx, which extends from the posterior nasal choanae to the caudal margin of the hard palate, (ii) velopharynx, extending from the cranial to caudal margin of the soft palate, (iii) oropharynx, or retroglossal segment, extending from the tip of the soft palate to the tip of the epiglottis, and (iv) hypopharynx, ranging from the cranial margin of the epiglottis to the glottis. The upper airway has been designed to accommodate several functional roles including the heating and humidification of air, respiration, speech, and swallowing. To accommodate these different functions, the upper airway is an intricate arrangement of soft (24 muscles and other soft tissues), cartilaginous (thyroid cartilage, epiglottis), and bony (hard palate, mandible, and hyoid bone) tissues.[38,39] Except for the posterior vertebral column providing some dorsal support, the upper airway has no bony or cartilaginous support, making it highly deformable and prone to collapse during sleep, which may lead to sleep-disordered breathing. The most deformable region of the

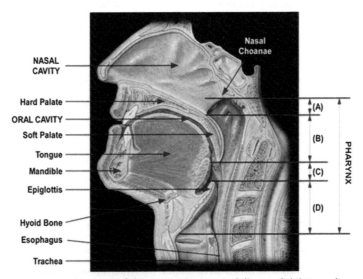

Fig. 5. Upper airway anatomy. Major areas of the upper airway are delineated: (*A*) Nasopharynx, (*B*) velopharynx, (*C*) oropharynx, and (*D*) hypopharynx. (*Adapted from* Clemente CD. Anatomy: a regional atlas of the human body. Baltimore (MD): Lippincott Williams & Wilkins; 1997; with permission.)

upper airway, and hence most prone to collapse, is the velopharynx, followed by the oropharynx.[40–43]

The major respiratory function of the upper airway is to permit air movement into and out of the lungs.[44] With the onset of inspiration, the upper airway is exposed to negative intraluminal pressure initiated by diaphragmatic contraction. A negative pressure reflex within the upper airway acts to stabilize the airway and prevent collapse through phasic activation of airway dilator muscles (eg, alae nasi and genioglossus) before the onset of diaphragmatic activity.[45] Phasic dilator muscle activity and preactivation delay increases with increasing negative airway pressure or increased central respiratory drive to maintain airway patency. Coordination of the upper airway muscle and thoracic pump muscle activity most likely occurs from the CRG, as discussed.[29]

Whether or not the upper airway collapses, particularly during sleep, depends on the transmural pressure across the upper airway (intraluminal pressure minus extraluminal pressure). Airflow through the upper airway can be modeled as a Starling resistor.[46–48] In this model, the presence of normal airflow, inspiratory flow limitation (partial airway obstruction), or complete airway obstruction depends on the relationship between the upstream pressure (ie, P_{us}), the critical pressure (P_{crit}), the collapsing pressure of the airway, and the downstream pressure (ie, tracheal pressure [P_{ds}]). When the P_{us} and P_{ds} pressure remain greater than the P_{crit} of the upper airway, non–flow-limited breathing is observed. When P_{ds} falls below the P_{crit}, partial airway obstruction with inspiratory flow limitation occurs. When the P_{crit} is greater than the P_{us} and P_{ds}, complete upper airway obstructions occurs. Several factors have been shown to increase the P_{crit} (ie, increase collapsibility), including reduced lung volumes,[49–52] resulting in reduced tracheal traction of the upper airway,[53] head/neck flexion,[54] supine posture,[55–58] and increased surface tension along the pharyngeal airway.[59]

THE UPPER AIRWAY AND SLEEP

A number of changes to the upper airway at sleep onset predispose it to collapse and can result in sleep-disordered breathing in some individuals. At the onset of sleep, there is a decrease in upper airway muscle activity,[60–62] which results in decreased upper airway compliance ("floppier" airway), smaller upper airway lumen size, and increased upper airway resistance.[63,64] Furthermore, the pharyngeal neurocompensatory reflexes,[23,30,65] which are triggered by negative intraluminal pressure, and ventilatory motor output, owing to loss of the wakefulness stimuli, are reduced.[66,67]

Lower Airway Anatomy and Physiology

The lower airway anatomy begins from the larynx and includes the airway and tissues from trachea to the lungs. The trachea is the largest portion of the lower airways that splits into 2 primary bronchi, which enter the lungs and divide into a hierarchy of smaller bronchial segments.[68] The trachea and bronchi are lined with cartilaginous rings to maintain their patency, where their role is to conduct air into the lungs and are referred to as conducting airways. The lower bronchi branch into the non-cartilaginous bronchioles. The bronchioles are referred to as transitional airways, because they are involved in both air conduction and gas exchange with the blood circulation. Gas exchange occurs in the alveoli, saclike structures that connect to bronchioles via alveolar ducts, by diffusion to the lung capillaries. The lungs are lined by the visceral pleura in apposition to the parietal pleural that lines the chest wall. The thoracic cage, which houses the lungs, consists of the ribs and respiratory muscles, which include the diaphragm, intercostal muscles, abdominal muscles, and accessory muscles, such as the sternocleidomastoid muscles and scalene muscles.[68,69]

Inspiration occurs when the CRG sends neural outflow to the diaphragm to contract and descend, creating a negative pleural pressure and intrathoracic pressure that generates a driving pressure. Accessory muscles and intercostal muscles elevate the chest wall and increase the anteroposterior diameter of the thoracic cage, thus increasing intrathoracic volume.[68] The extent to which the lungs inflate during respiration is determined by the compliance (Δ volume/Δ pressure) of the respiratory system. Respiratory system compliance is determined by the interaction between the inward, elastic recoil pressure of the lungs and the outward, recoil pressure of the chest wall.[70]

The natural resting lung volume, called the functional residual capacity (FRC), occurs when the elastic recoil pressures of the lungs and chest wall are in equilibrium. The lung volume after forced expiration from FRC is the residual volume. The difference between the FRC and residual volume is called the expiratory residual volume. Maximal inspiratory effort from FRC brings the lung to the total lung capacity. Both FRC and total lung capacity are reduced when supine compared with an upright or seated position.[71] The mechanisms for these reductions are owing to increases in transabdominal abdominal pressure and intrathoracic blood volume when supine. A reductions in the FRC when supine may contribute to impaired gas exchange owing to either increased work of breathing, increased ventilation-perfusion mismatch and/or a smaller oxygen reservoir. Anthropometry, sex, body posture, and neuromuscular tone contribute to changes in lung volumes.[72] Obesity can result in reduction in volumes that are most pronounced in the FRC and expiratory residual volume, although total lung capacity is relatively preserved.[73] Gender differences are apparent; men demonstrate a greater reduction in forced vital capacity than women.[74]

During rest, expiration is a neurally passive process, whereby the diaphragmatic relaxation and elastic recoil, increase intrathoracic pressure generating expiratory airflow. Increased respiratory demand requires recruitment of external intercostal and abdominal muscles to maintain sufficient airflow.[75] During non–flow-limited breathing, resistance to airflow is determined by the driving pressure between the upstream and downstream segments in the airway and inversely with airflow ($R = \Delta$ pressure/flow). During flow-limited breathing, whether expiratory or inspiratory, the airflow resistance is determined by the driving pressure between the upstream segment and the collapsing segment of the airway.[76]

Minute ventilation is a product of the respiratory rate (RR) and tidal volume (V_T). However, approximately one third of the V_T constitutes to ventilatory dead space, which does not contribute to effective ventilation, whereas the remaining two thirds contributes to effective V_A. The CRG is also important in determining respiratory timing. The respiratory cycle time (1/RR) can be divided into an inspiratory (T_I) and expiratory time components. The relative proportion of inspiratory to total respiratory cycle time (T_{TOT}) is referred to as the duty cycle (T_I/T_{TOT}) and is typically 30% to 45%. The duty cycle represents the proportion of time for gas exchange to occur during inspiration. Minute ventilation can also be defined as the product of the mean inspiratory flow (V_T/T_I, a measure of inspiratory drive) and the inspiratory duty cycle (T_I/T_{TOT}).[77]

Effects of Sleep on Lower Airway Physiology and Gas Exchange

Airway resistance
Airway resistance increases by about 230% during NREM sleep. The mechanism is owing to reduced tonic drive to the pharyngeal muscles with sleep onset.

Lung volume
In the supine position, FRC decreases from wake to sleep in nonobese subjects by approximately 0.2 to 0.5.[78,79] Postulated mechanisms for the

sleep-related decline in FRC include altered respiratory timing from the CRG, reduced chest wall and lung compliance, accumulated intrathoracic blood volume, and relative hypotonia of the diaphragm.[80] No known effects of age or sex have been reported to contribute to the sleep-related decline in lung volumes.

Minute ventilation
With sleep onset, V_T is reduced by 6% to 16% during NREM sleep and 25% during REM sleep.[81,82] The RR increases slightly, resulting in a rapid, shallow breathing pattern that is most prominent during REM sleep. The net effect, however, is that minute ventilation is reduced during NREM sleep (6%–7% reduction) and REM sleep (16% reduction) compared with wakefulness.[31] The effects of the reduction in ventilation combined with increases in upper airway resistance result in an increase in $Paco_2$ by 2 to 4 mm Hg and a decrease in Pao_2 by 3 to 9 mm Hg.[83,84]

Respiratory timing
During NREM sleep, mean inspiratory flow (V_T/T_I), a measure of respiratory drive, is similar to wakefulness. However, during REM sleep, mean inspiratory flow is reduced consistent with shallow breathing. The T_I/T_{TOT} remains similar during sleep and wakefulness.[31] Induction of upper airway obstruction with sleep onset, however, can have effects on respiratory timing. Specifically, induction of moderate upper airway obstruction results in increases in duty cycle by 97% to 140% and RR by 95% to 135% compared with non–flow-limited breathing. This change results in a 40% to 60% reduction in V_A, which can contribute to further hypoventilation, particularly in patients already compromised by chronic lung disease.[85]

SUMMARY

Respiration occurs owing to a complex interplay between the central nervous system, respiratory muscles, auxiliary components, and respiratory motor neurons. The initiation of sleep results in a withdrawal of the wakefulness stimuli and initiation of dynamic sleep processes that have diverse interactions with the respiratory system. The effect is to induce mild hypoventilation in the normal sleeping individual. For patients with chronic lung diseases or neuromuscular weakness, however, sleep represents a vulnerable state for worsening hypoventilation and contributes to respiratory failure. Understanding sleep-related changes in respiratory physiology will help in developing new therapies to prevent hypoventilation in susceptible populations.

REFERENCES

1. Mitchell RA, Berger AJ. Neural regulation of respiration. Am Rev Respir Dis 1975;111:206–24.

2. Horner RL. Respiratory physiology: central neural control of respiratory neurons and motoneurons during sleep. In: Kryger MH, Roth T, Dement WC, editors. Principles and practice of sleep medicine. 5th edition. St Louis (MO): Elsevier Saunders; 2011. p. 237–49.

3. Smith JC, Ellenberger HH, Ballanyi K, et al. Pre-Botzinger complex: a brainstem region that may generate respiratory rhythm in mammals. Science 1991;254:726–9.

4. Feldman JL, Del Negro CA. Looking for inspiration: new perspectives on respiratory rhythm. Nat Rev Neurosci 2006;7:232–42.

5. Smith JC, Abdala AP, Rybak IA, et al. Structural and functional architecture of respiratory networks in the mammalian brainstem. Philos Trans R Soc Lond B Biol Sci 2009;364:2577–87.

6. Mitchell GS. Back to the future: carbon dioxide chemoreceptors in the mammalian brain. Nat Neurosci 2004;7:1288–90.

7. Orem J, Lovering AT, Dunin-Barkowski W, et al. Tonic activity in the respiratory system in wakefulness, NREM and REM sleep. Sleep 2002;25:488–96.

8. Espana RA, Scammell TE. Sleep neurobiology from a clinical perspective. Sleep 2011;34:845–58.

9. Saper CB, Scammell TE, Lu J. Hypothalamic regulation of sleep and circadian rhythms. Nature 2005;437:1257–63.

10. Schwartz JR, Roth T. Neurophysiology of sleep and wakefulness: basic science and clinical implications. Curr Neuropharmacol 2008;6:367–78.

11. Joseph V, Pequignot JM, Van RO. Neurochemical perspectives on the control of breathing during sleep. Respir Physiol Neurobiol 2002;130:253–63.

12. White DP. Pathogenesis of obstructive and central sleep apnea. Am J Respir Crit Care Med 2005;172:1363–70.

13. Wellman A, White DP. Central sleep apnea and periodic breathing. In: Kryger MH, Roth T, Dement WC, editors. Principles and practice of sleep medicine. 5th edition. St Louis (MO): Elsevier Saunders; 2011. p. 1140–52.

14. Douglas NJ. Respiratory physiology: understanding the control of ventilation. In: Kryger MH, Roth T, Dement WC, editors. Principles and practice of sleep medicine. 5th edition. St Louis (MO): Elsevier Saunders; 2011. p. 250–8.

15. Verbraecken JA, De Backer WA. Upper airway mechanics. Respiration 2009;78:121–33.

16. Khoo MC. Determinants of ventilatory instability and variability. Respir Physiol 2000;122:167–82.

17. Slessarev M, Mardimae A, Preiss D, et al. Differences in the control of breathing between Andean highlanders and lowlanders after 10 days acclimatization at 3850 m. J Physiol 2010;588:1607–21.

18. Kumar P. Systemic effects resulting from carotid body stimulation-invited article. Adv Exp Med Biol 2009;648:223–33.

19. Kara T, Narkiewicz K, Somers VK. Chemoreflexes–physiology and clinical implications. Acta Physiol Scand 2003;177:377–84.

20. Smith CA, Nakayama H, Dempsey JA. The essential role of carotid body chemoreceptors in sleep apnea. Can J Physiol Pharmacol 2003;81:774–9.

21. Bulow K. Respiration and wakefulness in man. Acta Physiol Scand Suppl 1963;209:1–110.

22. Berthon-Jones M, Sullivan CE. Ventilation and arousal responses to hypercapnia in normal sleeping humans. J Appl Physiol Respir Environ Exerc Physiol 1984;57:59–67.

23. O'Donnell CP, Schaub CD, Haines AS, et al. Leptin prevents respiratory depression in obesity. Am J Respir Crit Care Med 1999;159:1477–84.

24. Duffin J. Measuring the ventilatory response to hypoxia. J Physiol 2007;584:285–93.

25. Hedemark LL, Kronenberg RS. Ventilatory and heart rate responses to hypoxia and hypercapnia during sleep in adults. J Appl Physiol Respir Environ Exerc Physiol 1982;53:307–12.

26. White DP, Douglas NJ, Pickett CK, et al. Hypoxic ventilatory response during sleep in normal premenopausal women. Am Rev Respir Dis 1982;126:530–3.

27. Malhotra A, Owens RL. What is central sleep apnea? Respir Care 2010;55:1168–78.

28. Dempsey JA, Smith CA, Przybylowski T, et al. The ventilatory responsiveness to CO(2) below eupnoea as a determinant of ventilatory stability in sleep. J Physiol 2004;560:1–11.

29. Jordan AS, White DP. Pharyngeal motor control and the pathogenesis of obstructive sleep apnea. Respir Physiol Neurobiol 2008;160:1–7.

30. Eckert DJ, Jordan AS, Merchia P, et al. Central sleep apnea: pathophysiology and treatment. Chest 2007;131:595–607.

31. Douglas NJ, White DP, Pickett CK, et al. Respiration during sleep in normal man. Thorax 1982;37:840–4.

32. Berthon-Jones M, Sullivan CE. Ventilatory and arousal responses to hypoxia in sleeping humans. Am Rev Respir Dis 1982;125:632–9.

33. Douglas NJ, White DP, Weil JV, et al. Hypercapnic ventilatory response in sleeping adults. Am Rev Respir Dis 1982;126:758–62.

34. Sullivan CE, Issa FG. Pathophysiological mechanisms in obstructive sleep apnea. Sleep 1980;3:235–46.

35. Gugger M, Molloy J, Gould GA, et al. Ventilatory and arousal responses to added inspiratory resistance during sleep. Am Rev Respir Dis 1989;140:1301–7.

36. Stanchina ML, Malhotra A, Fogel RB, et al. Genioglossus muscle responsiveness to chemical and mechanical stimuli during non-rapid eye movement sleep. Am J Respir Crit Care Med 2002;165:945–9.

37. Donner MW, Bosma JF, Robertson DL. Anatomy and physiology of the pharynx. Gastrointest Radiol 1985;10:196–212.

38. Strohl KP, Fouke JM. Dilating forces on the upper airway of anesthetized dogs. J Appl Physiol (1985) 1985;58:452–8.

39. Olsen GN, Weiman DS. Assessment of exercise oxygen consumption. Ann Thorac Surg 1988;46:483–4.

40. Isono S, Remmers JE, Tanaka A, et al. Static properties of the passive pharynx in sleep apnea. Sleep 1996;19:S175–7.

41. Isono S, Remmers JE, Tanaka A, et al. Anatomy of pharynx in patients with obstructive sleep apnea and in normal subjects. J Appl Physiol (1985) 1997;82:1319–26.

42. Ciscar MA, Juan G, Martinez V, et al. Magnetic resonance imaging of the pharynx in OSA patients and healthy subjects. Eur Respir J 2001;17:79–86.

43. Ryan B. Pneumothorax: assessment and diagnostic testing. J Cardiovasc Nurs 2005;20:251–3.

44. Ferris BG Jr, Mead J, Opie LH. Partitioning of respiratory flow resistance in man. J Appl Physiol 1964;19:653–8.

45. Horner RL. Motor control of the pharyngeal musculature and implications for the pathogenesis of obstructive sleep apnea. Sleep 1996;19:827–53.

46. Patil SP, Schneider H, Schwartz AR, et al. Adult obstructive sleep apnea: pathophysiology and diagnosis. Chest 2007;132:325–37.

47. Smith PL, Wise RA, Gold AR, et al. Upper airway pressure-flow relationships in obstructive sleep apnea. J Appl Physiol (1985) 1988;64:789–95.

48. Amatoury J, Kairaitis K, Wheatley JR, et al. Onset of airflow limitation in a collapsible tube model: impact of surrounding pressure, longitudinal strain, and wall folding geometry. J Appl Physiol (1985) 2010;109:1467–75.

49. Begle RL, Skatrud JB. Hyperinflation and expiratory muscle recruitment during NREM sleep in humans. Respir Physiol 1990;82:47–63.

50. Stanchina ML, Malhotra A, Fogel RB, et al. The influence of lung volume on pharyngeal mechanics, collapsibility, and genioglossus muscle activation during sleep. Sleep 2003;26:851–6.

51. Tagaito Y, Isono S, Remmers JE, et al. Lung volume and collapsibility of the passive pharynx in patients with sleep-disordered breathing. J Appl Physiol (1985) 2007;103:1379–85.

52. Squier SB, Patil SP, Schneider H, et al. Effect of end-expiratory lung volume on upper airway collapsibility in sleeping men and women. J Appl Physiol (1985) 2010;109:977–85.

53. Kairaitis K, Verma M, Amatoury J, et al. A threshold lung volume for optimal mechanical effects on upper airway airflow dynamics: studies in an anesthetized rabbit model. J Appl Physiol 2012;112:1197–205.

54. Isono S, Tanaka A, Tagaito Y, et al. Influences of head positions and bite opening on collapsibility of the passive pharynx. J Appl Physiol (1985) 2004;97:339–46.

55. Boudewyns A, Punjabi N, Van de Heyning PH, et al. Abbreviated method for assessing upper airway function in obstructive sleep apnea. Chest 2000;118:1031–41.

56. Penzel T, Moller M, Becker HF, et al. Effect of sleep position and sleep stage on the collapsibility of the upper airways in patients with sleep apnea. Sleep 2001;24:90–5.

57. Isono S, Tanaka A, Nishino T. Lateral position decreases collapsibility of the passive pharynx in patients with obstructive sleep apnea. Anesthesiology 2002;97:780–5.

58. Tagaito Y, Isono S, Tanaka A, et al. Sitting posture decreases collapsibility of the passive pharynx in anesthetized paralyzed patients with obstructive sleep apnea. Anesthesiology 2010;113:812–8.

59. Kirkness JP, Madronio M, Stavrinou R, et al. Relationship between surface tension of upper airway lining liquid and upper airway collapsibility during sleep in obstructive sleep apnea hypopnea syndrome. J Appl Physiol (1985) 2003;95:1761–6.

60. Wheatley JR, White DP. The influence of sleep on pharyngeal reflexes. Sleep 1993;16:S87–9.

61. Mezzanotte WS, Tangel DJ, White DP. Influence of sleep onset on upper-airway muscle activity in apnea patients versus normal controls. Am J Respir Crit Care Med 1996;153:1880–7.

62. Fogel RB, Trinder J, White DP, et al. The effect of sleep onset on upper airway muscle activity in patients with sleep apnoea versus controls. J Physiol 2005;564:549–62.

63. Tangel DJ, Mezzanotte WS, White DP. Influence of sleep on tensor palatini EMG and upper airway resistance in normal men. J Appl Physiol (1985) 1991;70:2574–81.

64. Wiegand L, Zwillich CW, Wiegand D, et al. Changes in upper airway muscle activation and ventilation during phasic REM sleep in normal men. J Appl Physiol (1985) 1991;71:488–97.

65. Mezzanotte WS, Tangel DJ, White DP. Mechanisms of control of alae nasi muscle activity. J Appl Physiol (1985) 1992;72:925–33.

66. Douglas NJ. Control of ventilation during sleep. Clin Chest Med 1985;6:563–75.

67. Henkel J, Holthaus M. Classical resonances in quantum mechanics. Phys Rev A 1992;45:1978–86.

68. Hienzer RC, Series F. Normal physiology of the upper and lower airways. In: Kryger MH, Roth T, Dement WC, editors. Principles and practice of sleep medicine. 5th edition. St Louis (MO): Elsevier Saunders; 2011. p. 259–68.

69. van LE, Dick TE. Intrinsic properties of pharyngeal and diaphragmatic respiratory motoneurons and muscles. J Appl Physiol (1985) 1992;73:787–800.

70. Papandrinopoulou D, Tzouda V, Tsoukalas G. Lung compliance and chronic obstructive pulmonary disease. Pulm Med 2012;2012:542769.

71. Watson RA, Pride NB. Postural changes in lung volumes and respiratory resistance in subjects with obesity. J Appl Physiol (1985) 2005;98:512–7.

72. Kirkness JP, Patil SP. Pathogenesis of obstructive sleep apnea in obesity. In: Dixon AE, Clerisme-Beaty EM, editors. Obesity and lung disease: a guide to management (respiratory medicine). New York: Springer; 2013.

73. Jones RL, Nzekwu MM. The effects of body mass index on lung volumes. Chest 2006;130:827–33.

74. Chen Y, Rennie D, Cormier YF, et al. Waist circumference is associated with pulmonary function in normal-weight, overweight, and obese subjects. Am J Clin Nutr 2007;85:35–9.

75. Bijaoui EL, Champagne V, Baconnier PF, et al. Mechanical properties of the lung and upper airways in patients with sleep-disordered breathing. Am J Respir Crit Care Med 2002;165:1055–61.

76. Boudewyns A, Schwartz AR, Van de Heyning PH. Upper airway collapsibility: measurement techniques and therapeutic implications. Acta Otorhinolaryngol Belg 2002;56:121–5.

77. Neder JA, Dal CS, Malaguti C, et al. The pattern and timing of breathing during incremental exercise: a normative study. Eur Respir J 2003;21: 530–8.

78. Hudgel DW, Devadatta P. Decrease in functional residual capacity during sleep in normal humans. J Appl Physiol Respir Environ Exerc Physiol 1984; 57:1319–22.

79. Ballard RD, Irvin CG, Martin RJ, et al. Influence of sleep on lung volume in asthmatic patients and normal subjects. J Appl Physiol (1985) 1990;68: 2034–41.

80. Casey KR, Cantillo KO, Brown LK. Sleep-related hypoventilation/hypoxemic syndromes. Chest 2007; 131:1936–48.

81. Skatrud JB, Dempsey JA. Airway resistance and respiratory muscle function in snorers during NREM sleep. J Appl Physiol (1985) 1985;59: 328–35.

82. Gould GA, Gugger M, Molloy J, et al. Breathing pattern and eye movement density during REM sleep in humans. Am Rev Respir Dis 1988;138: 874–7.

83. Naifeh KH, Kamiya J. The nature of respiratory changes associated with sleep onset. Sleep 1981;4:49–59.

84. Trinder J, Whitworth F, Kay A, et al. Respiratory instability during sleep onset. J Appl Physiol (1985) 1992;73:2462–9.

85. Schneider H, Krishnan V, Pichard LE, et al. Inspiratory duty cycle responses to flow limitation predict nocturnal hypoventilation. Eur Respir J 2009;33: 1068–76.

Sleep in Asthma

Wajahat H. Khan, MD[a], Vahid Mohsenin, MD[b],
Carolyn M. D'Ambrosio, MS, MD[c],*

KEYWORDS

- Sleep • Asthma • Nocturnal • Breathing • Dyspnea

KEY POINTS

- Understanding the mechanism of nocturnal asthma and the factors that exacerbate asthma during sleep would lead to better management of the condition.
- Normal sleep architecture changes with nocturnal asthma.
- The exact mechanisms for nocturnal exacerbation of asthma are not fully established.

EPIDEMIOLOGY

Many patients with asthma experience worsening of symptoms at night. A review of emergency room visits by Horn and colleagues[1] indicated that patients with respiratory symptoms were more likely to present to the emergency room between the hours of midnight and 8 AM That study further found that 40% of the calls to physicians from asthmatic patients occurred between 11 PM and 7 AM A greater proportion of asthma patients tend to die at night than those in the general population.[2,3] In a review of deaths related to asthma in Victoria, New Zealand, over a 1-year period, Robertson and colleagues[4] determined that 53% of the asthma exacerbations that led to death began between 6 PM and 3 AM

Understanding the mechanism of nocturnal asthma and the factors that exacerbate asthma during sleep would lead to better management of the condition.

Many patients with asthma experience nocturnal symptoms at some time in their lives and most experience them on a regular basis. In a large

survey of 7729 patients with asthma,[5] 74% reported experiencing nocturnal cough and wheeze at least once a week. The most studied causes and contributing factors to exacerbations of asthma at night include circadian changes in ventilation, airway responsiveness and inflammation, mucociliary clearance, ventilatory responses to hypercapnia and hypoxia, and hormone levels. This article is an update to that of D'Ambrosio and Mohsenin and Denjean and colleagues,[6,7] and reviews the normal physiologic changes that affect the lung during sleep and how those changes may contribute to nocturnal asthma.

PATHOPHYSIOLOGY
Flow Rates and Airway Resistance

Up to 90% of patients with asthma report some wheezing or cough at night.[8] Those symptoms may well be attributable to the functional changes that occur in ventilation during sleep. Normal subjects have sleep-related decreases in functional residual capacity (FRC), peak expiratory flow rate (PEFR), minute ventilation, and tidal volume.[9]

Disclosures: None.
[a] Department of Sleep Medicine, University of Pennsylvania, 3400 Spruce Street, Philadelphia, PA 19104, USA;
[b] Department of Pulmonary and Critical Care Medicine, Yale Center for Sleep Disorders, Yale University School of Medicine, 333 Cedar Street, New Haven, CT 06520, USA; [c] Department of Pulmonary, Critical Care and Sleep Medicine, The Center for Sleep Medicine, Tufts Medical Center, Tufts University School of Medicine, 800 Washington Street, Boston, MA 02111, USA
* Corresponding author.
E-mail address: cdambrosio@tuftsmedicalcenter.org

Clin Chest Med 35 (2014) 483–493
http://dx.doi.org/10.1016/j.ccm.2014.06.004
0272-5231/14/$ – see front matter © 2014 Elsevier Inc. All rights reserved.

Asthmatics have greater loss of FRC, PEFR, and tidal volume during sleep than normal subjects.

Several studies have found circadian changes in flow rates and airway resistance (**Fig. 1**). Hetzel and Clark[10] found a circadian change in PEFR in normal and asthmatic subjects. The lowest values for PEFR in both the normal and asthmatic subjects occurred in the early morning hours. The asthmatic subjects had much lower values than the normal subjects, indicating more severe bronchoconstriction.

To better define the site of increased airway resistance during sleep, Bellia and colleagues[11] examined 7 asthmatic patients and compared them with 4 normal adults. Upper and lower airway resistances were measured by placing catheters in the esophagus and supraglottic areas, with the measurement of airflow at the mouth using a tight-fitting mask. The lower airway resistance was calculated as the difference between total lung resistance and supraglottic resistance at a given lung volume. An increase in lower airway resistance was responsible for the decline in PEFR. The severity of the morning decrease in PEFR in the asthmatic subjects with nocturnal symptoms closely correlated with the higher values of lower airway resistance and its duration during sleep.[11]

Those findings were confirmed by Ballard and colleagues,[12] who studied 6 asthmatic patients with nocturnal symptoms and 4 control subjects overnight on 3 separate occasions. They measured lower airway resistance during sleep using a technique similar to that of Bellia and colleagues.[12] Each patient was studied during 1 night of normal sleep, 1 night awake, and 1 night after sleep deprivation. During the night of normal sleep, asthmatic patients had much greater airway resistance than the normal subjects. During the sleep prevention night, the airway resistance in the asthmatic group was lower by a factor of 2 but still higher than that of the controls. In the normal group, airway resistance did not change significantly between normal sleep and the sleep prevention night.

The studies on the effect of sleep stages on airway resistance are inconsistent, showing either no change,[12] an increase in stage N3 non–rapid eye movement (NREM) sleep,[13] or an increase in rapid eye movement (REM) sleep.[14] In a multivariate analysis of the relationship between sleep stages and sleep time and changes of airway resistance,[15] the latter part of sleep appears to be a more important determinant of increased airway resistance than the sleep stage.

The effects of sleep per se of worsening asthma and increased airway resistance are further supported by the work of Clark and Hetzel,[16] who studied asthmatic shift workers during rotating shifts with varying sleep schedules. They observed that their decline in PEFR was related to the change in sleep schedule as opposed to time of day.[16]

Spengler and Shea[17] have also addressed diurnal indices of pulmonary function. They studied 10 healthy individuals who remained awake in a semirecumbent position for 41 hours in a controlled environment with low light. They found circadian variations in forced expiratory volume in 1 second (FEV_1), cortisol, and core body temperature but not in PEFR.[17]

Bronchial Hyper-responsiveness

There is wide diurnal variation in bronchial hyper-responsiveness to histamine in asthmatic patients.[18] The variation in flow rates in a 24-hour period is related to changes in bronchial hyper-responsiveness in the subjects.[19] Several potential mechanisms exist for enhanced bronchial hyper-responsiveness in asthma, including enhanced parasympathetic tone, hormonal variations, and inflammation of the airways.

Parasympathetic System

The PEFR, specific airway conductance, and pulse rate were measured in a group of 7 asthmatic patients after an intravenous dose of atropine or placebo. The bronchoconstriction at 4 AM was almost completely reversed by atropine, suggesting a major role of the parasympathetic nervous system in nocturnal bronchoconstriction in asthma (**Fig. 2**).[20] The dose of atropine that completely blocked vagal activity in the bronchi was higher at 4 AM than at 4 PM. There was a strong correlation between pulse rate and PEFR at 4 AM and 4 PM, indicating increased vagal tone overnight. In the study, the changes in specific airway conductance were completely prevented at 4 AM

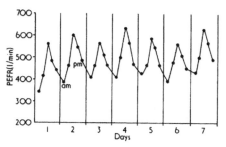

Fig. 1. Diurnal variation in peak expiratory flow rate in an asthmatic patient over four 24-hour periods. (*Adapted from* Soutar CA, Costello J, Ijaduola O, et al. Nocturnal and morning asthma. Thorax 1975;30:436; with permission.)

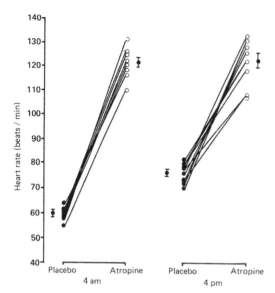

Fig. 2. The effect of atropine on the 4 AM and 4 PM peak expiratory flow rate in 10 patients with asthma. Atropine significantly improved the flow rate at 4 AM (P<.0001) and 4 PM (P<.04) when compared with placebo. (*From* Morrison JF, Pearson SB, Dean HG. Parasympathetic nervous system in nocturnal asthma. BMJ 1988;296:1427; with permission.)

by vagal blockade. That could be secondary to specific airway conductance being a more sensitive test for bronchomotor tone. The researchers were not able to completely block vagal activity to the bronchi by nebulized ipratropium bromide alone.[20,21]

Hormonal changes
The neuroendocrine system has also been a focus of attention as a possible contributor to nocturnal asthma. There are circadian variations in plasma cortisol and histamine concentrations, with the lowest values for cortisol at midnight and highest value for histamine at 4 AM in normal patients. The temporal relationship of lowest plasma cortisol concentration and dip in PEFR in asthmatic subjects has been shown.[22] Szefler and colleagues[22] measured plasma histamine, cortisol, cyclic adenosine monophosphate, and leukocyte β-adrenergic receptors in patients with asthma, both with and without nocturnal symptoms, and in normal subjects. In all groups, plasma histamine concentration was 2 times higher at 4 AM than at 4 PM There was no significant change in plasma cortisol, cyclic adenosine monophosphate, and epinephrine between the morning and evening measurements. Furthermore, when the circadian variations in plasma cortisol and histamine in normal subjects were compared with those of asthmatic patients, there were no significant differences.

These findings would not account for nocturnal exacerbations in some but not all asthmatics. That difference may be explained by receptor-binding affinity. Kraft and colleagues and Lewis[23,24] found a circadian glucocorticoid-binding affinity in patients with nocturnal asthma, but not in asthmatics without nocturnal symptoms or in control subjects. They found a reduced glucocorticoid-binding affinity at 4 AM in the nocturnal asthma subjects. They also found reduced steroid responsiveness in vitro by lymphocyte proliferation assays.

Barnes and colleagues[25] found that plasma histamine concentrations were significantly lower in normal subjects than asthmatic subjects at night. The increased histamine concentration was thought to be related to lower plasma epinephrine levels.

In the same study,[22] the mononuclear and polymorphonuclear leukocytes obtained at 4 AM from asthmatic subjects showed 33% lower β-adrenergic receptor density and had impaired response to isoproterenol infusion compared with those obtained at 4 PM

In an interventional study,[26,27] the infusion of low-dose levo-epinephrine resulted in decreased plasma histamine concentrations but no significant change in PEFR, suggesting a lack of cause-and-effect relationship between histamine and epinephrine levels and PEFR. Similarly, infusion of hydrocortisone in a group of 6 asthmatic patients at night prevented the early morning decrease in plasma cortisol levels but not the decrease in their PEFR.

These studies show that the variations in hormones and mediators may play a minor role in worsening of airway constriction at night in asthma.

Inflammatory changes
Inflammation of the airways is the main underlying mechanism of airway hyper-reactivity in asthma. Mohiuddin and Martin[28] evaluated the late asthmatic response after an allergen challenge and its relationship to nocturnal asthma. Ten patients with mild, stable asthma were given placebo or allergen inhalation in the morning and, on another day, again in the evening. The FEV_1 was measured soon after either the allergen or placebo was given and every hour for up to 12 hours after inhalation. Only 4 of the 10 patients had a late asthmatic response to the morning inhalation of allergen, but 9 of 10 patients had a late asthmatic response after the evening dose. Interestingly, the late asthmatic response after the evening dose occurred sooner, was more severe, and had a more prolonged effect on bronchoconstriction.

Bronchoalveolar lavage studies[29] of patients with nocturnal asthma show more intense inflammatory process in the airways, in the form of higher total leukocyte, neutrophil, and eosinophil counts at night than during the daytime (**Fig. 3**). Patients with asthma without nocturnal symptoms do not show increased inflammatory process at night compared with patients with nocturnal asthma. For all asthmatic patients, with and without nocturnal symptoms, however, the overnight decrease in PEFR correlates with the change in neutrophil and eosinophil counts.[29] This landmark study shows the role of an enhanced inflammatory process at night in worsening asthma.

Lung Volume Changes During Sleep

Lung volumes are shown to decrease during normal sleep. A study by Ballard and colleagues[9] defined the changes in FRC during sleep in normal human subjects and asthmatic patients. Using a horizontal volume-displacement body plethysmograph, they measured FRC in the supine and awake state and during sleep. Their results showed a decrease in FRC during sleep of 20% in normal subjects and 41% in asthmatic patients compared with awake and supine values (**Fig. 4**). The authors[9] postulated that the decrease in lung volume during sleep may be important in the development of nocturnal bronchoconstriction in asthmatic patients.

To test that hypothesis, the same group[30] studied ventilatory patterns during sleep in asthmatic patients while their lung volume was kept constant using a continuous negative pressure device—a poncho cuirass system—in a whole-body

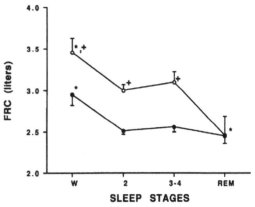

Fig. 4. Effect of different sleep stages on FRC in normal (*closed circle*) and asthmatic patients (*open circle*). Error bars, standard error (SE).* $P<.05$, wakefulness (W), and REM versus all other stages in asthmatics, and W versus all other stages in normal subjects; + $P<.05$, asthmatic patients versus normal subjects. (*From* Ballard RD, Irvin CG, Martin RJ, et al. Influence of sleep on lung volume in asthmatic patients and normal subjects. J Appl Physiol (1985) 1990;68:2034; with permission.)

plethysmograph. The subjects showed a decrease in FEV_1 during sleep despite the maintenance of a constant lung volume. The researchers[30] therefore concluded that the change in lung volume during sleep is not solely responsible for the decline in flow rates. Pulmonary capillary blood volume is found to be increased during sleep. To evaluate the role of increased pulmonary capillary volume in decreased functional residual capacity, Desjardin and associates[31] used diffusing capacity to estimate the pulmonary capillary blood volume in

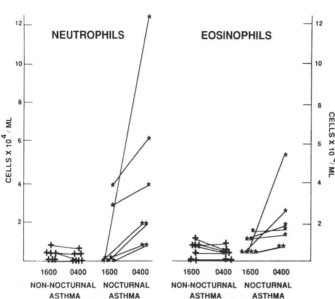

Fig. 3. The bronchoalveolar lavage neutrophils and eosinophils in patients with non-nocturnal and nocturnal asthma at 4 AM and 4 PM. The patients with nocturnal asthma had significantly higher neutrophil and eosinophil counts during early morning hours than in the afternoon ($P<.05$). (*From* Martin RJ, Cicutto LC, Smith HR, et al. Airway inflammation in nocturnal asthma. Am Rev Respir Dis 1991;143:351; Reprinted with permission of the American Thoracic Society. Copyright © 2014 American Thoracic Society.)

sleep. They studied a group of normal and asthmatic subjects with and without nocturnal symptoms. They found a decrease in FEV_1 overnight for the asthmatic patients with nocturnal worsening. Normal and asthmatic subjects without nocturnal symptoms did not have a significant decrease in overnight FEV_1 or pulmonary capillary blood volume compared with values obtained while awake and in the supine position. Conversely, the asthmatic patients with nocturnal worsening had a significant increase in measured pulmonary capillary blood volume not seen in the other subjects.[31] A decrease in FEV_1 may lead to more negative intrathoracic pressure, which, in turn, may lead to increased pulmonary capillary blood volume. The decline in FEV_1 is unlikely to be related to increased pulmonary capillary blood volume during sleep.

Sleep is associated with reduction in inspiratory muscle tonic activity.[32] The inspiratory intercostal muscles are inhibited more than the diaphragmatic muscle. This inhibition is more pronounced in REM than NREM sleep. The diminished inspiratory muscle tonic activity could, in part, explain the decrease in lung volume during sleep.

SUMMARY

The exact mechanism(s) for nocturnal exacerbation of asthma is not fully established. It is clear, however, that sleep per se, rather than clock time or circadian rhythm, has profound effects on airway function. There is an increase in bronchial inflammation and reactivity with concomitant increase in airway resistance and diminished airflow rates and functional residual capacity. These alterations are, in part, related to airway cooling, enhanced parasympathetic tone, allergen exposure, and some hormonal changes during sleep. Not all asthmatics, however, experience worsening of their asthma during sleep. This finding suggests a complex interplay among aforementioned factors and asthmatic persons (**Box 1**).

AROUSAL AND VENTILATORY RESPONSES

The ventilatory responses to hypoxia and hypercapnia are altered during sleep. That may have a significant bearing on the arousal responses to blood gas changes in nocturnal asthma during sleep. Under isocapnic conditions, 6 healthy men were studied at varying levels of hypoxia during sleep. The hypoxic ventilatory response was least during REM sleep and less in all stages of sleep compared with the awake state.[33,34]

The ventilatory response to hypercapnia is also of interest because patients with lung disease

---

> **Box 1**
> **Factors contributing to pathophysiology of nocturnal asthma**
>
> Increased airway resistance and diminished flow rates
> - Decreased inspiratory muscle activity
> - Decreased functional residual capacity
> - Airway cooling
>
> Increased bronchial hyper-reactivity
> - Enhanced parasympathetic tone
> - Bronchial inflammation
> - Increased circulating histamine

---

often have hypercapnia during sleep. In a study by Berthon-Jones and Sullivan,[33] normal male subjects had a 50% reduction in ventilatory response to hypercapnia during NREM sleep and a further reduction in REM sleep. In contrast, women had less blunting of the hypercapnic response in all stages of sleep.[33]

The effect of sleep deprivation on ventilatory responses to hypercapnia was studied by Schiffman and associates[35] in a group of men and women. They reported a significant impairment of the ventilatory response to hypercapnia after a night of sleep deprivation in 12 of the 13 subjects. To determine the arousal response to loaded breathing during sleep, the investigators[35] imposed an inspiratory load during normal sleep and after a period of sleep deprivation. Similar to the blunted hypercapnic and hypoxic responses during sleep, the arousal response to increasing respiratory resistance is markedly impaired.

White and colleagues[36] made a similar observation. The findings were confirmed by Grugger and colleagues,[37] who studied the ventilatory and arousal response to increased inspiratory resistance in normal men. The subjects were studied awake and during sleep, with increasing levels of inspiratory resistance, up to 10 cm $H_2O/L/s$, imposed on them. They showed that arousal response to the resistance was less during stages N3 sleep compared with stage 2 and REM sleep. No major change in ventilation was seen in that study.

In a similar study, Bellia and colleagues[13] found the peak and the longest period of bronchoconstriction occurred during stage N3 in asthmatic subjects.

Ballard and colleagues[38] further studied load detection in asthmatic subjects during sleep by inducing bronchoconstriction using methacholine inhalation. Each subject inhaled methacholine while awake, during normal sleep, and then during sleep after 36 hours of sleep deprivation. Lower airway resistance and inspiratory drive, as measured by occlusion pressure, were measured in all 3 occasions. Minute ventilation was well preserved despite bronchoconstriction in all 3 situations, mainly because of increased inspiratory drive. After sleep deprivation, the asthmatic subjects tolerated much greater bronchoconstriction and lower airway resistance before having an arousal or awakening. In contrast to previously mentioned studies, no correlation was found between sleep stages and arousal thresholds. These findings are relevant to the pathophysiology of nocturnal asthma and suggest the possibility of a vicious cycle of sleep deprivation and bronchospasm, with blunted arousal responses, that may help explain the increased morbidity and mortality of asthma at night.

SLEEP ARCHITECTURE

The human circadian sleep-wake cycle is entrained by light. After passing through the retinal ganglion cells, light blocks the sleep-promoting effects of melatonin in the suprachiasmatic nucleus of the brain.[39,40] Melatonin levels fluctuate throughout the 24-hour circadian period and regulate sleep. Although asthmatics are known to have poor sleep quality, there is little research on the effects of exogenous melatonin for sleep in asthmatic patients.

Interestingly, melatonin is found to enhance the production of inflammatory intermediates in several in vitro studies[39,41–43] and to enhance bronchial smooth muscle constriction in animal models.[44] To what extent melatonin has immunomodulating or bronchconstricting effects in humans is yet to be determined. In a randomized, double-blind, placebo-controlled study of 22 women with asthma, Campos and colleagues[45] evaluated the effects of exogenous melatonin. Participants were randomly assigned to receive either melatonin 3 mg 2 hours before bedtime or placebo. At the end of 4 weeks, melatonin treatment significantly improved subjective sleep quality. Furthermore, there were no differences in asthma symptoms, medication use, or PEFR between the 2 groups. Data are lacking concerning the long-term effects of melatonin in asthmatics.

Patients with nocturnal asthma symptoms are likely to have frequent arousals during sleep and report worse sleep quality. Forty percent of such patients wake each night with asthma symptoms, and 75% have problems with their asthma during sleep at least once a week.[5] In a laboratory study, 12 asthmatic volunteers with nocturnal symptoms were compared with 10 age-matched control subjects. Each subject slept in the sleep laboratory for 2 consecutive nights. The first night in the sleep laboratory was for the acclimatization of the subjects to the laboratory environment. The data from the second night of the sleep study indicated increased wake time, decreased mean sleep time, and increased number of awakenings in asthmatic subjects compared with normal subjects. There was no significant difference in sleep latencies, number of REM periods, or REM content. There was markedly less stage N3 sleep in the asthmatic group, however, and the difference was made up primarily by stage 2 sleep and, to a lesser extent, stage 1 sleep.[14]

Montplaisir and colleagues[46] reported a study on 12 asthmatic patients with fewer symptoms than the group studied by Kales and colleagues,[14] and again showed less total sleep time and sleep efficiency, with greater wake time after sleep onset compared with a group of 8 age-matched control subjects. They found no significant difference in percentages of sleep stages between the groups.

Sleep fragmentation and poor sleep quality are likely associated with asthma control and quality of life. In a cohort of 487 patients with asthma, Mastronarde and colleagues[47] found a correlation between sleep quality, asthma control, and quality of life. Furthermore, improvements in sleepiness and sleep quality were significantly associated with improvements in asthma control and quality of life.

In other studies,[48] daytime cognitive performance and objective overnight sleep quality were worse in patients with nocturnal asthma when compared with a control population. As has been shown previously, sleep deprivation can blunt ventilatory responses to hypoxia and hypercapnia in normal subjects.

OTHER PRECIPITATING FACTORS OF NOCTURNAL ASTHMA

Other possible contributing causes of nocturnal asthma include airway cooling, allergen exposure, decreased mucociliary transport and increased airway secretions, and gastroesophageal reflux disease (GERD).

Body and Airway Temperature

There is a decrease in core body temperature by 1.1°C between the hours of 2 AM and 4 AM. A study by Chen and colleagues[49,50] found that a decrease in body temperature of 0.7°C by cold exposure triggered an acute attack in most patients with asthma. To differentiate between the effects of core body temperature during sleep on airway tone regulation, as opposed to direct airway cooling, they had asthmatic subjects breathe warm, humidified air. They found that warm, humidified air prevented nocturnal bronchoconstriction even in the presence of lower core body temperature, suggesting a direct effect of cold air on airway tone. The beneficial effect of warm, humidified air appears to be related to its heat and water content.[51,52]

Mucociliary Transport and Airway Secretions

Because coughs are suppressed, airway secretions are increased during sleep. Martin and colleagues[19] made an observation in asthmatic subjects during bronchoscopy at 4 AM that there were more airway secretions and edema than at 4 PM in the same subjects. That area has not been studied thoroughly, however. There is evidence, however, that mucociliary transport is impaired during sleep in normal individuals. That was shown by Bateman and colleagues,[53] and Hasani and colleagues[54] using a radioaerosol technique to measure mucociliary transport.

Allergen Exposure

People are potentially exposed to allergens during sleep. It appears that late-phase response to allergen exposure is more pronounced in the evening hours than during the morning hours in asthmatic patients.[28] Some studies suggest that avoidance of allergen exposure can reduce the circadian changes in PEFR and the frequency and severity of asthma attacks.[55,56] However, in a systematic review of 23 controlled studies, Hammarquist and colleagues[57] found various efforts to reduce allergen exposure had no effect on asthma symptom scores or morning PEFR.

Gastroesophageal Reflux Disease

The association between asthma and GERD has been well established in several studies.[58–62] The prevalence of GERD in asthma has been estimated to be 34% to 89%, and 40% of patients have evidence for esophagitis.[62] In another study in patients with chronic cough,[63,64] 36% were found to have GERD as a cause for their cough symptoms. The mechanism of bronchoconstriction appears to be a vagal response to exposure of the lower esophagus to acidity. Actual aspiration of stomach contents appears to play a lesser role.[65]

Medical treatment of GERD is generally disappointing in improving asthma symptoms. In a double-blind, randomized, placebo-controlled, crossover study of 20 patients with asthma,[66] omeprazole, 40 mg daily for 4 weeks, did not change asthma symptoms, inhaled β-agonist use, or histamine bronchial responsiveness. In a more recent study,[67] 412 poorly controlled asthmatic patients were randomly assigned to receive either esomeprazole, 40 mg twice daily, or placebo. After 24 weeks, there was no symptom improvement in either the treatment or control group. On the other hand, surgical management of GERD is found to be effective in controlling the asthma symptoms. In a study comparing conservative treatment with antireflux surgery,[68] patients who had asthma and GERD were randomly assigned to 3 groups—cimetidine or placebo for 6 months and antireflux surgery. Antireflux surgery was superior to cimetidine or placebo in the elimination of respiratory symptoms. The beneficial effect of the antireflux surgery was documented up to 6 years later in 50% of the patients in the group.[68]

Sleep Apnea

Recent data suggest an association between obstructive sleep apnea and asthma.[69–73] Sleep apnea could cause exacerbation of asthma through several mechanisms. Treatment of sleep apnea with nasal continuous positive airway pressure also improves nocturnal and daytime symptoms of coexisting asthma.[51] The proposed mechanism for this beneficial effect of continuous positive airway pressure in asthma is elimination of chronic upper airway irritation by snoring and repeated apneas causing a neurally mediated reflex bronchoconstriction.[74] Another potential exacerbating factor of asthma is the higher incidence of gastroesophageal reflux in patients with sleep apnea. Acid irritation of the lower esophagus may cause vagally mediated reflex bronchoconstriction in addition to direct irritation of the airways by microaspiration. The intermittent hypoxia in sleep apnea may also potentiate bronchoconstriction. Several animal models have shown enhanced bronchial responsiveness to provocation in the setting of hypoxia.[75–77] Thus, the National Asthma Education and Prevention Expert Panel Report 3 has recommended that patients with poorly controlled asthma and symptoms of sleep-disordered (SDB) breathing be evaluated for sleep apnea.

In children, SDB has been linked to wheezing and asthma. It has also been identified as an independent risk factor for asthma severity. In a cohort of 108 asthmatic children age 4 to 18 years, Ross and colleagues[78] found those with SDB had a 3.62-fold increased odds of progressing to severe asthma at 1 year.

MANAGEMENT

Prevention

To minimize the exposure to allergens during sleep, the sleeping environment should be relatively free of dust and other organic allergens. The pillow and mattress should be encased in special covers. There should be sufficient ventilation and optimal humidity in the room. High-efficiency filtration systems are found to decrease allergen exposure.

Treatment

Long-acting β-agonist bronchodilators and inhaled corticosteroids

Many studies[79–82] find that inhaled long-acting β-agonists (LABA) have resulted in an improved morning FEV_1. Because of the risk of asthma-related death with LABA use,[83,84] inhaled corticosteroids, with or without a LABA, may be a more attractive treatment option. Weersink and colleagues[85] studied 46 subjects with nocturnal asthma. In a randomized, double-blind trial they compared fluticasone propionate, 250 μg, with salmeterol xinafoate, 50 μg, or the combination of the 2 drugs. Each treatment was administered via inhalation twice daily. They found the 3 treatment regimens were equally effective in improving circadian variations in PEFR, FEV_1 and bronchial hyper-responsiveness to methacholine.

Theophyllines

Sustained-release theophylline is used to treat nocturnal asthma. Rhind and colleagues[86] reported improvement in morning FEV_1 in asthmatic patients given sustained-release theophylline compared with placebo. The patients also had reduced daytime and nocturnal symptoms and reported improved sleep quality. Polysomnography, however, found increased wake time and reduction in NREM sleep while on theophylline.[86] Comparing twice-daily dosing of theophylline with the long-acting preparation given at 7 PM in patients with nocturnal asthma, Martin and colleagues[87] found that morning FEV_1 was significantly higher on the once-a-day regimen, with higher serum concentration of theophylline at night. Despite improvement in flow rates, there was no significant difference in sleep architecture between the 2 groups.

ANTICHOLINERGIC MEDICATIONS

As was described previously, increased vagal tone occurs at night in patients with nocturnal asthma. Coe and Barnes,[88] reported the effect of an inhaled anticholinergic drug, oxitropium bromide, on the morning FEV_1 decline. They found that the FEV_1 decline was reduced in a dose-dependent fashion with the use of inhaled oxitropium bromide. They concluded that the use of an anticholinergic inhaled medication may be of benefit in treating nocturnal asthma.

CORTICOSTEROIDS

Most patients with asthma should be treated with inhaled steroids. For those who require oral corticosteroids, evening dosing appears to be more effective in controlling nocturnal symptoms of asthma.[89]

REFERENCES

1. Horn CR, Clark TJ, Cochrane GM. Is there a circadian variation in respiratory morbidity. Br J Dis Chest 1987;81:248–51.
2. Douglas NJ. Asthma at night. Clin Chest Med 1985; 6:663–74.
3. Douglas NJ. Nocturnal asthma. QJM 1989;71: 279–89.
4. Robertson CF, Rubinfeld AR, Bowes G. Deaths from asthma in Victoria: a 12-month survey. Med J Aust 1990;152:511–7.
5. Turner-Warwick M. Epidemiology of nocturnal asthma. Am J Med 1988;85:6–8.
6. D'Ambrosio CM, Mohsenin V. Sleep in asthma. Clin Chest Med 1998;19(1):127–37.
7. Denjean A, Canet E, Praud JP, et al. Hypoxia-induced bronchial responsiveness in awake sheep: role of carotid chemoreceptors. Respir Physiol 1991;83:201–10.
8. Douglas NJ, Flenley DC. Breathing during sleep in patients with obstructive lung disease. Am Rev Respir Dis 1990;141:1053–70.
9. Ballard RD, Irvin CG, Martin RJ, et al. Influence of sleep on lung volume in asthmatic patients and normal subjects. J Appl Physiol (1985) 1990;68: 2034–41.
10. Hetzel MR, Clark TJ. Comparison of normal and asthmatic circadian rhythms in peak expiratory flow rate. Thorax 1980;35:732–8.
11. Bellia V, Visconti A, Insalaco G, et al. Validation of morning dip of peak expiratory flow as an indicator of the severity of nocturnal asthma. Chest 1988;94: 108–10.
12. Ballard RD, Saathoff MC, Patel DK, et al. Effect of sleep on nocturnal bronchoconstriction and ventilatory patterns in asthmatics. J Appl Physiol (1985) 1989;67:243–9.
13. Bellia V, Cuttitta G, Insalaco G, et al. Relationship of nocturnal bronchoconstriction to sleep stages. Am Rev Respir Dis 1989;140:363–7.
14. Kales A, Beall GN, Bajor GF, et al. Sleep studies in asthmatic adults: relationship of attacks to

sleep stage and time of night. J Allergy 1968;41: 164–73.

15. Shapiro CM, Catterall JR, Montgomery I, et al. Do asthmatics suffer bronchoconstriction during rapid eye movement sleep? BMJ 1986;292:1161–4.

16. Clark TJ, Hetzel MR. Diurnal variation of asthma. Br J Dis Chest 1977;71:87–92.

17. Spengler CM, Shea SA. Endogenous circadian rhythm of pulmonary function in healthy humans [Erratum in: Am J Respir Crit Care Med 2002;166(7):1005]. Am J Respir Crit Care Med 2000;162(3 Pt 1):1038–46.

18. DeVries K, Goei JT, Booj-Noord H, et al. Changes during twenty-four hours in the lung function and histamine activity in the bronchial tree in asthmatics and bronchitic subjects. Int Arch Allergy Immunol 1962;20:93–101.

19. Martin RJ, Cicutto LC, Ballard RD. Factors related to the nocturnal worsening of asthma. Am Rev Respir Dis 1990;141:33–8.

20. Morrison JF, Pearson SB. The effect of the circadian rhythm of vagal activity on bronchomotor tone in asthma. Br J Clin Pharmacol 1989;28:545–9.

21. Cattarall JR, Rhind GB, Whyte KF, et al. Is nocturnal asthma caused by changes in airway cholinergic activity? Thorax 1988;43:720–4.

22. Szefler SJ, Ando R, Cicutto LC, et al. Plasma histamine, epinephrine, cortisol, and leukocyte beta-adrenergic receptors in nocturnal asthma. Clin Pharmacol Ther 1991;49:59–68.

23. Kraft M, Vianna E, Martin RJ, et al. Nocturnal asthma is associated with reduced glucocorticoid receptor binding affinity and decreased steroid responsiveness at night. J Allergy Clin Immunol 1999;103:66–71.

24. Lewis DA. Sleep in patients with asthma and chronic obstructive pulmonary disease. Curr Opin Pulm Med 2001;7(2):105–12.

25. Barnes P, Fitzgerald G, Brown M, et al. Nocturnal asthma and changes in circulating epinephrine, histamine, and cortisol. N Engl J Med 1980;303: 263–7.

26. Soutar CA, Costello J, Ijaduola O, et al. Nocturnal and morning asthma. Thorax 1975;30:436–40.

27. Stewart IC, Rhind GB, Power JT, et al. Effect of sustained release terbutaline on symptoms and sleep quality in patients with nocturnal asthma. Thorax 1987;42:797–800.

28. Mohiuddin AA, Martin RJ. Circadian basis of the late asthmatic response. Am Rev Respir Dis 1990;142:1153–7.

29. Martin RJ, Cicutto LC, Smith HR, et al. Airways inflammation in nocturnal asthma. Am Rev Respir Dis 1991;143:351–7.

30. Martin RJ, Pak J, Irvin CG. Effect of lung volume maintenance during sleep in nocturnal asthma. J Appl Physiol (1985) 1993;75:1467–70.

31. Desjardin J, Sutarik JM, Suh BY, et al. Influence of sleep on pulmonary capillary volume in normal and asthmatic subjects. Am J Respir Crit Care Med 1995;152:193–8.

32. Ballard RD, Clover CW, White DP. Influence of non-REM sleep on inspiratory muscle activity and lung volume in asthmatic patients. Am Rev Respir Dis 1993;147:880–6.

33. Berthon-Jones M, Sullivan CE. Ventilation and arousal responses to hypercapnia in normal sleeping humans. J Appl Physiol (1985) 1984;57: 59–67.

34. Bogin RM, Ballard RD. Treatment of nocturnal asthma with pulse-release albuterol. Chest 1992; 102:362–6.

35. Schiffman PL, Trontell MC, Mazar MF, et al. Sleep deprivation decreases ventilatory response to carbon dioxide but not load compensation. Chest 1983;84:695–8.

36. White DP, Douglas NJ, Pickett CK, et al. Sleep deprivation and the control of ventilation. Am Rev Respir Dis 1983;128:984–6.

37. Grugger M, Molloy J, Gould GA, et al. Ventilatory and arousal responses to added inspiratory resistance during sleep. Am Rev Respir Dis 1989;140: 1301–7.

38. Ballard RD, Tan WC, Kelly PL, et al. Effect of sleep and sleep deprivation on ventilatory response to bronchoconstriction. J Appl Physiol (1985) 1990; 69:490–7.

39. Sutherland ER, Ellison MC, Kraft M, et al. Elevated serum melatonin is associated with the nocturnal worsening of asthma. J Allergy Clin Immunol 2003;112(3):513–7.

40. Czeisler CA, Allan JS, Strogatz SH, et al. Bright light resets the human circadian pacemaker independent of the timing of the sleep-wake cycle. Science 1986;233:667–71.

41. Garcia-Maurino S, Gonzalez-Haba MG, Calvo JR, et al. Melatonin enhances IL-2, IL-6, and IFN-gamma production by human circulating CD4+ cells: a possible nuclear receptor-mediated mechanism involving T helper type 1 lymphocytes and monocytes. J Immunol 1997;159:574–81.

42. Garcia-Maurino S, Pozo D, Carrillo-Vico A, et al. Melatonin activates Th1 lymphocytes by increasing IL-12 production. Life Sci 1999;65:2143–50.

43. Martins E Jr, Ligeiro de Oliveira AP, Fialho de Araujo AM, et al. Melatonin modulates allergic lung inflammation. J Pineal Res 2001;31:363–9.

44. Weekley LB. Influence of melatonin on bovine pulmonary vascular and bronchial airway smooth muscle tone. Clin Auton Res 1995;5:53–6.

45. Campos FL, da Silva-Júnior FP, de Bruin VM, et al. Melatonin improves sleep in asthma: a randomized, double-blind, placebo-controlled study. Am J Respir Crit Care Med 2004;170(9):947–51.

46. Montplaisir J, Walsh J, Malo JL. Nocturnal asthma: features of attacks, sleep and breathing patterns. Am Rev Respir Dis 1982;125:18–22.

47. Mastronarde JG, Wise RA, Shade DM, et al, American Lung Association Asthma Clinical Research Centers. Sleep quality in asthma: results of a large prospective clinical trial. J Asthma 2008;45(3):183–9.

48. Fitzpatrick MF, Engleman H, Whyte KF, et al. Morbidity in nocturnal asthma: sleep quality and daytime cognitive performance. Thorax 1991;46: 569–73.

49. Chen WY, Horton DJ. Airways obstruction in asthmatics induced by body cooling. Scand J Respir Dis 1978;59:13–20.

50. Chen WY, Horton DJ, Weiser PC. Airways obstruction induced by body cooling in asthmatics. Physiologist 1977;20:16.

51. Chan CS, Woolcock AJ, Sullivan CE. Nocturnal asthma: role of snoring and obstructive sleep apnea. Am Rev Respir Dis 1988;137:1502–4.

52. Chen WY, Chai H. Airway cooling and nocturnal asthma. Chest 1982;81:675–80.

53. Bateman JR, Pavia D, Clarke SW. The retention of lung secretions during the night in normal subjects. Clin Sci (Colch) 1978;55:523–7.

54. Hasani A, Agnew JE, Pavia D, et al. Effect of oral bronchodilators on lung mucociliary clearance during sleep in patients with asthma. Thorax 1993;48: 287–9.

55. Platts-Mills TA, Mitchell BB, Nock P, et al. Reduction of bronchial hyperreactivity during prolonged allergen avoidance. Lancet 1982;2:675–7.

56. Scherr MS, Peck LW. The effects of high efficiency air flow system on nighttime asthma attacks. W V Med J 1977;73:144–8.

57. Hammarquist C, Burr ML, Gotzsche PC. House dust mite control measures for asthma. Cochrane Database Syst Rev 2000;(4):CD001187. Oxford.

58. Martin ME, Grunstein MM, Larsen GL. The relationship of gastroesophageal reflux to nocturnal wheezing in children with asthma. Ann Allergy 1982;49:318–22.

59. Martin RJ. Nocturnal asthma. Clin Chest Med 1992; 13:533–50.

60. Martin RJ. Nocturnal asthma. Ann Allergy 1994;72: 5–10.

61. Mays EE. Intrinsic asthma in adults, association with gastroesophageal reflux. JAMA 1976;236: 2626–8.

62. Sontag SJ, O'Connell S, Khandelwal S. Most asthmatics have gastroesophageal reflux with or without bronchodilator therapy. Gastroenterology 1990;99:613–20.

63. Vaezi MF, Richter JE. Twenty-four hour ambulatory esophageal pH monitoring in the diagnosis of acid reflux-related chronic cough. South Med J 1997;90:305–11.

64. Van Keimpema AR, Ariaansz M, Raaijmakers JA, et al. Treatment of nocturnal asthma by addition of oral slow-release albuterol to standard treatment in stable asthma patients. J Asthma 1996; 33:119–24.

65. Harding SM, Schan CA, Guzzo MR, et al. Gastroesophageal reflux-induced bronchoconstriction, is microaspiration a factor? Chest 1995;108: 1220–7.

66. Teichtahl H, Yeomans ND, Kronborg IJ, et al. Adult asthma and gastro-oesophageal reflux: the effects of omeprazole therapy on asthma. Aust N Z J Med 1996;26:671–6.

67. Mastronard JG, Anthonise NR, Castro M, et al, The American Lung Association Asthma Clinical Research Centers. Efficacy of esomeprazole for treatment of poorly controlled asthma. N Engl J Med 2009;360:1487–99.

68. Larrain A, Carrasco E, Galleguillos F, et al. Medical and surgical treatment of nonallergic asthma associated with gastroesophageal reflux. Chest 1991; 99:1330–5.

69. Teodorescu M, Consens FB, Bria WF, et al. Correlates of daytime sleepiness in patients with asthma. Sleep Med 2006;7:607–13.

70. Ekici A, Ekici M, Kurtipek E, et al. Association of asthma-related symptoms with snoring and apnea and effect on health-related quality of life. Chest 2005;128:3358–63.

71. Janson C, De Backer W, Gislason T, et al. Increased prevalence of sleep disturbances and daytime sleepiness in subjects with bronchial asthma: a population study of young adults in three European countries. Eur Respir J 1996;9:2132–8.

72. Kalra M, Biagini J, Bernstein D, et al. Effect of asthma on the risk of obstructive sleep apnea syndrome in atopic women. Ann Allergy Asthma Immunol 2006;97:231–5.

73. Yigla M, Tov N, Solomonov A, et al. Difficult-to-control asthma and obstructive sleep apnea. J Asthma 2003;40:865–71.

74. Nadel JA, Widdicombe JG. Reflex effects of upper airway irritation on total lung resistance and blood pressure. J Appl Physiol (1985) 1962;17:861–5.

75. Alkhalil M, Schulman E, Getsy J. Obstructive sleep apnea syndrome and asthma: what are the links? J Clin Sleep Med 2009;5(1):71–8.

76. Vidruk EH, Sorkness RL. Histamine-induced reflex tracheal constriction is attenuated by hyperoxia and exaggerated by hypoxia. Am Rev Respir Dis 1985;132:287–91.

77. Ahmed T, Marchette B. Hypoxia enhances nonspecific bronchial reactivity. Am Rev Respir Dis 1985; 132:839–44.

78. Ross KR, Storfer-Isser A, Hart MA, et al. Sleep-disordered breathing is associated with asthma severity in children. J Pediatr 2012;160(5):736–42.

79. Fitzpatrick MF, Mackay T, Driver H, et al. Salmeterol in nocturnal asthma: a double blind, placebo controlled trial of a long acting inhaled beta-2 agonist. BMJ 1990;301:1365–8.

80. Neagley SR, White DP, Zwillich CW. Breathing during sleep in stable asthmatic subjects. Chest 1986; 90:334–7.

81. Petersdorf RA. Disturbance of heat regulation. In: Wintrobe MM, Thorn GW, Adams RD, et al, editors. Harrison's principles of internal medicine. 7th edition. New York: McGraw-Hill Book Co; 1974.

82. Veale D, Cooper BG, Griffiths CJ, et al. The effect of controlled-release salbutamol on sleep and nocturnal oxygenation in patients with asthma and chronic obstructive pulmonary disease. Respir Med 1994;88:121–4.

83. Weatherall M, Wijesinghe M, Perrin K, et al. Meta-analysis of the risk of mortality with salmeterol and the effect of concomitant inhaled corticosteroid therapy. Thorax 2010;65:39–43.

84. Nelson HS, Weis ST, Bleecker ER, et al, the SMART Study Group. The Salmeterol Multicenter Asthma Research Trial: a comparison of usual pharmacotherapy for asthma or usual pharmacotherapy plus salmeterol. Chest 2006;129(1):15–26.

85. Weersink EJ, Douma RR, Postma DS, et al. Fluticasone propionate, salmeterol xinafoate, and their combination in the treatment of nocturnal asthma. Am J Respir Crit Care Med 1997; 155(4):1241–6.

86. Rhind GB, Connaughton JJ, McFie J, et al. Sustained release choline theophyllinate in nocturnal asthma. BMJ 1985;291:1605–7.

87. Martin RJ, Cicutto LC, Ballard RD, et al. Circadian variations in theophylline concentrations and the treatment of nocturnal asthma. Am Rev Respir Dis 1989;139:475–8.

88. Coe CI, Barnes PJ. Reduction of nocturnal asthma by an inhaled anticholinergic drug. Chest 1986;90: 485–8.

89. Beam WR, Weiner DE, Martin MJ. Timing of prednisone and alterations of airways inflammation in nocturnal asthma. Am Rev Respir Dis 1992;146: 1524–30.

Cystic Fibrosis and Sleep

Eliot S. Katz, MD

KEYWORDS

- Sleep-disordered breathing • Hypoxemia • Respiratory insufficiency • Hypoventilation
- Noninvasive ventilation

KEY POINTS

- Patients with cystic fibrosis experience both sleep disruption and gas-exchange abnormalities during sleep.
- Symptomatically, cough and pain are reported in advanced stages of the disease in most individuals.
- Noninvasive ventilation and supplemental oxygen is frequently helpful in mitigating the adverse effects of nocturnal hypercapnia and hypoxemia.

INTRODUCTION

Cystic fibrosis (CF) pulmonary disease is characterized by chronic bacterial infection, gradual airway obstruction, and bronchiectasis, resulting in hypoxemia, hypercapnia, and increased work of breathing. In addition, CF has several features that adversely affect sleep including chronic cough, musculoskeletal pain, frequent defecation, gastrointestinal reflux, abdominal discomfort, and sometimes overnight enteral feeding. Medication usage and comorbid mood disorders may also contribute to the poor quality of sleep observed in CF. Many studies have reported considerable subjective sleep complaints with only modest objective polysomnographic changes. In general, sleep disruption or restriction has been associated with cardiovascular, metabolic, immune, and neurocognitive dysfunction. These abnormalities may exacerbate the CF-related insulin-dependent diabetes, pulmonary hypertension, frequent sinopulmonary infections, and mood disturbances. Poor sleep quality and excessive daytime sleepiness are commonly reported by CF patients and their caregivers, and correlate adversely with quality-of-life measures. In principle, treatment of gas-exchange abnormalities and sleep fragmentation could improve the quality of life and mitigate long-term complications of CF. This review focuses on the bidirectional interaction between sleep and CF.

SUBJECTIVE SLEEP DISTURBANCES

Most studies of subjective sleep quality in CF report disturbed sleep in more than 50% of patients, especially those with advanced lung disease.[1–3] Common sleep complaints include sleep-onset insomnia,[4] frequent awakenings, night cough, snoring, excessive daytime sleepiness, headaches, pain, frequent defecation,[4] anxiety, and reflux. Even when clinically stable, CF patients report more frequent awakenings with cough.[5] Longitudinal studies show that moderate to severe sleep complaints often persist over a period of years in 10% of CF patients.[6] In addition, CF patients are less likely to seek medical attention for their sleep problems than for their other concerns, and pulmonologists are most commonly consulted for their sleep complaints.[6] Sleep quality improves significantly following a hospitalization or rehabilitation admission (including intensive chest physical therapy, antibiotics, and nutritional counseling).

Disclosure: None.

Division of Respiratory Diseases, Department of Medicine, Boston Children's Hospital, Harvard Medical School, Mailstop 208, 300 Longwood Avenue, Boston, MA 02115, USA

E-mail address: eliot.katz@childrens.harvard.edu

Clin Chest Med 35 (2014) 495–504

http://dx.doi.org/10.1016/j.ccm.2014.06.005

Sleep complaints have been identified in both pediatric and adult CF patients. A population-based study of CF children between 0.5 and 5 years revealed that small and moderate to large sleep problems were present in 32% and 22%, respectively.[7] Parents also report that their children with CF have more morning sleepiness.[4] In older children and adolescents with CF (mean age 14.2 years), 44% complain of sleep-onset insomnia and 39% of sleep-maintenance insomnia, and 74% report excessive daytime sleepiness.[8] In a population-based study of adults with CF, excessive daytime sleepiness (EDS) as assessed with the Epworth Sleepiness Score was more common in CF patients than in control subjects (20% vs 7%).[9] Using the Pittsburgh Sleep Quality Index, adults with CF had poorer sleep quality in comparison with controls, which correlated with adverse quality-of-life measures.[9] Disturbed sleep quality is particularly common in CF patients awaiting transplant,[10] although there is a poor association with gas-exchange abnormalities.[1]

Pulmonary CF exacerbations in school-aged children[11] and adults[12] are usually accompanied by sleep disruption attributed primarily to coughing. Many patients report sleeping during the day as a consequence of inability to sleep at night.[11,12] Conversely, when describing improvement in their condition following the initiation of therapy, improvements in sleep were an important determinant of perceived exacerbation resolution.[11–13] Moreover, treatment of a CF pulmonary exacerbation results in decreases in sleepiness[14] and nocturnal cough.[15] However, one study reported that frequency of nocturnal cough did not significantly change following 14 days of antibiotics, despite clinical and spirometric improvement.[16]

Healthy individuals cough less than 1 time per hour, and rarely during sleep.[17] In patients with respiratory disorders, nocturnal coughing is typically observed during periods of wakefulness lasting at least 1 minute, rather than being associated with a brief arousal.[18] Nocturnal coughing was documented in more than 80% of children with CF, compared with a historical prevalence of 5% of healthy children.[16,17] Stable children with CF (mean age 12.8 years, forced expiratory volume in 1 second [FEV$_1$] 72%) were reported to cough 0.6 to 0.9 seconds per hour overnight, and this was more prevalent in those with more advanced lung disease.[19] Thus, although stable children with CF cough more than healthy children, the duration of this coughing is relatively brief. In a large questionnaire study (N = 99), 63% of CF patients reported that cough always or sometimes disrupted sleep,[20] and the severity was worse with decreasing FEV$_1$.[21]

The relationship between objective and subjective cough measures in children is modest.[15,22] Objective cough-recording devices have documented nocturnal cough in CF patients during a pulmonary exacerbation, often in the absence of patient-reported coughing.[16] CF patients cough at least 3 times more frequently during wakefulness in comparison with sleep.[16] Another group of clinically stable CF patients (mean age 26 years, FEV$_1$ 65%) reported 41 coughs per hour awake and 2 per hour asleep, with no correlation between objective and subjective cough rates.[21] The presence of cough resulting in fragmented sleep can impede the progression to rapid eye movement (REM) sleep.[23]

Between 40% and 60% of CF patients will complain of pain, frequently severe, which is associated with poor sleep quality.[5] In a retrospective study of chronic pain in CF patients older than 5 years who died, chronic pain was seen in 84% of patients including headaches (55%), chest pain (65%), back pain (19%), and abdominal pain (16%).[24] Of importance is that hypercarbia or hypoxia was reported to be the primary cause of headache, suggesting a potentially treatable condition. Opiate medications were used in more than 50% of patients, but no respiratory complications were reported.[24] Finally, a case of restless legs syndrome in a 22-year-old CF patient was reported with chronic hemoptysis and nonrestorative sleep, which resolved following iron supplementation.[25]

OBJECTIVE SLEEP QUALITY

Although subjectively poor sleep quality is common in CF patients, especially with advanced disease, most adult studies demonstrate only small objective abnormalities including lower sleep efficiency,[8,26] less REM sleep,[8,26] and an increased arousal index.[2,8,27] Children with CF also are reported to have lower sleep efficiency, reduced REM sleep, and increased electrocortical arousals compared with control children.[28] By contrast, infants with CF had a sleep architecture similar to that of healthy controls.[29] In addition, there are many polysomnographic studies in CF patients that have shown no or minimal differences in sleep architecture.[2,30,31] However, numerous studies document poor-quality sleep in the setting of CF pulmonary exacerbation.[14] Pulmonary exacerbations are associated with more wakefulness after sleep onset, less REM sleep, and more hypoxemia, which all improved significantly following approximately 2 weeks of inpatient therapy.[14] Most episodes of hypoxemia are not associated with arousal.[32]

Actigraphy has also been used to demonstrate subtle sleep disruption in many CF patients. Amin and colleagues[4] studied 44 clinically stable CF patients with mild to moderate lung disease (mean FEV_1 74%) using actigraphy for 5 days in a comparison with 40 control children. CF patients had lower sleep efficiency and more frequent nocturnal awakenings. Children with more severe pulmonary disease (lower FEV_1) had lower sleep efficiency and more nocturnal coughing. Of importance is that Amin and colleagues[4] studied stable CF patients and excluded CF patients with diabetes, tube feeding, antidepressant/hypnotic medication, and asthma, so this study may have underestimated the degree of sleep disruption in the CF population at large. These data indicate that CF children with mild to moderate lung disease in the absence of significant hypoxemia or hypercapnia still experience sleep disruption. Nevertheless, another study using actigraphy for 2 weeks demonstrated normal sleep duration, latency, and efficiency in CF, although sleep fragmentation was present and sleep quality was subjectively poor.[33] Sleep fragmentation was also worse in patients with a lower FEV_1.[33]

The multiple sleep latency test has been used to document EDS in a convenience sample of stable adult CF patients (n = 19, mean age 30 years, mean FEV_1 28%) with a mean sleep latency of 6.7 minutes, although the control group was also sleepy, at 4.6 minutes.[34] CF patients were also reported to have a decreased sleep efficiency (71% vs 93%), increased awakenings (4.2/h vs 2.4/h), and increased wakefulness after sleep onset (70 vs 20 minutes), Of note, these patients had no subjective sleepiness.[34] Nevertheless, there was an association between decreased sleep efficiency and decreased mood profile, including happiness.[34]

In general, sleep disruption is related to the severity of the pulmonary and gastrointestinal manifestations of CF. Sleep efficiency is correlated with the FEV_1,[8] and the degree of nocturnal desaturation.[26,35] However, the effect on sleep architecture of supplemental oxygen or positive pressure ventilation in hypoxemic CF patients has been inconsistent, with improvement in sleep quality in some studies[26,35,36] but not others.[37] Most studies show no significant difference in the obstructive or central apnea index between adults with CF and controls.[2,8] Night-to-night variability in polysomnographic studies have consistently shown minimal changes in respiratory parameters in patients with obstructive sleep apnea (OSA), although there is a first-night effect with regard to sleep architecture. Similarly, CF patients have similar gas-exchange metrics on 2 consecutive nights,[38,39] but have increased sleep efficiency on the second night.[38]

HYPOXEMIA DURING SLEEP

Nocturnal hypoxemia in CF precedes diurnal hypoxemia and is generally unrecognized symptomatically. Interestingly the magnitude of oxygen desaturation during sleep in CF has been reported to exceed that during exercise.[30,40] Documented oximetry monitoring is the most accurate modality for diagnosing sleep-related hypoxemia, and may be performed as an ambulatory study or as part of a laboratory-based comprehensive polysomnogram. There is no consensus on the definition of nocturnal desaturation that is clinically significant enough to warrant the use of supplemental oxygen. In general, significant hypoxemia is considered present if the blood oxygen saturation (SpO_2) is less than 90% for 10% of the total sleep time or if the minimal SpO_2 is less than 85%. Monitoring of oxygen saturation can reasonably be performed in the home setting, and a single night of data collection is sufficient.[41] Chronic hypoxemia has adverse effects on the pulmonary vasculature, leading to vasoconstriction, pulmonary hypertension, and, ultimately, right ventricular dysfunction. Chronic hypoxemia may also have adverse effects on metabolic (growth) and neurocognitive function.

Clinically significant chronic nocturnal hypoxemia is rarely observed in young children with CF,[27,28] but the nocturnal saturation may be statistically lower in comparison with controls (96.1% vs 97.3%).[42] Hypoxemia (SpO_2 <90% for >5% of the night) was not seen in 24 stable children with CF (mean age 9.5 years, FEV_1 >40%), although the nocturnal saturation was related to clinical and radiologic severity scores but not spirometry.[43] Thus, children with CF do tend to have lower SpO_2 and more frequent desaturations compared with control children, although this usually does not reach the consensus threshold for intervention. In infants with CF, oxygen desaturation during sleep was only observed during an acute respiratory infection.[29] In an older CF population of patients with an FEV_1 less than 60% (mean age 24 years, FEV_1 41% predicted), 18% spent greater than 10% of sleep with an SpO_2 less than 90%, and 11% had greater than 30% of sleep with SpO_2 less than 90%.[1] Hypoxemia in CF patients occurs primarily during REM sleep and has been associated with pulmonary hypertension.[32] Pulmonary hypertension is common in CF patients with advanced lung disease, and may be present even in young patients.[44] Despite these findings, there is no clear association between the severity of nocturnal hypoxemia and pulmonary hypertension in CF.[32]

Sleep is a vulnerable period for the respiratory system because of reductions in minute ventilation, lower lung volumes, increased upper airway resistance, and positional ventilation-perfusion mismatching.[45–47] CF patients are particularly vulnerable to hypoxemia during sleep, owing to their reduced baseline arterial oxygen pressure that develops overtime commensurate with parenchymal lung disease. In most individuals, the minute ventilation decreases by approximately 10% during sleep,[45] which has little effect on gas exchange in healthy individuals. However, in CF this reduction in ventilation may be increased to approximately 17%,[48] mostly related to decreased tidal volume, and frequently results in marked hypoxemia. This feature is particularly evident during REM sleep when the minute ventilation is lowest, upper airway resistance is highest, there are frequent central respiratory pauses, and lung volumes (and therefore oxygen reserve) are at a minimum.[23,32,36,37,47,49–52] Furthermore, at baseline, CF patients have considerable ventilation-perfusion mismatching[53] and are therefore closer to the steep-decline portion of the oxygen dissociation curve. Even the expected reduction in minute ventilation that occurs during sleep therefore poses a risk for marked reductions in oxygen saturation. Montgomery and colleagues[41] observed a small decrease in the awake oxygen saturation in 6 of 8 patients in the supine compared with the upright position. The redistribution of pulmonary blood flow toward the apices observed in the supine position may selectively affect CF patients with more extensive upper lobe disease.

Nocturnal hypoxemia is generally present when the FEV$_1$ is less than 64% or if the baseline oxygen saturation is less than 93% to 94%.[31,39,54] The amount of nocturnal desaturation most often has a modest correlation with both lung function and radiographic lung severity.[31,39,40,54,55] For CF patients with a resting SpO$_2$ between 94% and 97%, nocturnal desaturation is variable and cannot be reliably predicted based on any given threshold of clinical, radiographic, or spirometric criteria. For example, a cutoff for FEV$_1$ of less than 64% predicts a nocturnal oxygen saturation of less than 85% with sensitivity of 93% and specificity of 73%.[31] If the FEV$_1$ was greater than 65% predicted only 2 of 21 of CF patients were desaturated during sleep; if the FEV$_1$ was less than 65% predicted, 25 of 49 CF patients had nocturnal desaturation.[56] Thus, there is a modest correlation between pulmonary function and the onset of sleep-related hypoxemia.

The primary predictor of nocturnal hypoxemia is the resting awake oxygen saturation, with levels of 93% to 94% strongly predictive of nocturnal desaturation. Frangolias and Wilcox[56] observed that all CF patients (n = 7, mean age 27 years, FEV$_1$ 56%) with an awake SpO$_2$ of less than 93% desaturated (<90% for >5% of night) during sleep, and an awake SpO$_2$ greater than 98% excluded nocturnal desaturation. Crucially, significant oxygen desaturation during sleep may be present even with slightly low awake levels in the 94% to 96% range.[40] Significant oxygen desaturation was observed in 3 of 16 patients with an awake baseline SpO$_2$ of 94% or higher, indicating the need for screening patients without marked daytime desaturation.[55] The oxygen saturation nadir during exercise was not predictive for nocturnal hypoxemia[31] when stable or during pulmonary exacerbations.[57] Indeed, nocturnal desaturations were observed in 36% of CF patients with a baseline SpO$_2$ greater than 93%.[31] Other predictors of nocturnal desaturation include the evening or morning partial pressure of CO$_2$ (PCO$_2$).[55]

Nocturnal oxygen desaturations are commonly recognized during CF pulmonary exacerbations, with a substantial reduction after 10 days of therapy. Allen and colleagues[57] observed that at the time of pulmonary exacerbation, 38 of 45 CF patients (mean age 8.9 years) had significant nocturnal desaturation (≥5 minutes with a saturation ≥4% below baseline). Most patients improved after 10 days of antibiotic therapy, but 7 of 45 patients had no improvement and 34 of 45 had persistent desaturation on day 10 of treatment. Similarly, during pulmonary exacerbations, the CF patients most likely to desaturate have baseline FEV$_1$ less than 65% predicted.

HYPERCAPNIA DURING SLEEP

The central respiratory drive and respiratory muscle strength is generally normal in CF. Over time, progression of lung disease increases airway resistance and eventually results in alveolar hypoventilation, especially during sleep, exercise, or infection. Sleep is normally characterized by hypoventilation related to decreased drive to the upper and lower respiratory muscles. Nocturnal hypercapnia may be present without nocturnal hypoxemia or daytime gas-exchange abnormalities.[58] The measurement of end-tidal CO$_2$ is not accurate in the setting of CF lung disease because of poorly plateaued waveforms, and is further compromised with positive pressure ventilation. Transcutaneous CO$_2$ has been suggested as an alternative measure of nocturnal CO$_2$ retention, and has been shown to have a reasonable correlation with arterial CO_2 in some studies,[58] but resulted in an overestimate of 7 mm Hg in another study.[59] Most CF patients with nocturnal hypercapnia initially will have normal diurnal CO_2,[58] but all patients with diurnal hypercapnia will also have nocturnal hypercapnia.[58] In CF patients with an FEV_1 of less than 60% (mean age 24 years, FEV_1 41% predicted), 24% spent greater than 10% of sleep with a P_{CO_2} greater than 50 torr.[1]

Administration of supplemental oxygen in hypoxemic CF patients leads to hypercapnia in many instances,[36,60] in both REM and non-REM (NREM) sleep.[36] Moreover, in a study of 39 CF patients with hypoxemic respiratory failure (mean age 26 years, FEV_1 26% predicted), 13 patients developed hypercapnia requiring noninvasive ventilation (NIV) within a year.[60] Thus, hypercapnia may develop after initiating oxygen therapy by either suppression of the hypoxic drive or gradual progression of the underlying lung disease. A P_{CO_2} of 49 torr or more, but not FEV_1, is a risk factor for the development of hypercapnia within 1 year of starting oxygen therapy.[60] Of note, the development of hypercapnia was not associated with a steeper decline in FEV_1 following the initiation of oxygen therapy.[60]

OBSTRUCTIVE SLEEP APNEA

Increased upper airway resistance, including nasal obstruction, is a risk factor for OSA. CF is associated with a high incidence of chronic sinonasal disease including nasal polyps[61] and inflamed nasal mucosa on computed tomography.[62] A cross-sectional study of stable CF patients (mean age 8.4 years) revealed that subjectively 37% reported nasal obstruction and 44% mouth breathing, whereas objectively 28% had purulent discharge, 41% mucosal edema, and 14% polyps.[63] OSA is associated with considerable metabolic, cardiovascular, and neurocognitive morbidity. Even nonapneic snoring associated with hypercapnia has been associated with growth failure in a child with CF.[64] Moreover, growth delay and pulmonary dysfunction was reported in a child with CF related to OSA, which improved following treatment.[65]

The preponderance of evidence suggests that OSA is indeed very prevalent in children with CF, but remarkably not in adults with CF. Ramos and colleagues[66] evaluated 63 children with CF (out of a total clinic population of 85), and found that 56% had OSA syndrome (apnea index >1/h) and 26% had moderate to severe OSA (apnea index >5/h). OSA symptoms included mouth breathing during sleep (83%), difficulty breathing during sleep (70%), and snoring greater than 3 times per week (38%). Factors that predispose children with CF for OSA are similar to those in otherwise healthy children, including black race, over-jet, mouth breathing, and tonsillar hypertrophy.[66] Another study recruited an asymptomatic convenience sample of children with CF (mean age 5.3 years, FEV_1 79%) for comparison with a healthy control group. The CF patients had adenotonsillar hypertrophy (26%) and chronic rhinosinusitis (36%) that was not present in any of the control children. Polysomnographically, children with CF had reduced sleep efficiency (80% vs 88%), less REM sleep (12% vs 13%), and a higher arousal index (11% vs 8%) in comparison with control children.[28] Adenotonsillar hypertrophy was observed in 26% and chronic rhinosinusitis in 36%, and 5% had both. All but 1 of the children with otorhinolaryngologic abnormalities had OSA. OSA (defined by an apnea/hypopnea index [AHI] >2/h) was observed in 70% of children with CF and the average AHI was 7.3/h, compared with only 0.5/h for the control group.[28] In another study, OSA was most severe in 5- to 6-year-olds.[28] By contrast, a separate study of older children with CF (mean age 14 years, FEV_1 92%) demonstrated minimal OSA in this population.[27] In adult CF patients, the incidence of OSA has been consistently low in most polysomnographic series.[2,23,55]

SUPPLEMENTAL OXYGEN

Supplemental oxygen via nasal cannula is generally the first-line treatment of hypoxemia in patients with advanced CF lung disease because of its safety, ease of use, and excellent efficacy.[26] The threshold level of desaturation during sleep or wakefulness that necessitates supplemental oxygen in CF has not been established. At issue is balancing the risks of developing pulmonary hypertension related to nocturnal hypoxemia against the costs, psychological impact, logistical difficulties, discomfort, and potential for limiting mobility. Consensus guidelines in adult CF patients recommend supplemental oxygen "if oxygen saturation is less than 88% to 90% for ≥10% of the total sleep time."[67] The standard approach to mitigating the effects of nocturnal gas-exchange abnormalities during sleep in CF also includes maximizing therapy directed at airway clearance, bacterial superinfection, and comorbid asthma. This approach includes increasing chest physical therapy to enhance airway clearance including a session before bedtime, antibiotics, inhaled steroids, and bronchodilators.

Treatment of nocturnal hypoxemia aims to mitigate the adverse metabolic, cardiovascular, and neurocognitive effects that have been attributed to hypoxemia in other clinical settings. Most CF patients will develop pulmonary hypertension during their lifetime, and supplemental oxygen acutely decreases pulmonary artery pressure by 23%.[68] There is also an association between glucose intolerance and nocturnal desaturation in children with CF, but no clear causation or response to therapy has been established.[27] Supplemental oxygen improves oxygenation in both REM and NREM sleep, but as a consequence P_{CO_2} elevation often occurs, necessitating positive pressure.[26,36] Although supplemental oxygen may decrease the severity of pulmonary hypertension, most studies have shown no effect on cognition, sleep quality, exacerbation frequency, disease progression, or quality of life. However, a long-term randomized trial did report an improvement in school and work attendance in hypoxemic CF patients receiving nocturnal supplemental oxygen.[35] A meta-analysis evaluating sleep-architecture changes with and without supplemental oxygen demonstrated a slight decrease in REM sleep and a decreased sleep latency with treatment,[69] although other studies demonstrated no significant change.[26]

Despite the well-established benefit of supplemental oxygen in adults with severe hypoxemia in non-CF chronic obstructive pulmonary disease,[70] there is little evidence for improved mortality in the CF population. Zinman and colleagues[35] performed a randomized, double-blind, placebo-controlled trial of supplemental oxygen in 28 CF patients (mean age 22.5 years, FEV_1 36.5%) with a baseline awake O_2 partial pressure of less than 65 torr, with a follow-up analysis at 6 and 12 months. There was no significant difference in the hospitalization rate, exercise capability, disease progression, or mortality. However, the oxygen-treated group had significantly greater school or work attendance.[35] Perhaps these negative results arose because the study was too brief, had too few patients, and used oxygen only at night. Thus the optimal protocol for initiating supplemental oxygen in CF has not been established. Nevertheless, in 2009 the British Thoracic Society recommended that oxygen therapy "should be considered for hypoxic children with CF as a means to improve school attendance, and for those who obtain symptomatic relief."[71] General guidelines are to use sufficient supplemental oxygen to maintain saturations 93% or greater during acute exacerbations and 90% or greater over the long term in chronically hypoxemic patients.

Supplemental oxygen may suppress the hypoxic drive to breathe and, therefore, lead to further hypoventilation and CO_2 elevation. Two studies have reported the development of symptomatic hypercapnia following the initiation of supplemental oxygen in CF.[36,72] Insofar as end-tidal CO_2 levels are often inaccurate in the setting of CF, it is recommended to follow trends in the transcutaneous CO_2 and serum levels of bicarbonate during oxygen initiation.

NONINVASIVE VENTILATION

NIV is an option for CF patients with symptomatic nocturnal hypoventilation, which typically precedes daytime hypoventilation. NIV avoids the considerable morbidity associated with tracheostomy or an endotracheal tube. There is no consensus on the criteria for starting NIV in CF, but some investigators have recommended initiating therapy if there is a 10-torr increase in P_{CO_2} on supplemental oxygen, a 10-torr increase in P_{CO_2} during sleep, or an absolute P_{CO_2} of at least 60 torr.[60] Symptoms of nocturnal hypercapnia include dyspnea and headaches that may result in sleep fragmentation. A 6-week trial of NIV was reported to improve nocturnal P_{CO_2}, quality of life, and exercise performance.[72] NIV has also been reported to decrease morning headaches and to subjectively improve sleep quality.[73]

NIV can be delivered via nasal mask, oronasal mask, or intranasal cannulas, thereby avoiding the complications of a tracheostomy including infections, bleeding, and mucous plugging. Nasal masks enable speech, facilitate secretion clearance, and have a low dead space. However, nasal masks are unsuitable for many CF patients with increased nasal resistance. Oronasal masks are an effective substitute in mouthing breathing patients, but interfere with airway clearance, speech, and eating. The common side effects of NIV include irritation of the eyes, facial skin breakdown, and gastric distention. The facial symptoms can usually be remedied by adjusting the mask and headgear. The most serious complication of NIV is pneumothorax. Because the pressure levels in NIV for respiratory insufficiency in CF are higher than those used for OSA, there may be more side effects. Cross-sectional studies indicate that NIV is used in 7.6% of adults and 1.2% of children with CF.[74] NIV is typically started during a CF respiratory exacerbation.[74] In stable CF patients, diurnal hypercapnia is the primary indication for NIV.[74] The long-term impact of NIV on CF lung function is unknown.

Patients with advanced CF lung disease have an increased work of breathing, which can be reduced by 60% to 80% with NIV.[75–78] NIV decreases the inspiratory esophageal pressure swings and the diaphragmatic pressure–time product, both measures of respiratory effort.[75] Fauroux and colleagues[75] determined NIV pressure settings using invasive physiologic testing (esophageal manometry) in comparison with a visual analog comfort scale, and found that subjective comfort reports accurately reflected respiratory muscle unloading using pressure support ventilation. NIV results in a reduction in the degree of tachypnea, improved oxygenation, and subjective improvement of dyspnea, with excellent compliance.[79] However, despite symptomatic improvement, some studies did not demonstrate a decrease in Pco_2 with NIV.[78,80]

NIV increases the tidal volume and minute ventilation during sleep,[50] and therefore improves gas exchange and patient comfort.[50,75] In CF patients with advanced lung disease (mean age 26 years, FEV_1 32%), the minute ventilation decreased by 22% during REM sleep relative to wakefulness on room air, but only had a 14% reduction on NIV.[50] Short-term studies have shown that both proportional assist ventilation and pressure support ventilation are effective in improving subjective and objective respiratory insufficiency in CF, although the former required a lower mean airway pressure.[81] The use of NIV in the spontaneous mode without a backup rate resulted in a decrease in Pco_2 from 59 to 53 torr after 1 month.[60] Efrati and colleagues[73] also reported that the use of spontaneous-mode NIV in CF patients (mean age 25 years, FEV_1 16% predicted) was accompanied by a reduction in Pco_2 from 91 to 67 torr.

For dyspnea, the usual practice is to start bilevel ventilation with an inspiratory positive airway pressure (IPAP) of 10 to 12 cm H_2O and an expiratory positive airway pressure (EPAP) of 4 to 6 cm H_2O. The support levels are titrated upward toward IPAP 16 to 18 cm H_2O and EPAP 4 to 8 cm H_2O, in increments of 1 cm H_2O, until the dyspnea is relieved. The spontaneous pressure support mode is preferable initially, as respiratory drive is normal in CF and patients may adjust the tidal volume and rate to whatever feels most comfortable. When CO_2 elevation is extreme or if the spontaneous ventilation mode is insufficient to relieve symptoms, additional support may be provided using the "Timed" or "Assist Control" mode with a backup rate of 8 to 12 breaths per minute. If hypoxemia persists on NIV, supplemental oxygen is added to the circuit. Fauroux and colleagues[76] compared 2 methodologies for determining optimal NIV pressures in CF patients with advanced lung disease: invasive (esophageal pressure) versus noninvasive (respiratory rate, Spo_2, subjective comfort). Both methods improved the breathing pattern, but the invasive

technique was slightly more effective.[76] The methods were equally effective in improving gas exchange and decreasing the work of breathing, but the invasive technique was slightly better for patient-ventilator synchrony and comfort.[76] In general, the noninvasive technique should be the first line of therapy, with more invasive measures limited to patients with specific tolerance problems.

Single-night trials of NIV improve hypoxemia and hypercapnia but have little or no measurable effects on sleep architecture.[36,50] A placebo-controlled crossover 6-week trial of NIV, supplemental oxygen, and air in 8 CF patients (average age 37 years, FEV_1 35% predicted) demonstrated that NIV improved dyspnea, reduced nocturnal transcutaneous CO_2, and improved exercise performance.[72] However, there was no change in sleep architecture or daytime Pco_2.[72] Nevertheless, titration of NIV in the sleep laboratory is recommended to help select a properly fitting mask, establish the optimal pressure settings and backup rate, and evaluate ventilator triggering, sleep quality, gas exchange, respiratory rate, and patient comfort. During polysomnography, transcutaneous CO_2 monitoring validated with blood gases can be helpful in guiding the titration. A mask leak or irregular triggering of NIV may result in persistent gas-exchange abnormalities, increased work of breathing, and sleep fragmentation. NIV may also be used in patients requiring short-term daytime ventilator assistance during infectious exacerbations or in patients awaiting lung transplant,[77,79] although it interferes with feeding and speech.

Most CF patients with end-stage lung disease will tolerate NIV and report a subjective improvement in headaches and quality of sleep.[80] However, CF patients frequently report difficulty sleeping with NIV or report no subjective benefit, and therefore may refuse treatment.[74] The tolerance rate for NIV in trials of at least several weeks is generally greater than 60%, although the length of overnight use was reportedly as low as 4.3 hours per night.[72,78] The influence of NIV on long-term pulmonary function in CF patients with advanced lung disease is unknown. This question was addressed by a retrospective, observational study with a 1-year follow-up of CF patients treated with NIV compared with those without (matched for gender, mutation, and FEV_1).[82] In the year preceding NIV, the treated group had a more rapid decline in pulmonary function (−3% vs +2.6%), but after 1 year of NIV the decreases in FEV_1 were similar (−2.2% vs −2.3%), suggesting that there was a stabilization in the decline in pulmonary function on NIV.[82]

SUMMARY

Sleep is a vulnerable period for pulmonary function in CF patients with advanced lung disease. Subjective poor-quality sleep is frequently reported and is multifactorial, arising from pain, respiratory symptoms, hypoventilation, frequent defecation, depression, and medications that might disturb sleep. The influence of disturbed sleep on immune, metabolic, and cognitive function in CF has not been extensively studied, but may contribute to the considerable morbidity and mortality observed. Nocturnal hypoxemia occurs frequently in CF patients with advanced lung disease (FEV_1 <65%), but may also be seen in patients with milder lung disease. Hypoxemia is not usually associated with arousal from sleep and, therefore, may be unrecognized. As the lung disease progresses, hypercapnia and, eventually, dyspnea develop, which at least in the short term is responsive to NIV.

REFERENCES

1. Fauroux B, Pepin JL, Boelle PY, et al. Sleep quality and nocturnal hypoxaemia and hypercapnia in children and young adults with cystic fibrosis. Arch Dis Child 2012;97:960–6.
2. Perin C, Fagondes SC, Casarotto FC, et al. Sleep findings and predictors of sleep desaturation in adult cystic fibrosis patients. Sleep Breath 2012; 16(4):1041–8.
3. Sawicki GS, Sellers DE, Robinson WM. Self-reported physical and psychological symptom burden in adults with cystic fibrosis. J Pain Symptom Manage 2008;35:372–80.
4. Amin R, Bean J, Burklow K, et al. The relationship between sleep disturbance and pulmonary function in stable pediatric cystic fibrosis patients. Chest 2005;128:1357–63.
5. Flume PA, Ciolino J, Gray S, et al. Patient-reported pain and impaired sleep quality in adult patients with cystic fibrosis. J Cyst Fibros 2009; 8:321–5.
6. Sheehan J, Massie J, Hay M, et al. The natural history and predictors of persistent problem behaviours in cystic fibrosis: a multicentre, prospective study. Arch Dis Child 2012;97:625–31.
7. Ward C, Massie J, Glazner J, et al. Problem behaviours and parenting in preschool children with cystic fibrosis. Arch Dis Child 2009;94:341–7.
8. Naqvi SK, Sotelo C, Murry L, et al. Sleep architecture in children and adolescents with cystic fibrosis and the association with severity of lung disease. Sleep Breath 2008;12:77–83.
9. Bouka A, Tiede H, Liebich L, et al. Quality of life in clinically stable adult cystic fibrosis out-patients: associations with daytime sleepiness and sleep quality. Respir Med 2012;106:1244–9.
10. Burker EJ, Carels RA, Thompson LF, et al. Quality of life in patients awaiting lung transplant: cystic fibrosis versus other end-stage lung diseases. Pediatr Pulmonol 2000;30:453–60.
11. Abbott J, Holt A, Morton AM, et al. Patient indicators of a pulmonary exacerbation: preliminary reports from school aged children map onto those of adults. J Cyst Fibros 2012;11:180–6.
12. Abbott J, Holt A, Hart A, et al. What defines a pulmonary exacerbation? The perceptions of adults with cystic fibrosis. J Cyst Fibros 2009;8:356–9.
13. Bramwell EC, Halpin DM, Duncan-Skingle F, et al. Home treatment of patients with cystic fibrosis using the 'Intermate': the first year's experience. J Adv Nurs 1995;22:1063–7.
14. Dobbin CJ, Bartlett D, Melehan K, et al. The effect of infective exacerbations on sleep and neurobehavioral function in cystic fibrosis. Am J Respir Crit Care Med 2005;172:99–104.
15. Smith JA, Owen EC, Jones AM, et al. Objective measurement of cough during pulmonary exacerbations in adults with cystic fibrosis. Thorax 2006; 61:425–9.
16. Hamutcu R, Francis J, Karakoc F, et al. Objective monitoring of cough in children with cystic fibrosis. Pediatr Pulmonol 2002;34:331–5.
17. Munyard P, Bush A. How much coughing is normal? Arch Dis Child 1996;74:531–4.
18. Power JT, Stewart IC, Connaughton JJ, et al. Nocturnal cough in patients with chronic bronchitis and emphysema. Am Rev Respir Dis 1984;130: 999–1001.
19. van der Giessen L, Loeve M, de Jongste J, et al. Nocturnal cough in children with stable cystic fibrosis. Pediatr Pulmonol 2009;44:859–65.
20. Stenekes SJ, Hughes A, Grégoire MC, et al. Frequency and self-management of pain, dyspnea, and cough in cystic fibrosis. J Pain Symptom Manage 2009;38:837–48.
21. Kerem E, Wilschanski M, Miller NL, et al. Ambulatory quantitative waking and sleeping cough assessment in patients with cystic fibrosis. J Cyst Fibros 2011;10:193–200.
22. Chang B, Newman G, Carlin B, et al. Subjective scoring of cough in children: parent-completed vs child-completed diary cards vs an objective method. Eur Respir J 1998;11:462–6.
23. Stokes DC, McBride JT, Wall MA, et al. Sleep hypoxemia in young adults with cystic fibrosis. Am J Dis Child 1980;134:741–3.
24. Ravilly S, Robinson W, Suresh S, et al. Chronic pain in cystic fibrosis. Pediatrics 1996;98:741–7.
25. Hayes D. Restless leg syndrome manifested by iron deficiency from chronic hemoptysis in cystic fibrosis. J Cyst Fibros 2007;6:234–6.

26. Spier S, Rivlin J, Hughes D, et al. The effect of oxygen on sleep, blood gases, and ventilation in cystic fibrosis. Am Rev Respir Dis 1984;129:712–8.

27. Suratwala D, Chan JS, Kelly A, et al. Nocturnal saturation and glucose tolerance in children with cystic fibrosis. Thorax 2011;66:574–8.

28. Spicuzza L, Sciuto C, Leonardi S, et al. Early occurrence of obstructive sleep apnea in infants and children with cystic fibrosis. Arch Pediatr Adolesc Med 2012;166:1165–9.

29. Villa MP, Pagani J, Lucidi V, et al. Nocturnal oximetry in infants with cystic fibrosis. Arch Dis Child 2001;84:50.

30. Bradley S, Solin P, Wilson J, et al. Hypoxemia and hypercapnia during exercise and sleep in patients with cystic fibrosis. Chest 1999;116:647–54.

31. de Castro-Silva C, de Bruin VM, Cavalcante AG, et al. Nocturnal hypoxia and sleep disturbances in cystic fibrosis. Pediatr Pulmonol 2009;44: 1143–50.

32. Francis PW, Muller NL, Gurwitz D, et al. Hemoglobin desaturation: its occurrence during sleep in patients with cystic fibrosis. Am J Dis Child 1980;134: 734–40.

33. Jankelowitz L, Reid KJ, Wolfe L, et al. Cystic fibrosis patients have poor sleep quality despite normal sleep latency and efficiency. Chest 2005; 127:1593–9.

34. Dancey R, Tullis D, Heslegrave R, et al. Sleep quality and daytime function in adults with cystic fibrosis and severe lung disease. Eur Respir J 2002;19:504–10.

35. Zinman R, Corey M, Coates AL, et al. Nocturnal home oxygen in the treatment of hypoxemic cystic fibrosis patients. J Pediatr 1989;114:368–77.

36. Gozal D. Nocturnal ventilatory support in patients with cystic fibrosis: comparison with supplemental oxygen. Eur Respir J 1997;10:1999–2003.

37. Regnis JA, Piper AJ, Henke KG, et al. Benefits of nocturnal nasal CPAP in patients with cystic fibrosis. Chest 1994;106:1717–24.

38. Milross MA, Piper AJ, Norman M, et al. Night-to-night variability in sleep in cystic fibrosis. Sleep Med 2002;3:213–9.

39. Versteegh FG, Bogaard JM, Raatgever JW, et al. Relationship between airway obstruction, desaturation during exercise and nocturnal hypoxaemia in cystic fibrosis patients. Eur Respir J 1990;3: 68–73.

40. Coffey MJ, FitzGerald MX, McNicholas WT. Comparison of oxygen desaturation during sleep and exercise in patients with cystic fibrosis. Chest 1991;100:659–62.

41. Montgomery M, Wiebicke W, Bibi H, et al. Home measurement of oxygen saturation during sleep in patients with cystic fibrosis. Pediatr Pulmonol 1989;7:29–34.

42. Darracott C, McNamara PS, Pipon M, et al. Towards the development of cumulative overnight oximetry curves for children with cystic fibrosis. J Cyst Fibros 2004;3:S53.

43. Uyan ZS, Ozdemir N, Ersu R, et al. Factors that correlate with sleep oxygenation in children with cystic fibrosis. Pediatr Pulmonol 2007;42:716–22.

44. Ryland D, Reid L. The pulmonary circulation in cystic fibrosis. Thorax 1975;30:285–92.

45. Tabachnik E, Muller NL, Bryan AC, et al. Changes in ventilation and chest wall mechanics during sleep in normal adolescents. J Appl Physiol Respir Environ Exerc Physiol 1981;51:557.

46. Hudgel DW, Devadatta P. Decrease in functional residual capacity during sleep in normal humans. J Appl Physiol Respir Environ Exerc Physiol 1984; 57:1319–22.

47. Douglas J, White P, Pickett K, et al. Respiration during sleep in normal man. Thorax 1982;37:840–4.

48. Ballard RD, Sutarik JM, Clover CW, et al. Effects of non-REM sleep on ventilation and respiratory mechanics in adults with cystic fibrosis. Am J Respir Crit Care Med 1996;153:266–71.

49. Henderson-Smart DJ, Read DJ. Reduced lung volume during behavioral active sleep in the newborn. J Appl Physiol Respir Environ Exerc Physiol 1979; 46:1081.

50. Milross MA, Piper AJ, Norman M, et al. Low-flow oxygen and bilevel ventilatory support: effects on ventilation during sleep in cystic fibrosis. Am J Respir Crit Care Med 2001;163:129–34.

51. Tepper RS, Skatrud JB, Dempsey JA. Ventilation and oxygenation changes during sleep in cystic fibrosis. Chest 1983;84:388–93.

52. Muller NL, Francis PW, Gurwitz D, et al. Mechanism of hemoglobin desaturation during rapid-eye-movement sleep in normal subjects and in patients with cystic fibrosis. Am Rev Respir Dis 1980;121: 463–9.

53. Soni R, Dobbin CJ, Milross MA, et al. Gas exchange in stable patients with moderate-to-severe lung disease from cystic fibrosis. J Cyst Fibros 2008;7:285–91.

54. Smith DL, Freeman W, Cayton RM, et al. Nocturnal hypoxaemia in cystic fibrosis: relationship to pulmonary function tests. Respir Med 1994;88:537–9.

55. Milross MA, Piper AJ, Norman M, et al. Predicting sleep-disordered breathing in patients with cystic fibrosis. Chest 2001;120:1239–45.

56. Frangolias DD, Wilcox PG. Predictability of oxygen desaturation during sleep in patients with cystic fibrosis: clinical, spirometric, and exercise parameters. Chest 2001;119:434–41.

57. Allen B, Mellon F, Simmonds J, et al. Changes in nocturnal oximetry after treatment of exacerbations in cystic fibrosis. Arch Dis Child 1993;69:197–201.

58. Paiva R, Krivec U, Aubertin G, et al. Carbon dioxide monitoring during long-term noninvasive respiratory support in children. Intensive Care Med 2009;35:1068–74.

59. Pradal U, Braggion C, Mastella G. Transcutaneous blood gas analysis during sleep and exercise in cystic fibrosis. Pediatr Pulmonol 1990;8:162–7.

60. Dobbin CJ, Milross MA, Piper AJ, et al. Sequential use of oxygen and bi-level ventilation for respiratory failure in cystic fibrosis. J Cyst Fibros 2004;3: 237–42.

61. Hadfield PJ, Rowe-Jones JM, Mackay IS. The prevalence of nasal polyps in adults with cystic fibrosis. Clin Otolaryngol Allied Sci 2000;25:19–22.

62. Eggesbø B, Søvik S, Dølvik S, et al. CT characterization of inflammatory paranasal sinus disease in cystic fibrosis. Acta Radiol 2002;43:21–8.

63. Franco LP, Camargos PA, Becker HM, et al. Nasal endoscopic evaluation of children and adolescents with cystic fibrosis. Braz J Otorhinolaryngol 2009; 75:806–13.

64. Macdonald KD, McGinley BM, Brown DJ, et al. Primary snoring and growth failure in a patient with cystic fibrosis. Respir Care 2009;54:1727–31.

65. Hayes D. Obstructive sleep apnea syndrome: a potential cause of lower airway obstruction in cystic fibrosis. Sleep Med 2006;7:73–5.

66. Ramos RT, Salles C, Gregório PB, et al. Evaluation of the upper airway in children and adolescents with cystic fibrosis and obstructive sleep apnea syndrome. Int J Pediatr Otorhinolaryngol 2009;73: 1780–5.

67. Yankaskas JR, Marshall BC, Sufian B, et al. Cystic fibrosis adult care: consensus conference report. Chest 2004;125:1S–39S.

68. Davidson A, Bossuyt A, Dab I. Acute effects of oxygen, nifedipine, and diltiazem in patients with cystic fibrosis and mild pulmonary hypertension. Pediatr Pulmonol 1989;6:53–9.

69. Elphick HE, Mallory G. Oxygen therapy for cystic fibrosis. Cochrane Database Syst Rev 2013;(7): CD003884.

70. Cranston JM, Crockett AJ, Moss JR, et al. Domiciliary oxygen for chronic obstructive pulmonary disease. Cochrane Database Syst Rev 2005;(4):CD001744.

71. Balfour-Lynn IM, Field DJ, Gringras P, et al. BTS guidelines for home oxygen in children. Thorax 2009;64(Suppl 2):ii1–26.

72. Young AC, Wilson JW, Kotsimbos TC, et al. Randomised placebo controlled trial of non-invasive ventilation for hypercapnia in cystic fibrosis. Thorax 2008;63:72–7.

73. Efrati O, Modan-Moses D, Barak A, et al. Long-term non-invasive positive pressure ventilation among cystic fibrosis patients awaiting lung transplantation. Isr Med Assoc J 2004;6:527–30.

74. Fauroux B, Burgel PR, Boelle PY, et al. Practice of noninvasive ventilation for cystic fibrosis: a nationwide survey in France. Respir Care 2008;53: 1482–9.

75. Fauroux B, Pigeot J, Polkey MI, et al. In vivo physiologic comparison of two ventilators used for domiciliary ventilation in children with cystic fibrosis. Crit Care Med 2001;29:2097–105.

76. Fauroux B, Nicot F, Essouri S, et al. Setting of noninvasive pressure support in young patients with cystic fibrosis. Eur Respir J 2004;24:624–30.

77. Piper AJ, Parker S, Torzillo PJ, et al. Nocturnal nasal IPPV stabilizes patients with cystic fibrosis and hypercapnic respiratory failure. Chest 1992; 102:846–50.

78. Granton JT, Kesten S. The acute effects of nasal positive pressure ventilation in patients with advanced cystic fibrosis. Chest 1998;113:1013–8.

79. Caronia CG, Silver P, Nimkoff L, et al. Use of bilevel positive airway pressure (BIPAP) in end-stage patients with cystic fibrosis awaiting lung transplantation. Clin Pediatr (Phila) 1998;37:555–9.

80. Hill AT, Edenborough FP, Cayton RM, et al. Long-term nasal intermittent positive pressure ventilation in patients with cystic fibrosis and hypercapnic respiratory failure (1991-1996). Respir Med 1998;92: 523–6.

81. Serra A, Polese G, Braggion C, et al. Non-invasive proportional assist and pressure support ventilation in patients with cystic fibrosis and chronic respiratory failure. Thorax 2002;57:50–4.

82. Fauroux B, Le Roux E, Ravilly S, et al. Long-term noninvasive ventilation in patients with cystic fibrosis. Respiration 2008;76:168–74.

Sleep in Patients with Restrictive Lung Disease

Christine H.J. Won, MD, MS*, Meir Kryger, MD

KEYWORDS

- Restrictive lung disease • Interstitial lung disease • Sleep • Sleep-disordered breathing
- Hypoxemia

KEY POINTS

- Restrictive lung disease is associated with nocturnal pathophysiology, including sleep disturbances and breathing and oxygenation impairments during sleep.
- Sleep is disrupted because of changes in sleep architecture and comorbid sleep disorders.
- Sleep changes in restrictive lung diseases affect sleep quality and contribute to daytime fatigue in this population.
- Little is known about the impact of treatment of sleep disorders and sleep disruption on sleep quality and daytime complaints in restrictive lung disease.

Restrictive ventilatory defects occur from several pathologic mechanisms. Intrinsic lung disease such as pulmonary fibrosis and other interstitial lung disease (ILD) may cause reduced lung volumes as well as diffusion impairment. Restrictive ventilatory defects may also occur due to musculoskeletal abnormalities in the thoracic cage or due to respiratory muscle weakness from neuromuscular disease. In addition, obesity may cause significant restrictive lung physiology and lead to obesity hypoventilation syndrome (OHS). Restrictive lung disease is associated with nocturnal pathophysiology, including sleep disturbances and breathing and oxygenation impairments during sleep.

INTERSTITIAL LUNG DISEASE

Fatigue is a common complaint among patients with ILD. Sleep is disrupted due to respiratory pathophysiology such as nocturnal hypoxemia, changes in sleep architecture, and comorbid sleep disorders. These sleep changes in ILD affect sleep quality and contribute to daytime fatigue in this population.

Respiratory Physiology During Sleep

Sleep onset is normally characterized by reduced responsiveness to hypercapnia and hypoxemia, as well as reduced cortical and lung mechanic responsiveness. As a result, minute ventilation decreases from a reduction in tidal volume, whereas respiratory rate generally remains unchanged.[1,2] It is unclear whether patients with restrictive pathophysiology due to intrinsic lung disease experience a similar effect. During wakefulness, patients with ILD often have rapid, shallow breathing as a result of decreased lung compliance and a sensation of dyspnea due to afferent stimulation from vagal receptors.[3] Few studies suggest subjects with ILD may experience persistently elevated respiratory rates with shorter inspiratory and expiratory durations during sleep. The lack of change from wake to sleep state may be attributed to the maintenance of

Disclosures: None.
Section of Pulmonary, Critical Care and Sleep Medicine, Yale University School of Medicine, PO BOX 208057, 333 Cedar Street, New Haven, CT 06520-8057, USA
* Corresponding author.
E-mail address: christine.won@yale.edu

Clin Chest Med 35 (2014) 505–512
http://dx.doi.org/10.1016/j.ccm.2014.06.006
0272-5231/14/$ – see front matter Published by Elsevier Inc.

vagal-mediated reflexes causing hyperventilation during wakefulness.[4,5]

Others have found a significant reduction in respiratory rate with sleep onset in patients with ILD.[6] To eliminate the potential confounding of nocturnal hypoxemia on differences in ventilatory pattern in patients with ILD, Shea and colleagues[7] studied breathing patterns in patients with ILD whose oxygen saturations were maintained greater than 95% by breathing supplemental oxygen. During the wake state, respiratory frequency was higher and inspiratory and expiratory times were shorter among patients with ILD despite adequate oxygenation compared with normal subjects, supporting a respiratory stimulatory effect independent of hypoxemia during the daytime. During sleep, and specifically in slow wave sleep, however, there was no difference in the respiratory rate between normal controls and subjects with ILD, suggesting hyperventilatory responses during wakefulness are not maintained during sleep in subjects with ILD. Midgren and colleagues[8] similarly found greater hyperventilation reflected by reduced transcutaneous partial pressure of carbon dioxide ($Ptcco_2$) in patients with ILD compared with controls. However, during sleep, both controls and patients with ILD had comparable $Ptcco_2$, suggesting hyperventilation is ameliorated in patients with ILD during sleep.

The pattern of breathing may also be more inefficient and labored during sleep in patients with ILD. Hira and Sharma[9] showed through respiratory inductance plethysmography that patients with ILD produce similar tidal volume per rib cage and abdomen excursion during wakefulness. However, during sleep, patients with ILD required more excursion or effort per tidal volume compared with healthy controls.

Physiologically, respiratory muscles with the exception of the diaphragm become atonic during rapid eye movement (REM) sleep. Moreover, during phasic REM sleep, inspiratory drive is reduced. These normal physiologic changes are associated with only minor gas exchange abnormalities in healthy individuals; however, these changes may lead to profound hypoventilation and hypoxemia in patients with restrictive lung disease. It is not uncommon to observe sustained desaturations during REM sleep and pulse oximeter oxygen saturation (Spo_2) reaches a nadir of less than 70%.[5] Hypoxemia during REM sleep tends to be worse in those with more severe daytime hypoxemia.[4,5] The degree of desaturation during REM sleep is often more severe than that occurring during exercise.[5]

Nocturnal desaturation has been shown to be common in ILD and associated with worse clinical outcomes. Hira and Sharma[9] reported an average decline in Spo_2 of nearly 9% during sleep compared with approximately 4% among normal controls. Spo_2 reached a nadir by 10% to 16% in patients with ILD compared with 3% to 6% in healthy controls. Patients with ILD spent 17% of total sleep time with Spo_2 less than 85%, whereas none of the controls had such desaturations during sleep. Corte and colleagues[10] found that 37% of their subjects with ILD spent more than 10% of sleep with Spo_2 less than 90%. In their study, the desaturation index, defined as the number of desaturation events greater than 4%, was shown to be independently associated with mortality. Similarly, Medeiros and colleagues[11] found in a series of women with lymphangioleiomyomatosis that nocturnal hypoxemia (again defined as 10% total sleep time with Spo_2 <90%) occurred in 56% of patients and sleep time spent with Spo_2 less than 90% was associated with worse diffusion capacity and forced expiratory volume more than 1 second, as well as increased residual volume to total lung capacity ratio.

In contrast, McNicholas and colleagues[6] studied 7 patients with severe ILD and found none had significant complaints of sleep-disordered breathing (SDB), and, although 2 patients were found to have apneas, neither had greater than 3% desaturations associated with apneic episodes. The investigators concluded that nocturnal hypoxemia in this population is not severe and not of clinical relevance. However, Midgren[12] found nocturnal hypoxemia was in fact severe in patients with ILD, although to a lesser degree than that observed in patients with chronic obstructive lung disease. Similar to other studies, mean Spo_2 was reduced to a greater extent during REM sleep than during non-REM sleep in all 3 groups, although the difference was the least in the ILD group.

Sleep Architecture/Disturbances

Patients with ILD often have disrupted sleep and frequent arousals. Sleep in these patients is characterized by an increase in arousals, increased stage N1 and stage N2 sleep, and a decrease in stage N3 and REM sleep. Perez-Padilla and colleagues[4] showed stage N1 sleep comprised 33% of total sleep time in patients with ILD compared with 14% in controls. Sixty-five percent of patients with ILD did not have slow wave sleep, and not only was REM sleep delayed in onset but REM time was also only 12% of the total sleep time compared with 20% in healthy controls. There were also more frequent sleep stage shifts in the ILD group. Sleep architecture changes were more notable in those with daytime hypoxemia. Pascual and colleagues[13] showed similar patterns of sleep disruption and altered sleep architecture in patients with lung fibrosis awaiting lung transplantation. Several mechanisms potentially contribute to sleep fragmentation in patients with ILD, including hypoxemia, hypercapnia, cough, and other respiratory reflexes. Other causes of sleep disruption in patients with ILD may be related to esophageal dysmotility and reflux, which are common complications of some ILD-related disorders such as systemic sclerosis.[14] Finally, comorbid sleep disorders have been described in increasing frequency in patients with ILD.

Comorbid Sleep Disorders

Obstructive sleep apnea (OSA) and upper airway resistance syndrome have been shown to be common in ILD. Pihtili and colleagues[15] found 68% of 50 patients with ILD due to idiopathic pulmonary fibrosis (IPF), sarcoidosis, or scleroderma had OSA. OSA in this group was generally mild, with a mean apnea-hypopnea index (AHI) of 11 $\pm$ 12.5 events per hour. Patients in this study were not obese (mean body mass index [BMI], 25.9 $\pm$ 3.44 kg/m^2). More than half of these patients had predominantly REM-related sleep apnea. Both AHI and oxygen desaturations were worse with radiographically more severe disease. Lancaster and colleagues[16] studied 50 subjects with IPF and found OSA in 88%. In their study, the majority had moderate or severe OSA and BMI did not correlate strongly with AHI. However, the degree of restriction, as measured by total lung capacity on pulmonary function test, and impairment in diffusion capacity have shown to correlate with the severity of OSA.[17]

Comorbid sleep apnea in this patient population may worsen sleep quality and affect the course of lung disease. Comorbid OSA has shown to worsen sleep disturbances in ILD by reducing sleep efficiency and slow wave and REM sleep and increasing arousal index, thereby contributing to patients' complaints of fatigue.[15] Gastroesophageal reflux disease (GERD) is common in ILD possibly due to the effects of lung fibrosis on intrathoracic pressure, diaphragm function, and lower esophageal sphincter tone.[18] There is concern for GERD in the population with ILD because reflux may exacerbate respiratory symptoms and promote disease progression.[19] Although OSA has been implicated in GERD among healthy subjects,[20,21] OSA has yet to be implicated in promoting GERD in patients with ILD.[22] Finally, patients with ILD with OSA have worse estimated pulmonary artery pressures on echocardiogram than those without OSA, and positive airway pressure (PAP) improves this (**Fig. 1**).[23]

Other sleep disorders, including periodic limb movements in sleep (PLMS) and restless leg syndrome (RLS), have been observed in increasing frequency in those with ILD. In patients with ILD with these sleep disorders, sleep quality was worse, with increased arousal index and worse sleep efficiency that occurred in a dose-dependent manner to the number of limb movements per hour during sleep.[14]

Summary

As fibrotic lung disease progresses, the degree of nocturnal desaturation and breathing disorders worsen. Whether sleep architecture and sleep quality all progress in relation to the disease is unknown. Long-term evaluation of sleep and breathing in ILD is needed to determine whether sleep changes affect disease symptoms and course.

MUSCULOSKELETAL THORACIC DISEASE

Severe chest wall deformity may lead to a restrictive ventilatory defect with reduced total lung capacity, vital capacity, and functional residual capacity. These patients may have hypoxemia, hypercapnia, pulmonary hypertension, cor pulmonale, and chronic respiratory failure. Thoracic cage deformity alters chest wall mechanics and produces ineffective respiratory muscle mechanics. As a result, these patients may have increased work of breathing, diminished strength

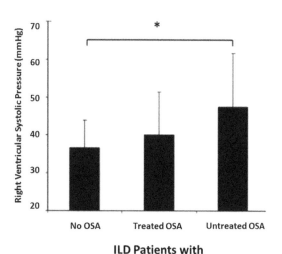

ILD Patients with

Fig. 1. Estimated pulmonary artery pressure is increased in patients with ILD and untreated OSA. * P value less than .05. (*Data from* Won C, Purvis T, Chun HJ. An overlap phenomenon exists with interstitial lung disease and obstructive sleep apnea. ATS abstracts. 2011.)

and endurance, and increased fatigue.[24] The supine position may have particular detrimental effects on breathing. Oxygen desaturations are common in the supine position. Positional hypoxemia may be worsened during sleep and particularly during REM sleep. Patients with musculoskeletal thoracic cage deformities may rely heavily on accessory respiratory muscles for ventilation. These patients are particularly vulnerable during REM sleep, when accessory muscles of breathing such as the intercostal muscles are inhibited by tonic hyperpolarization of spinal motor neurons.[25] These patients often develop hypoventilation, in contrast to those with restrictive lung disease due to parenchymal disease who develop hyperventilation. The inhibition of intercostal and accessory respiratory muscles during REM sleep may also cause a compensatory increase in diaphragmatic effort, leading to instability to the thoracic cage and paradoxic chest wall motion. This situation further contributes to hypoventilation, atelectasis, and abnormal distribution of inspired gas, leading to ventilation and perfusion mismatches.[25]

Patients with extrapulmonary restriction often develop reduced chemical drives to breathe and may hypoventilate during sleep and wakefulness. Persistent hypoventilation during sleep may lead to chronic hypercapnia and hypoxemia, with pulmonary arterial vasoconstriction, eventual vascular remodeling, and pulmonary hypertension and cor pulmonale. Hypoxemia and hypercapnia further impair respiratory muscle function,[26] increasing fatigability and accelerating the development of respiratory failure. A wide variety of abnormal breathing patterns has been reported and has included periodic breathing and central and obstructive apneas.[27] The cause of apneas is unclear; they may be due to sleep-related reduction in muscle tone in accessory muscles especially during REM sleep and alterations in control of breathing.

Patients with restrictive lung disease due to musculoskeletal deformities complain of disrupted nocturnal sleep, severe nocturnal and/or morning headaches, and symptoms of excessive daytime sleepiness (EDS). The headaches may be due to the increase in arterial partial pressure of carbon dioxide ($Paco_2$) during sleep. Patients with restrictive lung disease have frequent arousals from sleep associated with hypoxemia and hypercapnia. Stage N3 sleep and REM sleep as a proportion of total sleep time are reduced, whereas the proportions of stages N1 and N2 are increased.[25] These sleep disturbances may contribute to fatigue and worsen respiratory efforts. In fact, decreased sleep duration has been proposed as

a risk factor for the development of musculoskeletal thoracic cage abnormality, specifically degenerative lumbar scoliosis.[28] Li and colleagues[28] proposed sleep deprivation may lead to lowered bone mineral density and increased levels of interleukin-1, which in turn have been implicated in intervertebral disc degeneration and osteoporosis.

Nocturnal hypoxemia and hypercapnia may be treated with noninvasive positive pressure ventilation (NIPPV),[29] which may reduce work of breathing and allow respiratory muscles to rest during sleep. NIPPV may therefore improve daytime function. In addition, NIPPV provides positive end-expiratory pressure, which would improve alveolar recruitment and oxygenation, as well as eliminate obstructive apneas and hypopneas. Supplemental oxygen for those with sustained desaturations may prevent pulmonary vascular hypoxic vasoconstriction and pulmonary hypertension. Tracheostomy with positive pressure ventilation would be reserved for severe restrictive lung physiology and chronic respiratory failure. To date, there are little data regarding the effect on sleep these treatments may have in musculoskeletal restrictive lung disease.

NEUROMUSCULAR DISEASE

Respiratory muscle weakness may lead to significant restrictive ventilatory defect, hypoventilation, and respiratory failure. Many patients with neuromuscular disease die of respiratory failure due to severe diaphragmatic weakness or abnormalities in respiratory control. In normal subjects, during sleep upper airway resistance increases, chemosensitivity is reduced, and the wakefulness drive to breathe is lost, resulting in a slight reduction in ventilation. During REM sleep, ribcage and accessory breathing muscles are suppressed, particularly during bursts of eye movements, and breathing is irregular, rapid, and shallow, with a further decrease in ventilation.

In subjects with respiratory muscle weakness, sleep is fragmented, and similar to other restrictive lung diseases, there is shorter total sleep time, frequent arousals, increased stage 1 sleep, and reduction in REM sleep. SDB and nocturnal desaturations are common and the most severe during REM sleep. There may be significant hypoventilation and hypoxemia during REM sleep in those with diaphragmatic weakness or paralysis, because during REM sleep, the diaphragm remains the only stimulated respiratory muscle. Daytime respiratory function is weakly associated with nocturnal desaturation. Noninvasive ventilation improves sleep quality and breathing in subjects with respiratory muscle weakness. However, the optimal timing of initiation and its role in progressive neuromuscular diseases are unclear.

Myotonic Dystrophy

Myotonic dystrophy type 1 (DM1) is the most common adult-onset form of muscular dystrophy. DM1 is the neuromuscular condition with the most identified sleep disorders, including hypersomnia, central and obstructive sleep apneas, RLS, PLMS, and REM sleep dysregulation.[30] EDS is reported in 70% to 80% of patients and is the most frequent nonmuscular complaint in DM1. Different sleep-related findings may mimic several sleep disorders, including idiopathic hypersomnia and narcolepsy without cataplexy. For example, patients with DM1 may have sleep-onset REM periods, similar to that observed in narcolepsy. Ciafaloni and colleagues[31] examined postmortem samples of the temporal cortex of 38 patients with DM1. Among these patients, 7 of 13 patients who underwent polysomnography (PSG) and multiple sleep latency test (MSLT) showed reduced sleep latency and/or sleep-onset REM. However, the pathophysiologic mechanism for EDS and REM intrusion is likely distinct from that of narcolepsy because hypocretin levels in cerebrospinal fluid are not found to be abnormally low and these patients do not have consistent defects in hypocretin receptors.[31] Although to some degree subjective and objective daytime sleepiness may be associated with muscular impairment and sleep disturbance, it seems that EDS in patients with DM1 is caused by a primarily central process rather than by sleep fragmentation, SDB, or sleep-related movement disorders. EDS, for example, tends to persist despite successful treatment of SDB in patients with DM1.

Myotonic dystrophy type 2 (DM2), also called proximal myotonic myopathy, is rarer than DM1 and generally manifests with milder signs and symptoms. Descriptions of sleep in DM2 are less common than those reported for DM1. Chokroverty and colleagues[32] reported PSG data in patients with DM2 and showed increased arousals, decreased sleep efficiency, and increased alpha-delta sleep. Many patients also had OSA, paradoxic breathing, and absence of atonia during REM sleep. Patients were also noted to have dream enactment with absent atonia during REM sleep consistent with REM behavioral disorder (RBD). Romigi and colleagues[30] also described polysomnographic evidence of RBD in half of their patients with DM2. MSLT in several patients also showed reduced mean sleep latencies without sleep-onset REM periods. Lam and colleagues[33] reported a case-control study of 30 subjects with

genetically confirmed DM2 and 43 medical controls and surveyed sleep-related complaints of EDS, sleep quality, and fatigue. They also found significantly greater complaints of EDS, poor sleep quality, fatigue, and RLS complaints among patients with DM2, although they did not find greater frequency of OSA or RBD. The pathogenesis of sleep disturbance in patients with DM2 remains unknown. OSA may be related to upper airway muscle weakness and myotonia. In addition, abnormal central control of breathing and sleep-wake state due to brain stem abnormality may contribute to SDB, insomnia, and RBD. Whether sleep dysfunction in DM2 is of the same characteristic and severity as in DM1 is unknown.

Amyotrophic Lateral Sclerosis

Sleep disorders are common in neurodegenerative diseases such as Parkinson disease, multiple system atrophy (MSA), and amyotrophic lateral sclerosis (ALS). Cell loss in the respiratory center of the brain stem and dysfunction of bulbar and diaphragmatic muscles may increase the risk for SDB in MSA and ALS. The most common SDB in MSA is stridor, whereas in ALS, diaphragmatic weakness and nocturnal hypoventilation is most commonly experienced. As with other restrictive lung diseases, these patients are particularly vulnerable to having apneas and nocturnal hypoxemia during REM sleep when the diaphragm remains the only active respiratory muscle. Moreover, patients with ALS may experience progressive bulbar palsy leading to motor neuron degeneration that specifically impairs the glossopharyngeal nerve, vagus nerve, and hypoglossal nerve. In addition to difficulty with chewing, talking, and swallowing, patients may experience weak palatal control and tongue protrusion, and as a result be at risk for OSA. Nocturnal hypoxemia in this group may be associated with cognitive dysfunction, including poor memory and recall.[34] Moreover, stridor and nocturnal hypoventilation in MSA and ALS, respectively, are associated with increased mortality.

Fatigue is a common symptom reported in ALS. Patients with ALS have difficulties staying asleep, increased nocturia, and frequent nocturnal cramps. Other sleep disorders that have been described in patients with ALS include RBD and RLS.[35,36] Sleep efficiency is poor, and patients with ALS with sleep disturbances have worse functional disability as measured by the ALS Functional Rating Scale-Revised and Pittsburgh Sleep Quality Index, worse EDS as measured by Epworth Sleepiness Scale, and greater depression on Beck Depression Inventory.[37,38] When the disease progresses and a patient becomes locked in, they may lose their circadian rhythm for heart rate and body temperature and have greater fragmentation of stage N3 sleep without change in total stage N3 time.[39]

NIPPV may help patients with ALS improve oxygenation during sleep. However, whether NIPPV improves sleep quality, sleep efficiency, arousal index, and sleep architecture in patients with ALS is unclear.[40] Meanwhile, diaphragmatic pacing in patients with ALS has been shown to improve sleep efficiency and decrease arousal index, as well as treat REM-related apneas and hypopneas.[41] More research is necessary to investigate the impact of respiratory support on sleep.

OBESITY HYPOVENTILATION

OHS is defined by the clinical triad of obesity, daytime hypoventilation, and SDB. The mechanism by which obesity leads to hypoventilation is complex and not fully understood. Several mechanisms have been proposed in the pathogenesis of OHS, including abnormal respiratory system mechanics due to obesity, impaired central responses to hypercapnia and hypoxemia, SDB, and neurohormonal abnormalities.

SDB takes 2 forms in OHS. The most common form is OSA and occurs in the vast majority of patients with OHS (70%–90%). The second is central hypoventilation and accounts for the other 10% to 30% of SDB. In healthy individuals, there is mild hypoventilation and $Paco_2$ increases by 3 to 5 mm Hg. In patients with OHS, $Paco_2$ is often increased by greater than 10 mm Hg. Patients with OHS and OSA typically have severe OSA. They tend to demonstrate hypopneas rather than frank apneas with significant arterial oxygen desaturation. For those with central hypoventilation, patients often spend most of the sleep time hypoxemic (ie, arterial oxygen saturations <90%).[42]

Obese individuals breathe on the less compliant portion of the pressure-volume curve and require more work for ventilation. Severely obese individuals may also experience expiratory flow limitation with increased alveolar end-expiratory pressure due to incomplete expiration. This dynamic pulmonary hyperinflation overstretches the diaphragm and results in respiratory inefficiencies to increase the oxygen consumption dedicated to the work of breathing by 5-fold in severely obese individuals compared with nonobese persons.[43]

Only a minority of obese individuals develop OHS, suggesting there are other predisposing factors at work. There are likely individual differences in how respiratory muscles respond to respiratory mass loading. When individuals with OHS were compared with matched controls with similar degrees of obesity, subjects with OHS had worse lung compliance, functional residual capacity, chest wall compliance, and lung resistance. Although mechanical load may play an important role in the development of OHS, BMI may be an oversimplified measure of this mass-loading effect because it does not take into account among other things the distribution fat.[44,45]

Several observations suggest a deficit in the central ventilatory drive in patients with OHS. Obese persons with an intact central ventilatory response compensate for increased respiratory mechanical load and maintain eucapnia by generating greater diaphragmatic electromyogram activity, greater inspiratory intrathoracic pressures, and greater minute ventilation through increased respiratory rates.[46,47] Patients with OHS do not demonstrate this degree of compensation to CO_2 rebreathing or to hypoxemia. This central respiratory depression may result from maladaptation to SDB. Norman and colleagues[48] proposed a model explaining the transition of acute hypercapnia during SDB to daytime hypercapnia. They propose in this model that, in some individuals, the postapnea hyperventilation period is insufficient to completely eliminate the $Paco_2$ accumulated during an apneic event. As a result, $Paco_2$ accumulates steadily during the night and the kidneys may retain bicarbonate during sleep to buffer the ongoing respiratory acidemia. If the kidney's rate of bicarbonate excretion is slow, metabolic alkalemia may result at the end of the sleep period, and the patient compensates by hypoventilating during wake.

In patients with eucapnic SDB, acute hypoxemia acts as a respiratory stimulant and increases ventilatory drive at the termination of a respiratory event. Abrupt awakenings from sleep increase sympathetic signaling, which also stimulate postapneic hyperventilation. However, sustained hypoxemia acts as a neurocognitive depressant and may impair respiratory load sensation and respiratory arousal from sleep, leading to exaggerated apneic episodes and inadequate postevent ventilatory response.[49] Additional factors that may impair postapnea ventilation include blunted sympathetic stimulation and inadequate upper airway mechanoreceptor activation, leading to persistently increased upper airway resistance on awakening.

Treatment of SDB with PAP therapy or tracheostomy even without concomitant weight loss improves daytime hypoventilation in most patients with OHS. Mokhlesi and colleagues[50] found patients with OHS using PAP had significant improvements in $Paco_2$ and partial pressure of oxygen (Pao_2) with greater hours of usage per night, although the effect plateaued after 4.5 hours of PAP therapy. The rate of improvement for $Paco_2$ was nearly 2 mm Hg and for Pao_2 approximately 3 mm Hg per hour of PAP use. Furthermore, the need for supplemental oxygen during wakefulness decreased from 30% to 6% in those being treated with PAP. As short as 2 weeks of PAP therapy may improve hypercapnic and hypoxemic ventilatory responses.[51–53] However, PAP therapy does not reverse the underlying propensity for chronic hypoventilation, and hypercapnia recurs if patients with OHS stop using PAP.

SUMMARY

Patients with restrictive lung disease exhibit a wide range of sleep-related abnormalities, including breathing, movement, architecture, and circadian disorders. There are many unanswered questions regarding the role of sleep and the impact of sleep disorders and their treatment on intrapulmonary and extrapulmonary restrictive ventilatory disorders.

REFERENCES

1. Berthon-Jones M, Sullivan CE. Ventilatory and arousal responses to hypoxia in sleeping humans. Am Rev Respir Dis 1982;125:632–9.
2. Berthon-Jones M, Sullivan CE. Ventilation and arousal responses to hypercapnia in normal sleeping humans. J Appl Physiol Respir Environ Exerc Physiol 1984;57:59–67.
3. Dyspnea. Mechanisms, assessment, and management: a consensus statement. American Thoracic Society. Am J Respir Crit Care Med 1999;159:321–40.
4. Perez-Padilla R, West P, Lertzman M, et al. Breathing during sleep in patients with interstitial lung disease. Am Rev Respir Dis 1985;132:224–9.
5. Bye PT, Issa F, Berthon-Jones M, et al. Studies of oxygenation during sleep in patients with interstitial lung disease. Am Rev Respir Dis 1984;129:27–32.
6. McNicholas WT, Coffey M, Fitzgerald MX. Ventilation and gas exchange during sleep in patients with interstitial lung disease. Thorax 1986;41:777–82.
7. Shea SA, Winning AJ, McKenzie E, et al. Does the abnormal pattern of breathing in patients with interstitial lung disease persist in deep, non-rapid eye movement sleep? Am Rev Respir Dis 1989;139:653–8.
8. Midgren B, Hansson L, Eriksson L, et al. Oxygen desaturation during sleep and exercise in patients with interstitial lung disease. Thorax 1987;42:353–6.
9. Hira HS, Sharma RK. Study of oxygen saturation, breathing pattern and arrhythmias in patients of interstitial lung disease during sleep. Indian J Chest Dis Allied Sci 1997;39:157–62.
10. Corte TJ, Wort SJ, Talbot S, et al. Elevated nocturnal desaturation index predicts mortality in interstitial lung disease. Sarcoidosis Vasc Diffuse Lung Dis 2012;29:41–50.
11. Medeiros P Jr, Lorenzi-Filho G, Pimenta SP, et al. Sleep desaturation and its relationship to lung function, exercise and quality of life in LAM. Respir Med 2012;106:420–8.
12. Midgren B. Oxygen desaturation during sleep as a function of the underlying respiratory disease. Am Rev Respir Dis 1990;141:43–6.
13. Pascual N, Jurado B, Rubio JM, et al. Respiratory disorders and quality of sleep in patients on the waiting list for lung transplantation. Transplant Proc 2005;37:1537–9.
14. Prado GF, Allen RP, Trevisani VM, et al. Sleep disruption in systemic sclerosis (scleroderma) patients: clinical and polysomnographic findings. Sleep Med 2002;3:341–5.
15. Pihtili A, Bingol Z, Kiyan E, et al. Obstructive sleep apnea is common in patients with interstitial lung disease. Sleep Breath 2013;17:1281–8.
16. Lancaster LH, Mason WR, Parnell JA, et al. Obstructive sleep apnea is common in idiopathic pulmonary fibrosis. Chest 2009;136:772–8.
17. Mermigkis C, Stagaki E, Tryfon S, et al. How common is sleep-disordered breathing in patients with idiopathic pulmonary fibrosis? Sleep Breath 2010;14:387–90.
18. Raghu G, Freudenberger TD, Yang S, et al. High prevalence of abnormal acid gastro-oesophageal reflux in idiopathic pulmonary fibrosis. Eur Respir J 2006;27:136–42.
19. Zhang XJ, Bonner A, Hudson M, et al. Association of gastroesophageal factors and worsening of forced vital capacity in systemic sclerosis. J Rheumatol 2013;40:850–8.
20. Shepherd KL, James AL, Musk AW, et al. Gastro-oesophageal reflux symptoms are related to the presence and severity of obstructive sleep apnoea. J Sleep Res 2011;20:241–9.
21. Shepherd K, Hillman D, Holloway R, et al. Mechanisms of nocturnal gastroesophageal reflux events in obstructive sleep apnea. Sleep Breath 2011;15:561–70.
22. Pillai M, Olson AL, Huie TJ, et al. Obstructive sleep apnea does not promote esophageal reflux in fibrosing interstitial lung disease. Respir Med 2012;106:1033–9.
23. Won C, Purvis T, Chun HJ. An overlap phenomenon exists with interstitial lung disease and obstructive sleep apnea [abstract 17996]. In: American Thoracic Society. Denver, May 13–18, 2011.

24. Mezon BL, West P, Israels J, et al. Sleep breathing abnormalities in kyphoscoliosis. Am Rev Respir Dis 1980;122:617–21.

25. Guilleminault C, Kurland G, Winkle R, et al. Severe kyphoscoliosis, breathing, and sleep: the "quasimodo" syndrome during sleep. Chest 1981;79:626–30.

26. Esau SA. Hypoxic, hypercapnic acidosis decreases tension and increases fatigue in hamster diaphragm muscle in vitro. Am Rev Respir Dis 1989;139:1410–7.

27. Kiyan E, Okumus G, Cuhadaroglu C, et al. Sleep apnea in adult myotonic dystrophy patients who have no excessive daytime sleepiness. Sleep Breath 2010;14:19–24.

28. Li H, Liang C, Shen C, et al. Decreased sleep duration: a risk of progression of degenerative lumbar scoliosis. Med Hypotheses 2012;78:244–6.

29. Gonzalez C, Ferris G, Diaz J, et al. Kyphoscoliotic ventilatory insufficiency: effects of long-term intermittent positive-pressure ventilation. Chest 2003; 124:857–62.

30. Romigi A, Albanese M, Placidi F, et al. Sleep disorders in myotonic dystrophy type 2: a controlled polysomnographic study and self-reported questionnaires. Eur J Neurol 2014;21(6):929–34.

31. Ciafaloni E, Mignot E, Sansone V, et al. The hypocretin neurotransmission system in myotonic dystrophy type 1. Neurology 2008;70:226–30.

32. Chokroverty S, Bhat S, Rosen D, et al. REM behavior disorder in myotonic dystrophy type 2. Neurology 2012;78:2004.

33. Lam EM, Shepard PW, St Louis EK, et al. Restless legs syndrome and daytime sleepiness are prominent in myotonic dystrophy type 2. Neurology 2013;81:157–64.

34. Park SY, Kim SM, Sung JJ, et al. Nocturnal hypoxia in ALS is related to cognitive dysfunction and can occur as clusters of desaturations. PLoS One 2013;8:e75324.

35. Ebben MR, Shahbazi M, Lange DJ, et al. REM behavior disorder associated with familial amyotrophic lateral sclerosis. Amyotroph Lateral Scler 2012;13:473–4.

36. Lo Coco D, Piccoli F, La Bella V. Restless legs syndrome in patients with amyotrophic lateral sclerosis. Mov Disord 2010;25:2658–61.

37. Lo Coco D, La Bella V. Fatigue, sleep, and nocturnal complaints in patients with amyotrophic lateral sclerosis. Eur J Neurol 2012;19:760–3.

38. Lo Coco D, Mattaliano P, Spataro R, et al. Sleep-wake disturbances in patients with amyotrophic lateral sclerosis. J Neurol Neurosurg Psychiatry 2011;82:839–42.

39. Soekadar SR, Born J, Birbaumer N, et al. Fragmentation of slow wave sleep after onset of complete locked-in state. J Clin Sleep Med 2013;9:951–3.

40. Katzberg HD, Selegiman A, Guion L, et al. Effects of noninvasive ventilation on sleep outcomes in amyotrophic lateral sclerosis. J Clin Sleep Med 2013;9:345–51.

41. Gonzalez-Bermejo J, Morelot-Panzini C, Salachas F, et al. Diaphragm pacing improves sleep in patients with amyotrophic lateral sclerosis. Amyotroph Lateral Scler 2012;13:44–54.

42. Banerjee D, Yee BJ, Piper AJ, et al. Obesity hypoventilation syndrome: hypoxemia during continuous positive airway pressure. Chest 2007;131:1678–84.

43. Kress JP, Pohlman AS, Alverdy J, et al. The impact of morbid obesity on oxygen cost of breathing (VO(2RESP)) at rest. Am J Respir Crit Care Med 1999;160:883–6.

44. Lazarus R, Sparrow D, Weiss ST. Effects of obesity and fat distribution on ventilatory function: the normative aging study. Chest 1997;111:891–8.

45. Resta O, Foschino-Barbaro MP, Bonfitto P, et al. Prevalence and mechanisms of diurnal hypercapnia in a sample of morbidly obese subjects with obstructive sleep apnoea. Respir Med 2000;94:240–6.

46. Sampson MG, Grassino K. Neuromechanical properties in obese patients during carbon dioxide rebreathing. Am J Med 1983;75:81–90.

47. Lopata M, Onal E. Mass loading, sleep apnea, and the pathogenesis of obesity hypoventilation. Am Rev Respir Dis 1982;126:640–5.

48. Norman RG, Goldring RM, Clain JM, et al. Transition from acute to chronic hypercapnia in patients with periodic breathing: predictions from a computer model. J Appl Physiol (1985) 2006;100:1733–41.

49. Hlavac MC, Catcheside PG, McDonald R, et al. Hypoxia impairs the arousal response to external resistive loading and airway occlusion during sleep. Sleep 2006;29:624–31.

50. Mokhlesi B, Tulaimat A, Evans AT, et al. Impact of adherence with positive airway pressure therapy on hypercapnia in obstructive sleep apnea. J Clin Sleep Med 2006;2:57–62.

51. Han F, Chen E, Wei H, et al. Treatment effects on carbon dioxide retention in patients with obstructive sleep apnea-hypopnea syndrome. Chest 2001;119:1814–9.

52. Lin CC. Effect of nasal CPAP on ventilatory drive in normocapnic and hypercapnic patients with obstructive sleep apnoea syndrome. Eur Respir J 1994;7:2005–10.

53. Moura SM, Bittencourt LR, Bagnato MC, et al. Acute effect of nasal continuous positive air pressure on the ventilatory control of patients with obstructive sleep apnea. Respiration 2001;68:243–9.

Physiology of Sleep and Breathing Before and After Lung Transplantation

 CrossMark

Paola Pierucci, MD, Monique Malouf, FRACP*

KEYWORDS

- Lung transplant • Sleep disorders • OSA • CSA • SDB

KEY POINTS

- Disturbed respiratory physiology and sleep disordered breathing (SDB) are often undiagnosed in patients with end stage respiratory failure awaiting lung transplantation.
- SDB may persist or develop after LTx.
- Weight gain, gastrooesophageal reflux and immunosuppressive medications can trigger or aggravate SDB.

INTRODUCTION

Lung transplantation (LTX) during the course of the last 20 years has become an accepted life-saving modality of care for patients with end-stage pulmonary disease when maximal conventional medical therapies have not improved chances of survival.[1–7] There are several reasons for this: (1) improved surgical techniques; (2) appropriate timing for referral and transplant listing; (3) better management of patients in the immediate postoperative period after transplantation; (4) greater experience gained from large transplant centers that perform a larger volume of transplants have resulted in improved outcomes, survival, and quality of life (QOL). Overall, the improvements in treating intraoperative and perioperative complications with the identification of major risk factors such as infection, acute rejection, and earlier detection of bronchiolitis obliterans syndrome (BOS) have reduced mortality and morbidity.[1,8]

Sleep Disordered Breathing in LTX

Few publications have focused on sleep disordered breathing (SDB) before and after LTX. There are several conditions leading to LTX, including emphysema secondary to smoking and/or alpha1-antitrypsin deficiency, interstitial lung diseases, cystic fibrosis, and pulmonary hypertension either primary or secondary to congenital heart diseases. These conditions may all be associated with SDB (**Table 1**).

For the general population the association between weight gain and the presence of SDB has already been well described. In particular, people who initially had no or mild SDB are predicted to develop moderate to severe SDB, with significant weight gain. In patients already affected by SDB there is a strong relationship between weight gain and increased SDB severity.[9] An increased weight gain after transplantation can lead to the development of obstructive sleep apnea (OSA) in lung transplant recipients.[10]

DISTURBED RESPIRATORY PHYSIOLOGY DURING SLEEP AND SDB BEFORE LTX

As previously emphasized, several respiratory disorders are characterized by association with SDB, especially in their end-stage phase of their disease. This article reviews these in detail.

Disclosures: None.
Lung Transplant Unit, St Vincents Hospital, 390 Victoria Street, Darlinghurst, Sydney 2010, Australia
* Corresponding author.
E-mail address: mmalouf@stvincents.com.au

Clin Chest Med 35 (2014) 513–520
http://dx.doi.org/10.1016/j.ccm.2014.06.007

Table 1
Definitions of breathing alterations during sleep

Apnea	Obstructive breathing event with complete upper airways obstruction (residual air flow, 20% of the preceding period of stable breathing; ie, reduction in air flow at least 80%) Each event should last at least 10 s
Hypopnea	Obstructive breathing event with a reduction of airflow of at least 30%. Each event should last at least 10 s and be accompanied by a 3% oxygen saturation reduction or arousal
AHI	Number of apneas and hypopneas per hour of sleep Mild OSA: AHI 5–15 events/h Moderate OSA: AHI 15–30 events/h Severe OSA: AHI >30 events/h
RDI	Summarizes both the AHI and the RERA indices together

Abbreviations: AHI, apnea-hypopnea index; OSA, obstructive sleep apnea; RDI, respiratory disturbance index; RERA, Respiratory Effort–related Arousal.

Data from Berry RB, Brooks R, Gamaldo CE, et al, for the American Academy of Sleep Medicine. The AASM manual for the scoring of sleep and associated events: rules, terminology and technical specifications, version 2.0. Darion (IL): American Academy of Sleep Medicine; 2012. Available at: www.aasmnet.org.

Patients with Cystic Fibrosis

Disturbed breathing during sleep is common in patients with cystic fibrosis (CF), often as a result of progressive lung disease. Patients with CF may develop type 1 and 2 respiratory failure (RF) while awaiting LTX.[11] The hypoxia (type 1 RF) is related to the lack of functioning lung parenchyma in conjunction with chronic bronchopulmonary infections. The carbon dioxide retention leading to hypercapnic RF (type 2 RF) has complex causes, such as tenacious secretions, distorted lung architecture, and maximal use of respiratory and nonrespiratory muscles. All these problems may worsen during sleep, when the diaphragm is the only respiratory active muscle. During sleep, particularly during rapid eye movement (REM) sleep, nocturnal episodes of hypoventilation occur frequently, causing desaturation and consequently hypercapnia, which increases the morbidity associated with hypercapnia such as morning headaches and worsening of RF resulting in pulmonary hypertension and heart failure.[12] The use of noninvasive positive pressure ventilation (NIPPV) has been shown to be of benefit in end-stage RF in patients with CF and is often used as a bridge to transplantation.[13] NIPPV in this population has been shown to improve arterial blood gas values and decrease dyspnea. The improvement is caused by the augmentation of ventilation by means of the delivery of pressure/volume during inspiration and expiration and therefore improving minute ventilation through the inspiratory positive airway pressure (IPAP) and the expiratory positive airway pressure (EPAP). The difference between IPAP and EPAP is the pressure support delivered to the patient. Although the IPAP helps by supporting the inspiratory effort and decreases the muscles' workload, the EPAP acts by recruiting and distending the collapsed alveoli, increasing the functional residual capacity, and improving gas exchange through the alveolar/capillary barrier. Moreover, NIPPV is noninvasive, can be used intermittently, and it is well tolerated in hospital and at home. Most patients reported improvements with reduction in headache, improved quality of sleep, and increased activities of daily living after its sustained use.[14,15]

PATIENTS ON WAITING LIST FOR LTX

Few investigators have studied the quality of sleep of patients on the waiting list for LTX, and therefore the numbers of patients analyzed are small. In these studies a significantly poorer quality of sleep was observed compared with the control group. There was a greater predominance of non-REM stage 1 and 2 sleep, more fragmented sleep patterns with more phase changes per hour, and a greater average time of wakefulness between sleep periods. No statistically significant differences were found in terms of increased apnea-hypopnea index (AHI) in the group of patients on the LTX waiting list compared with the controls. However, this finding could be confounded by most of the patients requiring oxygen overnight for severe hypoxia.[16]

In our experience among all patients on the LTX waiting list who had received a polysomnography (PSG) study on room air (80 patients), about 40% had altered respiratory physiology during sleep or SDB (32 patients). We defined SDB either as a respiratory disturbance index (RDI) of greater than or equal to 10 or greater than or equal to 10% of total sleep time (TST) with arterial oxygen saturation (Sao_2) less than or equal to 90% in the presence of awake Sao_2 greater than or equal to 90% or both. In more detail, 24 of 32 patients (40%) had severe hypoxemia during sleep. Eighteen of 32 (38%) had RDI less than 10 per hour and had more than 10% of TST spent under oxygen saturations of 90%; 14 of 32 (44%) had an RDI greater than 10; 8 of these 32 (25%) had both greater than 10% of TST with a saturation less than 90% and RDI greater than 10. Moreover, 30 patients underwent PSG with oxygen supplementation and 9 of them had SDB, whereas 7 underwent PSG on noninvasive ventilation (NIV) and only 1 had SDB. There was no association between the underlying diagnosis and the presence of SDB. The survival on the waiting list was not affected by the results found in the diagnostic group. Pretransplant survival was not affected by the known presence or absence of adverse respiratory physiology during sleep. The emphysema subgroup was analyzed in a separate subgroup and their survival was not affected by nocturnal respiratory physiologic compromise. Overall, the presence of disordered respiratory physiologic status did not affect posttransplant survival.[17]

RESPIRATORY PHYSIOLOGIC CHANGES AFTER TRANSPLANTATION

The advent of heart and LTX gave scientists the unique opportunity to study the pattern of breathing with complete absence of vagal afferents from the lungs. Studies conducted on mammals before the LTX showed that, in most mammals, proprioceptive pulmonary vagal afferents determine the frequency and the amplitude of the ventilation. Without that feedback, breathing became increasingly slow, deep, and more variable. The same studies performed on healthy humans did not show such a robust agreement compared with results found in mammals. Different techniques were used to achieve a reversible vagal block, and these were never selective for pulmonary innervations (bilateral anesthetic blockade, aerosolized anesthetics, airway anesthesia). Therefore evidence-based results to assess this outcome were not obtained until LTX became an option for patients.[18]

The surgical LTX operation consists of preservation of the upper four-fifths of recipients' tracheal innervation and recurrent laryngeal nerves, whereas sympathetic heart and lung connections are sacrificed. Studies were performed in heart and lung/lung transplant recipients and focused on the breathing pattern and its variability during awake and sleep. Although patients after LTX develop respiratory disturbance during sleep, results failed to find any significant correlation between respiratory disturbance during sleep and the effect of chronic pulmonary denervation as a cause for their emergence.[19]

QUALITY OF LIFE/QUALITY OF SLEEP AFTER LTX

A robust body of literature has focused on global QOL after transplantation. A recent review reported evidence of improvement in QOL in these patients during the first 6 months after the transplantation, continuing up to 1 year. After the first year, for most patients, the benefits became more evident, whereas for a small group of patients these outcomes were negatively affected by the onset of BOS and other morbidities. These data also show that anxiety, depression, and other psychosocial morbidities are prevalent in lung transplant recipients and may have a negative impact on QOL and sleep.[20,21]

SDB AND SEVERE HEART DISEASES BEFORE AND AFTER HEART TRANSPLANTATION

Most of the ideas regarding the link between SDB and end-stage diseases have come from the heart failure experience. There is strong evidence linking cardiovascular diseases and sleep disorders. OSA is significantly associated with the risk of stroke and death from any cause and the association is independent of other risk factors.[22] In addition, patients affected by severe heart failure often have SDB.[23] Thus, apneas and hypopneas (with or without Cheyne-Stokes respiration) are common during end-stage heart diseases.[24] Most research that has documented a correlation between sleep disorders and transplant has come from the heart transplant experience. Sleep disorders are responsible for sleep disruption by arousal because of development of hypoxemia, which may play a role in worsening of cardiac dysfunction, and this is correlated with the findings that patients with severe cardiac dysfunction seem to have a high prevalence of sleep apnea. Often OSA is not diagnosed before heart transplantation (HTX), whereas the prevalence has been documented in some series to be as high as 45% in patients waiting for HTX.[25] Therefore the risks associated with sleep apnea need to be considered after HTX. Although OSA may be part of the multifactorial causes leading to heart failure before and after HTX, several reports suggest that OSA should be considered as a potential cause of graft failure in heart transplant recipients and should be identified as a preexisting abnormality during transplant work-up for patients with heart failure.[26–28]

SDB AFTER LTX

Following the findings in the heart transplant population, few studies have explored the prevalence of SDB after LTX.

What Are the Changes Before and After LTX in Terms of SDB?

In our study 25 of 38 (65.8%) patients had room air studies both before and after LTX. Underlying diagnoses for this group (n = 25) were emphysema n = 10, pulmonary fibrosis n = 5, CF n = 7, bronchiectasis n = 1, eosinophilic granulomatous disease n = 1, and congenital heart disease/Eisenmenger n = 1. Our findings showed that 11 of 25 (44%) patients who received PSG before LTX had SDB. After the LTX, 5 of 11 patients persisted to be symptomatic for SDB. Four of the 14 patients who before LTX were not affected by SDB developed new SDB after LTX, so that a total of 9 patients had SDB after LTX (**Fig. 1**).

There was a statistically significant improvement in sleep oxygenation after lung transplantation both in minimum sleep oxygen saturation and percentage of TST with $SaO_2 \leq 90\%$ (SaO_2 91.5% ± standard deviation [SD] 4.7% vs 96.0% ± SD 1.85% before and after LTX respectively; mean change of 5.5%, 95% confidence interval, 3.4–7.6; $P<.001$). No difference was found in the sleep efficiency, arousal index, and sleep stage percentage (**Box 1**).

As a consequence in the post-LTX period, there was a marked reduction in ventilatory support requirements, although ventilation was still necessary for 11 patients (NIV, n = 1; continuous positive airway pressure [CPAP], n = 10).

Among these patients 10 continued to use CPAP and 1 required bilevel. The reasons for this novel emergence of SDB was postulated to be posttransplant central fat accumulation caused by corticosteroid therapy, and increased body mass index (BMI) resulting in OSA.[17] Naraine and colleagues found that the percentage of SDB was higher with 63% of patients studied affected by SDB when using a cutoff of AHI greater than 10 per hour and 83% when the AHI was greater than 5 per hour. However, no data before LTX were available for this series. In this SDB population OSA was observed in 38% and central seep apnea (CSA) in 25%. Subjects with SDB were older, had been transplanted more recently, were more likely to be on cyclosporine, and had better lung function than subjects without SDB.[10]

Box 1
Comparison of PSG performed on room air before and after LTX in 25 recipients

Parameter	Pre-LTX PSG	Post-LTX PSG	P Value
TST (minutes)	333.7 ± 7	349.7 ± 5	.9
Sleep efficiency (%)	76.9 ± 2	77.1 ± 10.4	.96
Arousal index	19.9 ± 11.6	19.9 ± 13.7	.98
Overall RDI	8.48 ± 10.8	11.9 ± 18.5	.3
Sleep Stage (%)			
1	8.6 ± 5.9	8.0 ± 8.6	.9
2	57.8 ± 10	60.1 ± 11.3	.3
3	8.8 ± 4.8	9.1 ± 10.9	.9
4	7.8 ± 7	4.75 ± 4.9	.09
NREM (%)	81.9 ± 7.6	85.5 ± 6.0	.8
REM (%)	18.1 ± 7.6	17.5 ± 6.0	.8
Sleep O_2 saturation	91.5 ± 4.7	96.0 ± 1.85	<.001

Abbreviation: NREM, non-REM.

COMORBIDITIES CORRELATED WITH SDB AFTER LTX

SDB and Gastroesophageal Reflux Disease After LTX

The presence of gastroesophageal reflux disease (GORD) is common in patients after LTX.[29–31] GORD may occur as a preoperative condition or is potentially induced by immunosuppressive drugs (eg, calcineurin inhibitors) or iatrogenic vagal nerve injury at surgery. Interstitial lung diseases secondary to connective tissue disorders or idiopathic pulmonary fibrosis as well as CF have all been associated with GORD.[32–35] It has also been suggested that GORD leading to pulmonary aspiration may be one of the key factors promoting posttransplant chronic graft dysfunction or BOS.[36–38]

The presence of SDB may aggravate the risk of pulmonary aspiration, because OSA is known to

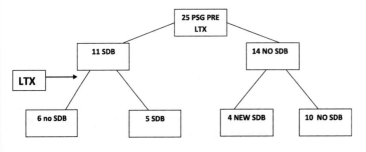

Fig. 1. The scheme for SDB found on room air PSG before and after LTX.

increase the severity and frequency of GORD symptoms. The nocturnal period represents a highly vulnerable period for pulmonary aspiration of stomach contents because sleep is commonly associated with decreased upper esophageal sphincter tone, reduced esophageal acid clearance, and increased esophageal acid contact time. An increased proximal acid migration and increased pharyngeal and lung aspiration are consequently especially noted after LTX.[39–43]

The use of therapies to reduce the prevalence of GORD must be considered. Such therapies include elevation of the upper part of the bed and antireflux therapies such as selective proton pump inhibitors, histamine H2 antagonists, cytoprotective agents, antidopaminergics, and prokinetics. Ph probe and esophageal manometry should be routinely performed in all patients after LTX. In addition, if maximum therapy does not result in relief of GORD symptoms, then a surgical procedure such as a Nissen fundoplication should be considered.[44,45]

SDB and Increased Weight After LTX

Significant weight gain after transplantation has already been described in recipients of kidney, liver, and heart transplants and consequential emergence of SDB.[46–51] The same also applies to LTx recipients. Studies have observed that 1-year weight gain in a cohort of lung transplant recipients was similar to that observed in other solid organ recipients. In particular, the median weight change during the first year after transplantation was greater than 10%, and was more evident in patients with previous suppurative (CF or bronchiectasis) and obstructive lung diseases such as emphysema.[52–54] The mechanisms underlying posttransplant weight gain are still unclear and require further study. As in the general population, obesity is frequently associated with increased risks of hypertension, diabetes mellitus, and coronary artery disease. A higher incidence of complications similarly occur early and late after transplantation in obese patients, such as SDB, infections, diabetes, cardiovascular diseases, deconditioning, increased length of stay in hospital, and increased use of NIV after transplantation.

Although the literature lacks long-term follow-up for lung transplant recipients with SDB, in our series of patients weight gain was evident but there was no significant statistical correlation with the presence of SDB. Pre-LTX baseline BMI was 22.8 ± 4.6 and post-LTX BMI increased to 24.3 ± 4.7 ($P = .9$).[17] In other series an upward trend was found in patients with increased BMI

and sleep obstructive event index. In those series as well as in ours, weight gain after transplantation had increased by 18%. This result predicts an approximate 32% increase in both the AHI and the odds of subsequently developing moderate to severe SDB.[10]

The increase in the BMI has led not just to the presence of OSA but also to an increase in complications for procedures requiring sedation, such as bronchoscopies, routinely performed after transplantation.[55] Often these patients require a laryngeal mask or endotracheal intubation during these procedures.[56] Moreover, patients with SDB had also higher systolic blood pressure than those without SDB.[10]

SDB and Immunosuppressive Drugs

Another factor that may contribute to weight gain and SDB after transplantation is the use of immunosuppressive drugs, especially corticosteroids. During the first year after transplantation, recipients receive the largest amount of corticosteroids, because the incidence of acute rejection within the first 6 to 12 months is the greatest.[57]

The mineral corticoid activity of a steroid may lead to salt and water retention, which can result in weight gain and hypertension. The typical adipose deposition with these medications is truncal, particularly in the facial and neck regions (classic Cushing). This localization of fat in these areas has been recognized in the literature as being associated with the onset or worsening of sleep disorders, particularly OSA. Fat deposition in patients with OSA is usually observed in those areas of the soft palate surrounding the collapsible segment of the pharynx, whereas in equally obese control subjects without OSA the fat is mainly concentrated in the posterior-lateral palatal zones.[58]

A contribution to the increased adipose mass that is seen after LTx, may be due to immunosuppressive medications such as cyclosporine and prednisolone, which can increase fluid retention, edema, and weight increase. Moreover, it can induce impaired insulin release and peripheral insulin resistance in genetically susceptible individuals.[59] If patients are already overweight at the time of transplantation, it is possible that altered insulin release and sensitivity may influence the weight gain after transplantation as well.[60] Cyclosporine has been associated with the presence of CSA in a small cohort of patient after transplantation.[10] In addition, tacrolimus, an alternate calcineurin inhibitor, can induce hyperglycemic conditions such as diabetes mellitus and therefore weight gain.[59,60]

SDB and Type of Surgical Cut

The LTX-associated chest pain caused by the surgical procedure may have an impact on the quality and architecture of sleep but at the present time no studies have explored this issue. Less invasive surgical procedures (minithoracotomy) that avoid the sternum cut (clamshell) could minimize pain-related issues and facilitate greater chest expansion during sleep in early posttransplant patients. Further studies are required to explore these correlations.

SUMMARY

Disturbed respiratory physiology and SDB are often underdiagnosed in patients waiting for LTX.

It seems clear that most of the diseases that lead to end-stage RF requiring LTX may be associated with SDB. The use of oxygen or NIV needs to be considered after diagnostic PSG. NIV should be considered as an initial treatment option in patients with CF and type 2 RF, because a growing body of literature now supports its use and it has been validated as a bridge to the LTX. Of equal importance is the quality of sleep in these patients and its improvement during NIV use while on the waiting list for LTX. Although the physiology of breathing changes after LTX (because of the implantation of new lungs) as a result of marked improvement of oxygen saturations during the sleep, the presence of SDB can persist after the procedure or occur de novo if previously not present. In some patients with chronic RF the typical breathing abnormality during sleep is hypoventilation rather than obstructive or central sleep apnea as in CF. Other comorbidites may also contribute to the development of SDB, such as increased weight after the transplantation caused by better health status as a result of the reversed catabolic status that is associated with respiratory cachexia. During the first year after LTX the use of corticosteroids may have a role in increased weight gain because of related truncal fat accumulation leading to OSA. Other relevant factors such as GORD need to be considered. If undiagnosed, such factors can trigger or aggravate the presence of SDB and can lead to graft dysfunction and development of BOS.

Therefore further research is warranted to confirm the prevalence of SDB in patients before and after LTX and to explore their quality of sleep and with the aim to improve their QOL.

REFERENCES

1. Reitz BA, Wallwork JL, Hunt SA, et al. Heart and lung transplantation: successful therapy for patients with pulmonary vascular disease. N Engl J Med 1982;306:557–64.
2. Harringer W, Haverich A. Heart and heart-lung transplantation: standards and improvements. World J Surg 2002;26:218–25.
3. Spratt P, Glanville AR, MacDonald P, et al. Heart/Lung transplantation in Australia: early results of the St Vincent's program. Transplant Proc 1990; 22:2141–2.
4. Whyte RI, Robbins RC, Altinger J, et al. Heart-lung transplantation for primary pulmonary hypertension. Ann Thorac Surg 1999;67:937–42.
5. Barlow CW, Robbins RC, Moon MR, et al. Heart-lung versus double-lung transplantation for suppurative lung disease. J Thorac Cardiovasc 2000; 119:466–76.
6. Cohen L, Littlefield C, Kelly P, et al. Predictors of quality of life and adjustment after lung transplantation. Chest 1998;113:633–44.
7. Finlen Copeland CA, Vock DM, Pieper K, et al. Impact of lung transplantation on recipient quality of life: a serial, prospective, multicenter analysis through the first posttransplant year. Chest 2013; 143(3):744–50.
8. Glanville AR, Estenne M. Indications, patient selection and timing of referral for lung transplantation. Eur Respir J 2003;22(5):845–52.
9. Peppard PE, Young T, Palta M, et al. Longitudinal study of moderate weight change and sleep-disordered breathing. JAMA 2000;284(23):3015–21.
10. Naraine VS, Bradley TD, Singer LG. Prevalence of sleep disordered breathing in lung transplant recipients. J Clin Sleep Med 2009;5(5):441–7.
11. Shennib H, Noirclerc M, Ernst P. Double-lung transplantation for cystic fibrosis. The Cystic Fibrosis Transplant Study Group. Ann Thorac Surg 1992; 54(1):27–31.
12. Davis PB, di Sant'Agnese PA. Assisted ventilation for patients with cystic fibrosis. JAMA 1978; 239(18):1851–4.
13. Hodson ME, Madden BP, Steven MH, et al. Noninvasive mechanical ventilation for cystic fibrosis patients–a potential bridge to transplantation. Eur Respir J 1991;4(5):524–7.
14. Hill AT, Edenborough FP, Cayton RM, et al. Long-term nasal intermittent positive pressure ventilation in patients with cystic fibrosis and hypercapnic respiratory failure (1991-1996). Respir Med 1998; 92(3):523–6.
15. Caronia CG, Silver P, Nimkoff L, et al. Use of bilevel positive airway pressure (BIPAP) in end-stage patients with cystic fibrosis awaiting lung transplantation. Clin Pediatr (Phila) 1998;37(9):555–9.
16. Pascual N, Jurado B, Rubio JM, et al. Respiratory disorders and quality of sleep in patients on the waiting list for lung transplantation. Transplant Proc 2005;37(3):1537–9.

17. Malouf MA, Milrose MA, Grunstein RR, et al. Sleep-disordered breathing before and after lung transplantation. J Heart Lung Transplant 2008;27(5): 540–6.

18. Shea SA, Horner RL, Banner NR, et al. The effect of human heart-lung transplantation upon breathing at rest and during sleep. Respir Physiol 1988; 72(2):131–49.

19. Sanders MH, Costantino JP, Owens GR, et al. Breathing during wakefulness and sleep after human heart-lung transplantation. Am Rev Respir Dis 1989;140(1):45–51.

20. Singer JP, Singer LG. Quality of life in lung transplantation. Semin Respir Crit Care Med 2013; 34(3):421–30.

21. Singer JP, Chen J, Blanc PD, et al. A thematic analysis of quality of life in lung transplant: the existing evidence and implications for future directions. Am J Transplant 2013;13(4):839–50. http://dx.doi.org/10.1111/ajt.12174.

22. Yaggi HK, Concato J, Kernan WN, et al. Obstructive sleep apnea as a risk factor for stroke and death. N Engl J Med 2005;353(19):2034–41.

23. Villa M, Lage E, Quintana E, et al. Prevalence of sleep breathing disorders in outpatients on a heart transplant waiting list. Transplant Proc 2003;35(5): 1944–5.

24. Javaheri S, Parker TJ, Liming JD, et al. Sleep apnea in 81 ambulatory male patients with stable heart failure. Types and their prevalences, consequences, and presentations. Circulation 1998;97(21):2154–9.

25. Nkere UU, Hall MC, Corris PA, et al. Sleep apnoea/hypopnoea syndrome: a potential cause of graft failure following heart transplantation. Eur J Cardiothorac Surg 1998;13(2):203–5.

26. Klink ME, Sethi GK, Copeland JG, et al. Obstructive sleep apnea in heart transplant patients. A report of five cases. Chest 1993;104(4):1090–2.

27. Hayes D Jr, Kirkby S, Splaingard ML, et al. Sleep-disordered breathing after combined heart-lung transplantation. Am J Respir Crit Care Med 2012; 186(6):569–70.

28. Collop NA. Cheyne-Stokes ventilation converting to obstructive sleep apnea following heart transplantation. Chest 1993;104(4):1288–9.

29. Shepherd KL, Chambers DC, Gabbay E, et al. Obstructive sleep apnoea and nocturnal gastroesophageal reflux are common in lung transplant patients. Respirology 2008;13(7):1045–52.

30. Young LR, Hadjiliadis D, Davis RD, et al. Lung transplantation exacerbates gastroesophageal reflux disease. Chest 2003;124(5):1689–93.

31. Hadjiliadis D, Duane Davis R, Steele MP, et al. Gastroesophageal reflux disease in lung transplant recipients. Clin Transplant 2003;17(4):363–8.

32. Pearson JE, Wilson RS. Diffuse pulmonary fibrosis and hiatus hernia. Thorax 1971;26(3):300–5.

33. Mays EE, Dubois JJ, Hamilton GB. Pulmonary fibrosis associated with tracheobronchial aspiration. A study of the frequency of hiatal hernia and gastroesophageal reflux in interstitial pulmonary fibrosis of obscure etiology. Chest 1976;69(4): 512–5.

34. Feigelson J, Girault F, Pecau Y. Gastro-oesophageal reflux and esophagitis in cystic fibrosis. Acta Paediatr Scand 1987;76(6):989–90.

35. Tobin RW, Pope CE 2nd, Pellegrini CA, et al. Increased prevalence of gastroesophageal reflux in patients with idiopathic pulmonary fibrosis. Am J Respir Crit Care Med 1998;158(6):1804–8.

36. Boehler A, Kesten S, Weder W, et al. Bronchiolitis obliterans after lung transplantation: a review. Chest 1998;114(5):1411–26.

37. Estenne M, Maurer JR, Boehler A, et al. Bronchiolitis obliterans syndrome 2001: an update of the diagnostic criteria. J Heart Lung Transplant 2002;21(3): 297–310. Available at: http://www.ncbi.nlm.nih.gov/pubmed?term=EganJ%5BAuthor%5D&cauthor=true&cauthor_uid=11897517J.

38. D'Ovidio F, Aramini B. Bronchiolitis obliterans in lung transplantation. In: Meyer K, Glanville AR, editors. Gastroesophageal reflux and aspiration in chronic lung allograft dysfunction and bronchiolitis obliterans syndrome: detection and treatment. Respiratory medicine. Series editor: Sharon IS. Round. 2013. p. 219–35.

39. Eastwood PR, Katagiri S, Shepherd KL, et al. Modulation of upper and lower esophageal sphincter tone during sleep. Sleep Med 2007;8(2):135–43.

40. Orr WC, Elsenbruch S, Harnish MJ, et al. Proximal migration of esophageal acid perfusions during waking and sleep. Am J Gastroenterol 2000; 95(1):37–42.

41. Huxley EJ, Viroslav J, Gray WR, et al. Pharyngeal aspiration in normal adults and patients with depressed consciousness. Am J Med 1978;64(4): 564–8.

42. Ing AJ, Ngu MC, Breslin AB. Obstructive sleep apnea and gastroesophageal reflux. Am J Med 2000; 108(Suppl 4a):120S–5S.

43. Green BT, Broughton WA, O'Connor JB. Marked improvement in nocturnal gastroesophageal reflux in a large cohort of patients with obstructive sleep apnea treated with continuous positive airway pressure. Arch Intern Med 2003;163(1):41–5.

44. Davis RD Jr, Lau CL, Eubanks S. Improved lung allograft function after fundoplication in patients with gastroesophageal reflux disease undergoing lung transplantation. Thorac Cardiovasc Surg 2003;125(3):533–42. Available at: http://www.ncbi.nlm.nih.gov/pubmed?term=MessierRH%5BAuthor%5D&cauthor=true&cauthor_uid=12658195J.

45. Cantu E 3rd, Appel JZ 3rd, Hartwig MG, et al. Early fundoplication prevents chronic allograft

dysfunction in patients with gastroesophageal reflux disease. Ann Thorac Surg 2004;78(4): 1142–51 [discussion: 1142–51].

46. Johnson CP, Gallagher-Lepak S, Zhu YR, et al. Factors influencing weight gain after renal transplantation. Transplantation 1993;56(4):822–7.

47. Gonyea JE, Anderson CF. Weight change and serum lipoproteins in recipients of renal allografts. Mayo Clin Proc 1992;67(7):653–7.

48. Palmer M, Schaffner F, Thung SN. Excessive weight gain after liver transplantation. Transplantation 1991;51(4):797–800.

49. Stegall MD, Everson G, Schroter G, et al. Metabolic complications after liver transplantation. Diabetes, hypercholesterolemia, hypertension, and obesity. Transplantation 1995;60(9):1057–60.

50. Everhart JE, Lombardero M, Lake JR, et al. Weight change and obesity after liver transplantation: incidence and risk factors. Liver Transpl Surg 1998; 4(4):285–96.

51. Baker AM, Levine TB, Goldberg AD, et al. Natural history and predictors of obesity after orthotopic heart transplantation. J Heart Lung Transplant 1992;11(6):1156–9.

52. Singer LG, Brazelton TR, Doyle RL, et al. Weight gain after lung transplantation. J Heart Lung Transplant 2003;22(8):894–902.

53. Matsuoka H, Arai T, Mori M, et al. A p38 MAPK inhibitor, FR-167653, ameliorates murine bleomycin-induced pulmonary fibrosis. Am J Physiol Lung Cell Mol Physiol 2002;283(1):L103–12.

54. Lucey EC, Ngo HQ, Agarwal A, et al. Differential expression of elastin and alpha 1(I) collagen mRNA in mice with bleomycin-induced pulmonary fibrosis. Lab Invest 1996;74(1):12–20.

55. Chhajed PN, Glanville AR. Management of hypoxemia during flexible bronchoscopy. Clin Chest Med 2003;24(3):511–6.

56. Chhajed PN, Aboyoun C, Malouf MA, et al. Prophylactic nasopharyngeal tube insertion prevents acute hypoxaemia due to upper-airway obstruction during flexible bronchoscopy. Intern Med J 2003; 33(7):317–8.

57. Hopkins PM, Aboyoun CL, Chhajed PN, et al. Prospective analysis of 1235 transbronchial lung biopsies in lung transplant recipients. J Heart Lung Transplant 2002;21:1062–7.

58. Horner RL, Mohiaddin RH, Lowell DG, et al. Sites and sizes of fat deposits around the pharynx in obese patients with obstructive sleep apnoea and weight matched controls. Eur Respir J 1989; 2(7):613–22. Available at: http://www.ncbi.nlm.nih.gov/pubmed?term=HopkinsPM%5BAuthor%5D&cauthor=true&cauthor_uid=12823679.

59. Thompson ML, Flynn JD, Clifford TM. Pharmacotherapy of lung transplantation: an overview. J Pharm Pract 2013;26(1):5–13. http://dx.doi.org/10.1177/0897190012466048.

60. Hopkins PM, McNeil K. Evidence for immunosuppression in lung transplantation. Curr Opin Organ Transplant 2008;13(5):477–83. http://dx.doi.org/10.1097/MOT.0b013e32831040bf.

Sleep and Breathing in Congestive Heart Failure

David Rosen, MD[a],*, Francoise Joelle Roux, MD, PhD[b], Neomi Shah, MD, MPH[a]

KEYWORDS

- Heart failure • Sleep apnea • Obstructive sleep apnea • Central sleep apnea
- Cheyne-Stokes respiration • Sleep-disordered breathing • CPAP • BPAP

KEY POINTS

- Sleep apnea is a common and underdiagnosed comorbidity of heart failure.
- Untreated sleep apnea is an independent risk factor for increased mortality in heart failure.
- Heart failure and sleep apnea are interrelated in that one disease can cause the other and vice versa.
- Noninvasive positive pressure ventilation is the mainstay of therapy for sleep apnea in heart failure.

INTRODUCTION

Heart failure (HF) is one of the most prevalent and costly diseases in the United States.[1] Sleep apnea (SA) is now recognized as a common, yet under-diagnosed, comorbidity of HF.[2] Much investigation on the relationship between these two disorders has occurred already to help elucidate why they frequently occur together, what effect their coexistence has on patients' morbidity and mortality, and how to best manage them when they coincide. This article discusses the unique qualities that SA has when it occurs in HF and explains the underlying pathophysiology that illuminates why SA and HF frequently occur together. The authors provide an overview of the treatment options for SA in HF and discuss the relative efficacies of these treatments. Of note, because of a paucity of data on SA in HF with preserved ejection fraction (HFpEF), the authors' discussion of HF only refers to HF with reduced EF unless otherwise specified. In addition, the term SA is used as a broad term referring to any

of its subtypes, be it central SA (CSA), obstructive SA (OSA), or the occurrence of both together.

SLEEP CHARACTERISTICS IN HF WITHOUT SA

Irrespective of the presence of a primary sleep disorder, nocturnal symptoms of HF alone can interfere with sleep quality. Cough is a well-established cause of sleep dysfunction[3] and can be a manifestation of HF-related pulmonary edema. In addition, angiotensin-converting enzyme (ACE) inhibitors are a class I recommended medication for the treatment of HF[4]; 10% to 20% of patients treated with this medication will develop an ACE inhibitor–induced cough.[5] Orthopnea and nocturia are common symptoms of HF, and they also cause sleep dysfunction. The effect of these symptoms on sleep quality was objectively measured by Java-heri[6] in a single-center prospective study of patients with HF in whom polysomnography was obtained without screening for symptoms of SA. In the subset of patients with no SA (n = 32, mean

[a] Pulmonary Medicine, Montefiore Medical Center, 111 E 210 Street, Bronx, NY 10467, USA; [b] Connecticut Multispecialty Group, Division of Pulmonary, Critical Care and Sleep Medicine, 85 Seymour Street, Suite 923, Hartford, CT 06106, USA
* Corresponding author. 44 Godwin Avenue, Suite 201, Midland Park, NJ 07432.
E-mail address: davidrosenmd@gmail.com

Clin Chest Med 35 (2014) 521–534
http://dx.doi.org/10.1016/j.ccm.2014.06.008
0272-5231/14/$ – see front matter © 2014 Elsevier Inc. All rights reserved.

apnea-hypopnea index [AHI] = 2/h), the percentage of light sleep (N1) was elevated at 34% of the total sleep time. There was complete absence of deep sleep (N3, or slow wave sleep); the arousal index was elevated at 15/h. These patients also corroborated that the sleep measured on the night of their polysomnogram (PSG) was typical of a night's sleep at home. In 2003, Arzt and colleagues[7] compared polysomnography data in a HF cohort with a non-HF community sample cohort. In the subgroup of patients with HF with an AHI less than 5, they had statistically significantly increased sleep-onset latency and wake after sleep onset as compared with the control group. They also had significantly reduced rapid-eye-movement sleep and sleep efficiency, with an average of 1.2 hours less sleep per night.

DIAGNOSIS OF SA

To diagnose SA, patients must undergo a PSG. It typically includes measurements of various activities during sleep, including heart rate, pulse oximetry, abdominal movement, chest wall movement, airflow through the nose and mouth, electroencephalographic activity, and leg movements. These measurements allow for the detection of hypoxemia during sleep and apneas and hypopneas, among other things. An apnea or hypopnea is defined as the complete or partial cessation of airflow for 10 seconds or more, respectively. Apneas and hypopneas are further characterized into central and obstructive subtypes. An obstructive apnea (OA) or hypopnea occurs when there is pharyngeal obstruction to airflow caused by collapse of the pharyngeal muscles at some point along the upper airway. The PSG will indicate persistent or increasing thoracoabdominal effort despite the lack of airflow. In contrast, a central apnea or hypopnea occurs when there is an absence or decrease of respiratory effort along with the cessation of airflow.[8] The total number of apneas and hypopneas that occur during a PSG are added together and divided by the total amount of time patients slept during the PSG to give the AHI. The AHI indicates the average number of respiratory events that occur per hour. SA is diagnosed when there is an abnormally high AHI. An AHI less than 5 is normal, between 5 and 14 indicates mild SA, between 15 and 29 is moderate SA, and 30 or more is severe SA. When most of the respiratory events are caused by obstruction of airflow, the SA is called OSA. When most of the respiratory evens are caused by a lack of breath initiation, the SA is called CSA.[8] AHI and hypoxemia are not only helpful in diagnosing and categorizing SA but their resolution with therapy can help also objectively determine treatment response.

SA IN THE SETTING OF HF
Epidemiology and Mortality of CSA in HF

In the general population, CSA is rare in that its prevalence in the general population is less than 1%,[9] which is starkly different than the prevalence of OSA. However, in the HF population, CSA prevalence can range from 21%[10] to 37%.[11] There is uncertainty as to whether CSA incurs a mortality risk in HF. There are several studies that argue for[12,13] and against[14,15] this assertion, though they are limited in that they are single centered with small sample sizes and there is no uniformity between them in how they diagnose CSA, define CSA, and in their inclusion/exclusion criteria (for example, whether patients with CSA on noninvasive positive pressure ventilation [NIPPV] are allowed in the study).[16] Nevertheless, most studies indicate an independent association of CSA with increased mortality in HF.

CSA and Cheyne-Stokes Respiration in HF

CSA is actually a broad term that encompasses several different disorders. The condition that causes CSA in patients with HF is called Cheyne-Stokes respiration (CSR).[17] It is a periodic breathing pattern whereby hyperpneic breaths gradually decrease into hypopneas and/or apneas in a crescendo-decrescendo fashion. This cycle of breathing periods lasts anywhere from 30 seconds to 2 minutes.

CSR occurs in HF via several derangements to homeostatic processes. Pulmonary congestion will stimulate vagal nerve fibers in the alveolar wall called J receptors, which cause a hyperventilatory response.[18] In addition, for reasons unknown, the apneic threshold remains close to the resting P_{CO_2} in HF. Therefore, any slight decrease in P_{CO_2} can bring it to less than the apneic threshold and cause an apnea. Once the apnea occurs, it continues until peripheral and central chemoreceptors can sense the P_{CO_2} has returned to an appropriate level. As a result of reduced cardiac output, the circulation time is increased. Therefore, the peripheral and central P_{CO_2} chemoreceptors incur a lag in sensing changes in P_{CO_2}.[19] This lag partially explains why peripheral and central chemoreceptors will overshoot in their hyperventilatory response to a high P_{CO_2} or undershoot their hypoventilatory response to a low P_{CO_2}[20] and, thus, perpetuate the cycle. Aside from J receptor stimulation, other events that may initiate the CSR cycle include hyperventilatory responses from hypoxemia[21] or upper airway obstruction[22] or impaired diffusing capacity (**Fig. 1**).[23]

Epidemiology of OSA in HF

OSA is exceedingly prevalent in the United States. It is estimated that among the Western population, 24% of men and 9% of women have SA.[24] Among patients with HF, the prevalence of OSA was reported to be 11% in a study by Javaheri and colleagues,[25] which consisted of 81 cardiology clinic patients who had an left ventricular EF (LVEF) less than 45%. In this study, the mean AHI in the OSA group was in the severe range (36 ± 10 per hour). Patients with OSA tended to be heavier and had a higher prevalence of snoring compared with those without OSA. A subsequent study by Sin and colleagues[26] consisted of a larger group of consecutive patients with congestive heart failure (CHF) (n = 450; n = 382 [85%] men) with a mean LVEF of 27.3 ± 15.6%. Using an AHI cutoff of 10 per hour of sleep, the prevalence of OSA in this group was 37% (n = 168). Similar to Javaheri's study mentioned above[25], the mean AHI for the OSA group was in the severe range.

Like most patients with OSA, those with OSA and HF are heavier, snore frequently, and also are more likely to be men than women. Unlike most patients with OSA, excessive daytime sleepiness is not commonly reported in patients with OSA with HF. This finding suggests that OSA in HF may be less likely to present with sleepiness compared with OSA without HF.[25] This point was further investigated by Arzt and colleagues[27] when they compared patients with HF with those from a community sample, for any given severity of OSA. They found that patients with OSA and HF have less total sleep time compared with patients with OSA without HF. Despite having shorter sleep duration, patients with OSA with HF had lower mean Epworth Sleepiness Scores for all categories of SA severity compared with patients with OSA without HF. They concluded that the lack of subjective sleepiness cannot be used as a consistent symptom for ruling out OSA in patients with HF.

Besides clinic-based studies, there is evidence from population-based cohorts that also confirms an independent association between OSA and HF. As suggested by cross-sectional data from the Sleep Heart Health Study,[28] OSA (defined as an AHI ≥11/h) was associated with a 2.38 relative increase in the likelihood of having HF after adjusting for confounding variables. Recently published *prospective* data from the sleep heart health study reported on the relationship between OSA and incident HF. A total of 1927 men and 2495 women aged 40 years and older and free of HF at baseline were followed for a mean duration of 8.7 years. In this study, men with severe OSA were 58% more likely to have incident HF than those with an AHI less than 5.[29]

Mortality in Patients with Coexisting OSA and HF

Limited studies exist that have assessed the impact of OSA on mortality. Wang and colleagues[30] conducted a prospective study of patients with HF (n = 164, LVEF ≤45%). Each study participant underwent sleep testing, and the investigators assessed mortality in patients with untreated (AHI ≥15/h) and patients with mild

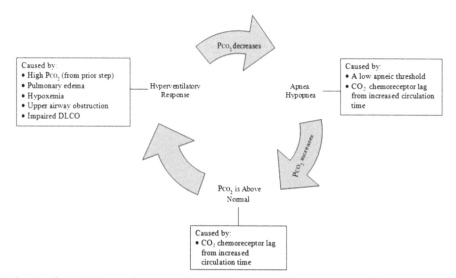

Fig. 1. Mechanism for initiation and perpetuation of CSR. DLCO, diffusing capacity of carbon monoxide.

or no OSA (AHI <15/h). Patients were followed forward in time (max 7.3 years, mean 2.9 years ±2.2). The death rate in patients with untreated OSA was significantly higher compared with the group with mild to no OSA (8.7 vs 4.2 deaths per 100 patient-years, P = .029). No deaths were noted in the small group of patients (n = 14) with OSA who were on treatment (**Fig. 2**).

THE HF AND SA POSITIVE FEEDBACK LOOP

It is likely that HF and SA can actually become enmeshed in a positive feedback loop whereby the presence of one of these diseases promotes the second disease, which in turn promotes the first disease. The authors review the evidence supporting both directions of this assertion.

How HF Can Cause and Worsen SA

The prevailing hypothesized pathophysiologic mechanism supporting the theory that HF causes SA is based on the changes that occur when an individual with HF transitions from an upright position during the day to a recumbent position at night. This transition causes a shift of interstitial fluid from the lower extremities to other areas of the body, including the neck and lungs. The upsurge of interstitial fluid in the neck causes narrowing of the pharynx, thereby increasing the risk of developing obstructive apneic events. The buildup of fluid in the pulmonary interstitium leads to pulmonary congestion and causes patients to experience dyspnea. This dyspnea produces a hyperventilation response, which then sets off central apneic events. More specifically, it leads to the periodic breathing pattern of CSR (see earlier discussion regarding the pathophysiology of CSR).[31]

Multiple studies have shown that the application of lower body positive pressure in awake healthy subjects can increase their neck circumference,[32–34] which supports the hypothesis that changing from an upright to a recumbent position can increase the risk of an OA. Yumino and colleagues[35] demonstrated this phenomenon in male patients with HF by measuring the relationship between changes in leg fluid volume (LFV) and AHI during a nighttime PSG.[35] They studied 57 consecutive male patients with HF with no prior treatment of SA. They found a statistically significant inverse correlation between the change in LFV and the change in neck circumference. In addition, there was a significant inverse correlation between the change in LFV and AHI. They also studied the effects of the application of continuous positive airway pressure (CPAP) during a second PSG for those with predominantly OSA (AHI ≥15 with majority events from obstruction). They found that CPAP significantly reduced the patients' neck circumference change as compared with their prior PSG without CPAP. This finding led to their

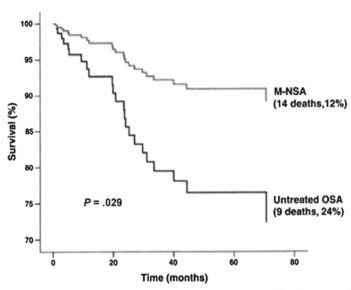

Fig. 2. Multivariable Cox proportional hazards survival plots for patients with mild to no sleep apnea (M-NSA) versus untreated OSA. Multivariable Cox proportional hazards plots showing worse survival of patients with HF with untreated OSA than in those with M-NSA (hazard ratio = 2.81, P = .029) after adjusting for significant confounders (LVEF, New York Heart Association functional class, and age). The adjusted survival curves are shown at the average values of these confounders. (*Data from* He J, Neal B, Gu D, et al. International collaborative study of cardiovascular disease in Asia: design, rationale, and preliminary results. Ethn Dis 2004;14(2):260–8.)

novel proposition for an additional mechanistic benefit of CPAP. In addition to its pneumatic splinting of the upper airway, they posited CPAP improves OSA by preventing buildup of fluid in the neck. They also demonstrated a dose-response relationship between the change in LFV when recumbent and progression from no SA to OSA and from OSA to CSA. They suggested that as the change in LFV increases, the fluid shift causes pulmonary congestion to reach a threshold whereby hyperventilation and resultant CSA occur. This finding also explains the observation that the type of SA in the setting of HF can vary over time between obstructive-predominant and central-predominant. Thus, on a night when someone is particularly volume overloaded, this might promote more CSA because of worsened pulmonary edema. On a night with less volume overload, there might be less pulmonary edema but still some neck soft tissue edema from rostral fluid shifts causing OSA. Ryan and colleagues[36] found evidence to support this hypothesis when they evaluated patients in the control arm of the Continuous Positive Airway Pressure for Central Sleep Apnea and Heart Failure (CANPAP) trial (see section entitled "*CPAP in CSA and HF (CSA/HF)*" for more on this trial) who had both follow-up sleep studies and EF measurements (n = 98). These patients had CSA and were being conservatively managed with HF therapy. Eighteen of these patients converted spontaneously to OSA predominant sleep-disordered breathing on follow-up assessment. The conversion group had a statistically significantly greater improvement in LVEF (2.8% vs −0.07%) and a significantly greater reduction in lung-to-ear circulation time (−7.6 s vs 0.6 s) when compared with the nonconversion group. These findings show a convincing association between the reduction in circulation time and a transition from CSA to OSA (**Box 1**).

How OSA Can Cause and Worsen HF

HF is the result of a complex interplay of multiple compensatory mechanisms in response to chronically reduced cardiac output. These mechanisms include neurohormonal processes, ventricular remodeling, and the Frank-Starling mechanism. Although these processes serve to bolster mean arterial pressure (MAP) and, thus, tissue perfusion in the short run, they eventually lead to a cascade of structural and neurohormonal changes that entangle into a vicious cycle of worsening HF.[37] There has been much investigation as to how OSA can promote the initiation and continuation of many of these harmful compensatory processes.

Hemodynamic effects of OSA

During an OA event, there is thoracoabdominal respiratory effort on a closed pharynx, which creates negative intrathoracic pressure (NITP).[38] This NITP results in deleterious effects on LV afterload, which impairs cardiac contractility by reducing coronary blood flow and increasing oxygen demand[37] and reduces stroke volume and cardiac output.[39]

In those with HF, the NITP created and the afterload increase during an OA event is significantly greater as compared with those without HF. Bradley and colleagues[38] corroborated this when they simulated OAs in 9 men with HF by having them perform the Mueller maneuver. They studied its effects on intrathoracic pressure as measured by an esophageal manometer and on afterload as measured by LV transmural pressure. Compared with a control group, the decrease of intrathoracic pressure and increase in afterload was significantly greater in those with HF. In addition, the amount of time it took for the stroke volume to return to baseline was increased in the HF group. Theoretically, NITP will also increase right ventricular (RV) preload, and the hypoxemic response to an OA will cause hypoxic pulmonary vasoconstriction, thereby increasing RV afterload. This increase in RV afterload can lead to the development of RV distention and leftward septal displacement, thereby impairing LV filling.[40] However, although this is a cogent hypothesis, it is still unclear if OSA alone is a significant cause of pulmonary hypertension and cor pulmonale.[41]

Sympathetic nervous system activation

A decrease in SV and MAP leads to the stimulation of the sympathetic nervous system, which leads to the release of catecholamines and increased cardiac output.[42] This increased sympathetic nervous system activation (SNA) is one of the processes that leads to HF. OAs can contribute to SNA in a variety of ways. Carbon dioxide retention, a byproduct of apnea, causes central nervous system (CNS) acidification, which

---

Box 1
Harmful effects of OSA on the heart

1. Increased LV afterload
2. Increased sympathetic nervous system activation
3. Generation of proinflammatory reactive oxygen species
4. Promotion of arrhythmia

then activates the CNS' central respiratory controller, which then increases sympathetic tone.[43] The decrease in MAP that accompanies an OA stimulates carotid sinus baroreceptors, which respond by increasing SNA.[44] Both chronic and acute intermittent hypoxia stimulates peripheral chemoreceptors that increase SNA.[45] Fletcher and colleagues[46] demonstrated that denervation blocks of peripheral chemoreceptors blocks the hypertensive response associated with SNA.

Chronic intermittent hypoxia (CIH) can also increase the sensitivity of chemoreceptors to a given hypoxic stimulus. Meaning, someone with CIH will have a larger degree of SNA when exposed to an acute hypoxic stimulus as compared to someone who does not experience CIH.[47] This phenomenon of increased chemoreceptor sensitivity has been shown to occur in HF patients as well.[48] The arousal from sleep that occurs at the termination of an apneic event also increases SNA.[49] Spaak and colleagues[50] compared muscle sympathetic nerve activity in patients with HF with SA with patients with HF without SA and demonstrated that the SA cohort had higher sympathetic nerve activity.

Generation of reactive oxygen species

CIH causes episodic tissue hypoxia followed by reoxygenation, which leads to the formation of various reactive oxygen species (ROS) that are known to promote the development of cardiovascular disease[51] and LV dysfunction.[52] Human studies have demonstrated the elevation of ROS in the setting of OSA[53] as well as a reduction of ROS with the initiation of CPAP.[54] When exposed to CIH, animal studies have demonstrated the nicotinamide adenine dinucleotide phosphate (NADPH) oxidase family of enzymes producing ROS in the carotid body.[55] The development of ROS is mediated by particular enzymes and transcription factors that are upregulated in the setting of CIH. These enzymes include NADPH oxidase, xanthine oxidase, and uncoupled nitric oxide synthase. The involved transcription factors include nuclear factor κB (NF-κB) and the hypoxia inducible factor (HIF) family of transcription factors.

NF-κB production has been demonstrated to increase in the setting of CIH, and this transcription factor is known to lead to the production of inflammatory cytokines.[56] In addition, CIH has been shown to increase production of HIF-1 alpha in animal studies.[57]

Aside from promoting inflammation, ROS reduce nitric oxide levels, thus causing vascular endothelial dysfunction by limiting vasodilatory capability. This process promotes the development of hypertension.[58]

Electrophysiologic abnormalities

Frequent and uncontrolled arrhythmias play a role in the development of cardiomyopathy and HF via various mechanisms. They can promote ventricular dyssynchrony, tachycardia-induced cardiomyopathy, and hemodynamic impairment.[59]

There are multiple studies showing an association between arrhythmia and OSA in humans. Using data from the Sleep Heart Health Study,[60] Mehra and colleagues[61] compared the prevalence of nocturnal arrhythmias during nighttime PSG in those with severe OSA with a matched non-OSA cohort. They calculated separate prevalences for atrial fibrillation (AF), nonsustained ventricular tachycardia (NSVT), bigeminy, quadrigeminy, and complex ventricular ectopy. In each of these categories, the severe OSA cohort had a significantly higher prevalence of the arrhythmia. The starkest differences were in the NSVT and AF category, whereby the severe OSA cohort had approximately 4 times the prevalence compared with the non-OSA cohort. Untreated OSA has been shown to increase the risk of AF recurrence after cardioversion, and treatment with CPAP can lower the rate of recurrence.[62] Serizawa and colleagues[63] reported increased discharge of implantable cardioverter-defibrillator in patients with HF with sleep-disordered breathing as compared with those without it. Gupta and colleagues[64] discovered a univariate association between the presence of OSA and prolonged QRS. There was also a dose-response worsening of QRS prolongation in those with more severe OSA. In their multivariate analysis, the association remained significant in women but not in men.

There are several factors that can account for the increased risk of arrhythmia in OSA. As mentioned earlier, OSA can increase sympathetic tone, which has been shown to promote atrial arrhythmia by causing electrophysiologic derangements in the atrium.[65] Myocardial stretch and ventricular remodeling are promoted by OSA, and these factors also contribute to the development of arrhythmia.[66] Myocardial ischemia may also be contributing as this has been shown to promote AF in dogs.[67] Inflammatory cytokines, produced in the setting of OSA by ROS, are also arrhythmogenic.[68]

TREATMENT OF SA IN THE SETTING OF HF

NIPPV, the mainstay of treatment of SA, is discussed in a separate section. See **Table 1** for a summary of treatment options for coexistent SA and HF.

Table 1
Treatment options for coexistent sleep apnea and heart failure

	CSA	OSA
Conservative OSA therapy (weight loss, avoid supine sleep, etc.)	–	+
Optimal Heart Failure Management	+	+
NIPPV		
CPAP	+	+
BPAP	+	+
ASV	+	
Nocturnal Oxygen	+	+/–
Exercise	+/–	+/–
CRT	+	–
Heart Transplant	+	–
Theophylline	+/–	–
Acetazolamide	+	–

"–": Insufficient evidence to support this treatment modality.

"+": Evidence demonstrates a benefit for this treatment modality.

"+/–": A full recommendation for this treatment option is prevented by either conflicting evidence, limited evidence, or limited therapeutic effect.

Conservative Therapies

The usual lifestyle and behavioral recommendations for the treatment of OSA also apply to those with HF. Namely, supine sleep, sedating medications, and sedating substances like alcohol should be avoided. In those that are obese, weight loss is encouraged.[69] Optimal HF management will also help in treating SA. This management of course includes the usage of a beta-blocker, ACE inhibitor, behavioral interventions to promote euvolemia, and use of diuretics.

Diuresis

As mentioned earlier, there has been significant study of how fluid shifts from the legs to the neck and lungs on nighttime transition to a recumbent position can influence the occurrence of both obstructive and central sleep apneic events. The hypothetical intervention to combat this process is, of course, optimal management of volume status. Bucca and colleagues[70] sought to corroborate this theory when they performed a study of the effects of diuresis on 15 consecutive patients with severe OSA, HFpEF, obesity, and pulmonary edema. The patients were given furosemide and spironolactone for 3 days and had their AHI and oropharyngeal junction (OPJ) area

(among other things) assessed before and after the intervention. The AHI was reduced from an average of 74.9 to 57.17/h, and the OPJ increase and weight reduction was also significant. In patients with CSA, the mainstay of therapy is also diuresis, as these apneic events are thought to be predicated on the presence of significant pulmonary edema.[71]

Exercise

Exercise training, a class I recommended therapy for patients with HF,[4] may or may not improve sleep apnea. Ueno and colleagues[72] evaluated the effects of a 4-month exercise program (1 hour of exercise 3 times a week) on the severity of sleep apnea in 8 patients with OSA and 9 with CSA. The exercise program significantly improved the AHI in the OSA cohort but not in the CSA cohort. Yamamoto and colleagues[73] had the opposite findings in their nonrandomized trial of a 6-month exercise program in 10 patients with HF and OSA. They compared their findings with a control group of 8 patients with HF and OSA who refused to partake in the exercise program. At the completion of the program, central apneic events were significantly reduced, but obstructive events were unchanged.

Cardiac Resynchronization Therapy

There has also been study into whether the more invasive HF therapies help SA. Lamba and colleagues[74] performed a meta-analysis of the benefits of cardiac resynchronization therapy (CRT) on SA. The analysis included effects on CSA, OSA, and overall SA. The CSA group had a significant reduction of AHI by 13.05. The OSA subgroup had no significant change, despite the documented improvement in LVEF. The overall SA group had a mean AHI reduction of 9.63. The improvement of CSA with CRT further supports the hypothesis that CSA depends on the presence of pulmonary edema. With the improvement of LVEF seen in CRT, pulmonary edema is prevented and the CSR process of hyperventilation and hypocapnia is avoided.

Heart Transplant

Heart transplant will attenuate, but not fully resolve, CSA. Mansfield and colleagues[75] demonstrated a decrease in AHI from 28 to 7/h in 13 patients with CSA receiving a heart transplant. Thus, despite the normalization of LVEF in these patients, the CSR process will persist. This finding opposes the hypothesis that CSA depends wholly on the presence of pulmonary edema.

Medications

Theophylline has been shown to improve CSA in patients with HF. It is thought that the underlying mechanisms for its benefit are based on its action as a CNS respiratory stimulant.[76] Javaheri and colleagues[77] performed a randomized, double-blinded crossover study of the effects of theophylline on 15 patients with HF and CSA. They were given placebo for 5 days, and after a 1-week washout they were given theophylline for 5 days. Surprisingly, the patients were given inpatient cardiac monitoring during each phase of the study. They had a PSG on day 5 of each phase. During the theophylline phase, the AHI was significantly reduced from 47/h to 18/h. This AHI reduction was caused by a reduction in central apneic events and hypopneas, as there was no change in obstructive apneic events. There were no significant differences in ventricular arrhythmias; but one patient had a supraventricular arrhythmia, and they comment that this "may or may not have been due to the drug."[77] Other studies have replicated this finding,[78] but they lack in that their treatment period and sample size are brief. Without stronger supportive data, the medication has not been regularly used out of the concern for the risk of arrhythmia.

Acetazolamide is a drug that is known to improve idiopathic CSA[79] and central apnea at high altitude.[80] There is one small study that shows it also benefits CSA in HF. Javaheri[81] performed a double-blind placebo-controlled crossover study on 12 male patients with HF and CSA. They were given acetazolamide or placebo 1 hour before bedtime for 6 nights. The acetazolamide group had a mean reduction in AHI from 55 to 34/h and also indicated improved subjective sleep quality on a questionnaire. The trial was limited in that it did not evaluate long-term efficacy of the medication on other HF parameters (LVEF, and so forth). In patients who require a diuretic for euvolemia, these data suggest an additional advantage for using this particular diuretic.

Oxygen

For treatment of OSA, nocturnal oxygen is an option for those who cannot tolerate any NIPPV. It has a theoretic benefit of preventing desaturation related to OAs, but it has not been studied specifically in the HF population. In the general population, nocturnal oxygen does improve AHI and resolve nocturnal hypoxemia, but it does so less efficaciously than NIPPV.[82] In addition, unlike NIPPV, it does not attenuate the hypertensive response to an apneic event,[83] thus supporting the concept that factors other than hypoxemia play a role in the deleterious effects of the apneic events. Moreover, patients with OSA treated with oxygen actually have a longer apnea-hypopnea duration.[82]

For treatment of CSA, nocturnal oxygen has shown more positive results. Hanly and colleagues[84] studied 9 patients with CSA and severe HF and found that 1 night of carbon dioxide supplementation reduced AHI from 30.0 to 18.9/h. Javaheri and colleagues[85] had a similar overall reduction of AHI in 36 patients (49/h to 29/h), but there was no significant change in the number of ventricular arrhythmias. Andreas and colleagues[86] demonstrated that 1 week of nocturnal oxygen in patients with severe HF with evidence of CSR events on a PSG led to an improvement in exercise tolerance and cognitive function but no change in daytime symptoms. Sasayama and colleagues[87] performed the longest trial of nighttime oxygen therapy in patients with HF with CSA. This trial was a multicenter, unblinded randomized controlled trial (RCT) of oxygen versus usual breathing in 51 patients. At the end of the treatment period, the treatment group had a significant improvement in quality of life and New York Heart Association functional class. There was no significant change in EF or cardiac event rates. Blackshear and colleagues[88] raise the concern that the lack of blinding with prior trials makes the findings of any benefit of oxygen to be suspect. They briefly discussed in a correspondence their preliminary findings in a 3-month-long crossover double-blind placebo-controlled trial of oxygen supplementation in 22 patients with HF, two-thirds of which with CSR and one-third without. Although the CSR subgroup had a significant improvement in oxygenation and AHI, none of the other HF parameters showed any improvement. However, they do concede that their small sample size may be underpowered to find a benefit.

Other Therapies for OSA

Mild OSA can be treated with a mandibular advancement device, and there has been some investigation as to its efficacy in the HF population; but this trial could not clearly delineate whether the SA was predominantly OSA or CSA.[89] A recently developed therapy for OSA that involves placing a one-way valve in the nostrils to generate positive pressure in the pharynx generated some interest, as it seems to be a much simpler and cheaper way to apply positive pressure to the upper airway.[90] However, a newly published RCT did not show it to be any better than placebo for the treatment of moderate to severe OSA.[91]

CPAP FOR THE TREATMENT OF SA IN HF

CPAP has been shown to have a beneficial impact on surrogate markers of CHF severity. For example, it reduces neck circumference while recumbent,[35] reduces the generation of ROS,[54] reduces the rate of recurrence of AF,[62] and reduces the cardiac sympathetic tone.[92]

CPAP in OSA and HF (OSA/HF)

Whether to treat OSA in patients with HF who do not have excessive daytime sleepiness is a challenging question. As mentioned earlier, there have been a multitude of small nonrandomized studies demonstrating CPAP's benefit in combating pathophysiologic processes that can cause HF. This finding would suggest that CPAP should be given to nonsleepy patients with OSA/HF. However, RCTs demonstrating a benefit in this population are small with limited follow-up. In fact, RCTs addressing this question in nonsleepy patients with OSA *without HF* are also lacking. Barbé and colleagues[93] were the first to address this particular question with a large multicenter RCT of more than 700 patients, published in 2012. They evaluated CPAP versus no intervention in patients with an AHI greater than 20 and epworth sleepiness scale less than 10. They found no statistically significant difference in incidence of hypertension or cardiovascular disease (CVD) events. However, their follow-up of 4.1 years is a relatively short period of time for the cardiovascular effects of OSA to lead to a cardiovascular event. In addition, the analysis was intention to treat; 36% of the patients used CPAP for less than 4 hours. Thus, this large nonadherent group may have diluted the dose-dependent effects of CPAP. In support of this finding, the frequency of incident hypertension and CVD events trended toward significance (*P* value .2), and the frequency of this end point in the adherent subgroup was statistically significant (*P* value .04). Therefore, this trial may also lend support to the notion of treating nonsleepy patients with OSA/HF. The question is very important, as patients with OSA/HF are more often nonsleepy as compared with patients with general OSA[7]; it is these patients in particular who have higher sympathetic nervous system activity as compared with the sleepy patients with HF/OSA.[94]

There have been multiple studies of CPAP's effects on various end points in HF and OSA (for example, quality of life, mortality, LVEF), and the results have been mixed. These results may be partially caused by the wide variability in trial designs, length of follow-up, particular choice of NIPPV (for example, auto-titrating CPAP or fixed-

pressure CPAP), and inclusion/exclusion criteria for study participation.[40] However, overall, the data do seem to suggest a benefit to giving CPAP to these patients. Small randomized trials with a brief follow-up have shown patients with HF/OSA treated with CPAP will have improvements in blood pressure, AHI, and LVEF.[95,96] No trials as of yet have shown a statistically significant survival benefit for the use of CPAP in OSA/HF, though some have trended toward a benefit.[30] Kasai and colleagues[97] demonstrated that CPAP will lengthen the time to hospitalization for HF in 65 patients with HF/OSA compared with 23 patients who declined treatment. There was also a dose-response relationship for this end point in that the more compliant group had an even longer time to hospitalization.

CPAP in CSA and HF (CSA/HF)

Sin and colleagues[98] conducted an RCT on 66 patients with HF, 29 of whom had CSA. In the CSA subgroup, there was a significant improvement in LVEF on 3-month follow-up; there was a significantly reduced event rate of either mortality or cardiac transplantation. The CANPAP trial[99] was a multicenter, investigator-blinded RCT of 258 patients with HF with severe CSA. The treatment group had a significant improvement in LVEF, AHI, serum norepinephrine levels, and 6-minute walk test results after 3 months. However, in the clinical end points of quality of life and hospitalizations, there was no difference. In addition, there was no significant difference in transplant-free survival. In a post hoc analysis of the subgroup that had normalization of AHI with CPAP (defined as AHI <15), they found a statistically significant transplant-free survival. This finding suggests that in those patients who have a favorable improvement of AHI with CPAP, it is an effective treatment with a mortality benefit. Overall, CPAP in the HF/CSA population seems to have modest, but not impressive, benefits.

OTHER NIPPV OPTIONS FOR THE TREATMENT OF CSA IN HF
Bilevel Positive Airway Pressure in CSA and HF (CSA/HF)

In those patients with CSA/HF who did not normalize their AHI with CPAP, the next logical step in therapy was bilevel positive airway pressure (BPAP). Dohi and colleagues[100] treated 20 consecutive patients with CSA/HF with CPAP. Of those 20, 9 were CPAP nonresponders and so were treated with BPAP. The CPAP nonresponders had their AHI brought from a baseline mean of 54.4/h to 30.3/h with CPAP titration and finally to 8.4/h with BPAP titration. The CPAP responders had a mean AHI of 7.4/h after titration. In a 6-month follow-up, both groups had significantly improved LVEF and B-type natriuretic peptide (BNP). Other small studies showed similar results.[101,102]

Adaptive Servo-Ventilation in CSA and HF (CSA/HF)

Another modality called adaptive servo-ventilation (ASV) has largely supplanted BPAP in the treatment of CSA/HF, as it is more efficacious in abolishing central apneic events. It is able to vary its given pressure support based on patients' effort to ventilate in the prior breath. If the machine senses hyperventilation, it will provide little to no pressure support; in periods of hypoventilation, it will provide high amounts of pressure support. This manner serves to keep patients' respiratory rate steady and for their airflow to be maintained at a steady amplitude and peak.[103] There have been small RCTs showing superior LVEF and AHI improvement for ASV as compared with CPAP.[104,105] A more recent RCT by Randerath and colleagues[106] compared ASV with CPAP in HF and complex OSA, which is a combination of CSA and OSA. In this study, there was a better reduction of AHI in the ASV arm and a significant reduction of BNP in the ASV arm only; neither arm had a significant LVEF change. There has been 1 small RCT comparing BPAP with ASV in CSA/HF,[107] and it showed no significant change in AHI or EF. Of note, some of the patients with HF had HFpEF, a population that has not been heavily studied for sleep-disordered breathing.

Overall, ASV has shown some promising results in the treatment of SA in HF. However, like BPAP and CPAP, a clear survival benefit has not yet been established in this population. CPAP is the only modality that has data to suggest its compliant usage bestows a mortality benefit. Thus, current clinical practice is to treat patients with CSA/HF with CPAP and to switch to ASV if CPAP is unable to reduce the AHI to less than 15. There are, however, large clinical trials in effect that are evaluating whether ASV treatment confers a mortality benefit.[108]

REFERENCES

1. He J, Neal B, Gu D, et al. International collaborative study of cardiovascular disease in Asia: design, rationale, and preliminary results. Ethn Dis 2004; 14(2):260–8.
2. Khayat R, Small R, Rathman L, et al. Sleep-disordered breathing in heart failure: identifying and treating an important but often unrecognized comorbidity in heart failure patients. J Card Fail 2013;19(6):431–44.
3. Lee KK, Birring SS. Cough and sleep. Lung 2010; 188(1):91–4.
4. Yancy CW, Jessup M, Bozkurt B, et al. 2013 ACCF/AHA guideline for the management of heart failure: a report of the American College of Cardiology Foundation/American Heart Association Task Force on Practice Guidelines. J Am Coll Cardiol 2013; 62(16):e147–239.
5. Dicpinigaitis PV. Angiotensin-converting enzyme inhibitor–induced cough: ACCP evidence-based clinical practice guidelines. Chest 2006;129(Suppl 1):169S–73S.
6. Javaheri S. Sleep dysfunction in heart failure. Curr Treat Options Neurol 2008;10(5):323–35.
7. Arzt M, Young T, Finn L, et al. Sleepiness and sleep in patients with both systolic heart failure and obstructive sleep apnea. Arch Intern Med 2006; 166(16):1716–22.
8. Quan SF, Gillin JC, Littner MR, et al. Sleep-related breathing disorders in adults: recommendations for syndrome definition and measurement techniques in clinical research. Sleep 1999;22(5):667–89.
9. Bixler EO, Vgontzas AN, Ten Have T, et al. Effects of age on sleep apnea in men: I. Prevalence and severity. Am J Respir Crit Care Med 1998;157(1): 144–8.
10. Yumino D, Wang H, Floras JS, et al. Prevalence and physiological predictors of sleep apnea in patients with heart failure and systolic dysfunction. J Card Fail 2009;15(4):279–85.
11. Javaheri S. Sleep disorders in systolic heart failure: a prospective study of 100 male patients. The final report. Int J Cardiol 2006;106(1):21–8.
12. Corra U, Pistono M, Mezzani A, et al. Sleep and exertional periodic breathing in chronic heart failure: prognostic importance and interdependence. Circulation 2006;113(1):44–50.
13. Javaheri S, Shukla R, Zeigler H, et al. Central sleep apnea, right ventricular dysfunction, and low diastolic blood pressure are predictors of mortality in systolic heart failure. J Am Coll Cardiol 2007; 49(2):2028–34.
14. Andreas S, Hagenah G, Moller C, et al. Cheyne-Stokes respiration and prognosis in congestive heart failure. Am J Cardiol 1996;78(11):1260–4.
15. Roebuck T, Solin P, Kaye DM, et al. Increased long-term mortality in heart failure due to sleep apnoea is not yet proven. Eur Respir J 2004;23(5):735–40.
16. Yumino D, Bradley TD. Central sleep apnea and Cheyne-Stokes respiration. Proc Am Thorac Soc 2008;5(2):226–36.
17. Javaheri S. Sleep-related breathing disorders in heart failure. In: Mann DL, editor. Heart failure: a companion to Braunwald's heart disease. Philadelphia: WB Saunders; 2004. p. 471–87.

18. Xie A, Skatrud JB, Puleo DS, et al. Apnea-hypopnea threshold for CO2 in patients with congestive heart failure. Am J Respir Crit Care Med 2002; 165(9):1245–50.

19. Jahaveri S. Central sleep apnea. Clin Chest Med 2010;31(2):235–48.

20. Chenuel B, Smith C, Skatrud J, et al. Increased propensity of apnea in response to acute elevations in left atrial pressure during sleep in the dog. J Appl Physiol (1985) 2006;101(1):76–83.

21. Fanfulla F, Mortara A, Maestri R, et al. The development of hyperventilation in patients with chronic heart failure and Cheyne-Stokes respiration: a possible role of chronic hypoxia. Chest 1998; 114(4):1083–90.

22. Sahlin C, Svanborg E, Stenlund H, et al. Cheyne-Stokes respiration and supine dependency. Eur Respir J 2005;25(5):829–33.

23. Szollosi I, Thompson BR, Krum H, et al. Impaired pulmonary diffusing capacity and hypoxia in heart failure correlates with central sleep apnea severity. Chest 2008;134(1):67–72.

24. Young T, Palta M, Dempsey J, et al. The occurrence of sleep-disordered breathing among middle-aged adults. N Engl J Med 1993;328(17): 1230–5.

25. Javaheri S, Parker T, Liming J, et al. Sleep apnea in 81 ambulatory male patients with stable heart failure: types and their prevalences, consequences, and presentations. Circulation 1998;97(21):2154–9.

26. Sin DD, Fitzgerald F, Parker JD, et al. Risk factors for central and obstructive sleep apnea in 450 men and women with congestive heart failure. Am J Respir Crit Care Med 1999;160(4):1101–6.

27. Arzt M, Young T, Finn L, et al. Association of sleep-disordered breathing and the occurrence of stroke. Am J Respir Crit Care Med 2005;172(11):1447–51.

28. Shahar E, Whitney CW, Redline S, et al. Sleep-disordered breathing and cardiovascular disease: cross-sectional results of the sleep heart health study [comment]. Am J Respir Crit Care Med 2001;163(1):19–25.

29. Gottlieb DJ, Yenokyan G, Newman AB, et al. Prospective study of obstructive sleep apnea and incident coronary heart disease and heart failure: the sleep heart health study. Circulation 2010;122(4): 352–60.

30. Wang H, Parker JD, Newton GE, et al. Influence of obstructive sleep apnea on mortality in patients with heart failure. J Am Coll Cardiol 2007;49(15): 1625–31.

31. White LH, Bradley TD. Role of nocturnal rostral fluid shift in the pathogenesis of obstructive and central sleep apnoea. J Physiol 2013;591(Pt 5): 1179–93.

32. Shiota S, Ryan CM, Chiu KL, et al. Alterations in upper airway cross-sectional area in response to lower body positive pressure in healthy subjects. Thorax 2007;62(10):868–72.

33. Su MC, Chiu KL, Ruttanaumpawan P, et al. Lower body positive pressure increases upper airway collapsibility in healthy subjects. Respir Physiol Neurobiol 2008;161(3):306–12.

34. Chiu KL, Ryan CM, Shiota S, et al. Fluid shift by lower body positive pressure increases pharyngeal resistance in healthy subjects. Am J Respir Crit Care Med 2006;174(12):1378–83.

35. Yumino D, Redolfi S, Ruttanaumpawan P, et al. Nocturnal rostral fluid shift: a unifying concept for the pathogenesis of obstructive and central sleep apnea in men with heart failure. Circulation 2010; 121(14):1598–605.

36. Ryan C, Floras J, Logan A, et al. Shift in sleep apnoea type in heart failure patients in the CANPAP trial. Eur Respir J 2010;35(3):592–7.

37. Loscalzo J, Libby P, Epstein J. Basic biology of the cardiovascular system. In: Longo DL, Fauci AS, Kasper DL, et al, editors. Harrison's principles of internal medicine. 18th edition. New York: McGraw-Hill; 2012. p. 1798–810.

38. Bradley TD, Hall MJ, Ando S, et al. Hemodynamic effects of simulated obstructive apneas in humans with and without heart failure. Chest 2001;119(6): 1827–35.

39. Kemp CD, Conte JV. The pathophysiology of heart failure. Cardiovasc Pathol 2012;21(5):365–71.

40. Kasai T, Bradley TD. Obstructive sleep apnea and heart failure: pathophysiologic and therapeutic implications. J Am Coll Cardiol 2011;57(2):119–27.

41. Javaheri S, Javaheri S, Javaheri A. Sleep apnea, heart failure, and pulmonary hypertension. Curr Heart Fail Rep 2013;10(4):315–20.

42. Chaggar PS, Malkin CJ, Shaw SM, et al. Neuroendocrine effects on the heart and targets for therapeutic manipulation in heart failure. Cardiovasc Ther 2009;27(3):187–93.

43. Guyenet PG, Stornetta RL, Abbott SB, et al. Central CO2 chemoreception and integrated neural mechanisms of cardiovascular and respiratory control. J Appl Physiol 2010;108(4):995–1002.

44. Morgan BJ, Denahan T, Ebert TJ. Neurocirculatory consequences of negative intrathoracic pressure vs. asphyxia during voluntary apnea. J Appl Physiol 1993;74(6):2969–75.

45. Weiss JW, Liu Y, Huang J. Physiological basis for a causal relationship of obstructive sleep apnoea to hypertension. Exp Physiol 2007;92(1):21–6.

46. Fletcher EC, Lesske J, Culman J, et al. Sympathetic denervation blocks blood pressure elevation in episodic hypoxia. Hypertension 1992;20(5):612–9.

47. Greenberg HE, Sica AL, Batson D, et al. Chronic intermittent hypoxia increases sympathetic responsiveness to hypoxia and hypercapnia. J Appl Physiol 1999;86(1):298–305.

48. Bradley TD, Tkacova R, Hall MJ, et al. Augmented sympathetic neural response to simulated obstructive apnoea in human heart failure. Clin Sci (Lond) 2003;104(3):231–8.

49. Schneider H, Schaub CD, Chen CA, et al. Effects of arousal and sleep state on systemic and pulmonary hemodynamics in obstructive apnea. J Appl Physiol 2000;88(3):1084–92.

50. Spaak J, Egri ZJ, Kubo T, et al. Muscle sympathetic nerve activity during wakefulness in heart failure patients with and without sleep apnea. Hypertension 2005;46(6):1327–32.

51. Dumitrascu R, Heitmann J, Seeger W, et al. Obstructive sleep apnea, oxidative stress and cardiovascular disease: lessons from animal studies. Oxid Med Cell Longev 2013;2013:234631.

52. Chen L, Einbinder E, Zhang Q, et al. Oxidative stress and left ventricular function with chronic intermittent hypoxia in rats. Am J Respir Crit Care Med 2005;172(7):915–20.

53. Jordan W, Cohrs S, Degner D, et al. Evaluation of oxidative stress measurements in obstructive sleep apnea syndrome. J Neural Transm 2006;113(2):239–54.

54. Yokoe T, Minoguchi K, Matsuo H, et al. Elevated levels of C-reactive protein and interleukin-6 in patients with obstructive sleep apnea syndrome are decreased by nasal continuous positive airway pressure. Circulation 2003;107(8):1129–34.

55. Peng YJ, Nanduri J, Yuan G, et al. NADPH oxidase is required for the sensory plasticity of the carotid body by chronic intermittent hypoxia. J Neurosci 2009;29(15):4903–10.

56. Garvey JF, Taylor CT, McNicholas WT. Cardiovascular disease in obstructive sleep apnoea syndrome: the role of intermittent hypoxia and inflammation. Eur Respir J 2009;33(5):1195–205.

57. Prabhakar NR, Kumar GK, Nanduri J. Intermittent hypoxia augments acute hypoxic sensing via HIF-mediated ROS. Respir Physiol Neurobiol 2010;174(3):230–4.

58. Carlson JT, Rangemark C, Hedner JA. Attenuated endothelium-dependent vascular relaxation in patients with sleep apnoea. J Hypertens 1996;14(5):577–84.

59. Lee GK, Klarich KW, Grogan M, et al. Premature ventricular contraction-induced cardiomyopathy: a treatable condition. Circ Arrhythm Electrophysiol 2012;5(1):229–36.

60. Quan SF, Howard BV, Iber C, et al. The sleep heart health study: design, rationale, and methods. Sleep 1997;20(12):1077–85.

61. Mehra R, Benjamin EJ, Shahar E, et al. Association of nocturnal arrhythmias with sleep-disordered breathing: the Sleep Heart Health Study. Am J Respir Crit Care Med 2006;173(8):910–6.

62. Kanagala R, Murali NS, Friedman PA, et al. Obstructive sleep apnea and the recurrence of atrial fibrillation. Circulation 2003;107(2):2589–94.

63. Serizawa N, Yumino D, Kajimoto K, et al. Impact of sleep-disordered breathing on life-threatening ventricular arrhythmia in heart failure patients with implantable cardioverter-defibrillator. Am J Cardiol 2008;102(8):1064–8.

64. Gupta S, Cepeda-Valery B, Romero-Corral A, et al. Association between QRS duration and obstructive sleep apnea. J Clin Sleep Med 2012;8(6):649–54.

65. Allesie M, Ausma J, Schotten U. Electrical, contractile and structural remodeling during atrial fibrillation. Cardiovasc Res 2002;54(2):230–46.

66. Franz MR, Cima R, Wang D, et al. Electrophysiological effects of myocardial stretch and mechanical determinants of stretch-activated arrhythmias. Circulation 1992;86(3):968–78.

67. Sinno H, Derakhchan K, Libersan D, et al. Atrial ischemia promotes atrial fibrillation in dogs. Circulation 2003;107(14):1930–6.

68. Aviles RJ, Martin DO, Apperson-Hansen C, et al. Inflammation as a risk factor for atrial fibrillation. Circulation 2003;108(24):3006–10.

69. Epstein LJ, Kristo D, Strollo PJ, et al. Clinical guideline for the evaluation, management, and long-term care of obstructive sleep apnea in adults. J Clin Sleep Med 2009;5(3):263–76.

70. Bucca CB, Brussino L, Battisti A, et al. Diuretics in obstructive sleep apnea with diastolic heart failure. Chest 2007;132(2):440–6.

71. Kasai T. Sleep apnea and heart failure. J Cardiol 2012;60(2):78–85.

72. Ueno LM, Drager LF, Rodrigues AC, et al. Effects of exercise training in patients with chronic heart failure and sleep apnea. Sleep 2009;32(5):637–47.

73. Yamamoto U, Mohri M, Shimada K, et al. Six-month aerobic exercise training ameliorates central sleep apnea in patients with chronic heart failure. J Card Fail 2007;13(10):825–9.

74. Lamba J, Simpson CS, Redfearn DP, et al. Cardiac resynchronization therapy for the treatment of sleep apnoea: a meta-analysis. Europace 2011;13(8):1174–9.

75. Mansfield DR, Solin P, Roebuck T, et al. The effect of successful heart transplant treatment of heart failure on central sleep apnea. Chest 2003;124(5):1675–81.

76. Javaheri S, Evers JA, Teppema LJ. Increase in ventilation caused by aminophylline in the absence of changes in ventral extracellular fluid pH and PCO2. Thorax 1989;44(2):121–5.

77. Javaheri S, Parker TJ, Wexler L, et al. Effect of theophylline on sleep-disordered breathing in heart failure. N Engl J Med 1996;335(8):562–7.

78. Hu K, Li Q, Yang J, et al. The effect of theophylline on sleep-disordered breathing in patients with stable chronic congestive heart failure. Chin Med J 2003;116(11):1711–6.

79. DeBacker WA, Verbraecken J, Willemen M, et al. Central apnea index decreases after prolonged treatment with acetazolamide. Am J Respir Crit Care Med 1995;151(1):87–91.

80. Hackett PH, Roach RC, Harrison GL, et al. Respiratory stimulants and sleep periodic breathing a high altitude: almitrine versus acetazolamide. Am Rev Respir Dis 1987;135(4):896–8.

81. Javaheri S. Acetazolamide improves central sleep apnea in heart failure: a double-blind, prospective study. Am J Respir Crit Care Med 2006;173(2):234–7.

82. Mehta V, Vasu TS, Phillips B, et al. Obstructive sleep apnea and oxygen therapy: a systematic review of the literature and meta-analysis. J Clin Sleep Med 2013;9(3):271–9.

83. Schneider HJ, Schaub CD, Chen CA, et al. Neural and local effects of hypoxia on cardiovascular responses to obstructive apnea. J Appl Physiol 2000;88(3):1093–102.

84. Hanly PJ, Millar TW, Steljes DG, et al. The effect of oxygen on respiration and sleep in patients with congestive heart failure. Ann Intern Med 1989;111(1):777–82.

85. Javaheri S, Ahmed M, Parker TJ, et al. Effects of nasal O2 on sleep-related disordered breathing in ambulatory patients with stable heart failure. Sleep 1999;22(8):1101–6.

86. Andreas S, Clemens C, Sandholzer H, et al. Improvement of exercise capacity with treatment of Cheyne-Stokes respiration in patients with congestive heart failure. J Am Coll Cardiol 1996;27(6):1486–90.

87. Sasayama S, Izumi T, Matsuzaki M, et al. Improvement of quality of life with nocturnal oxygen therapy in heart failure patients with central sleep apnea. Circ J 2009;73(7):1255–62.

88. Blackshear JL, Safford R, Fredrickson P, et al. Scientific letter: a double-blind, randomised, placebo-controlled, 3-month crossover trial of night-time oxygen therapy in advanced systolic heart failure. Heart 2012;98(19):1468–9.

89. Eskafi M. Sleep apnoea in patients with stable congestive heart failure: an intervention study with a mandibular advancement device. Swed Dent J Suppl 2004;168:1–56.

90. Rosenthal L, Massie CA, Dolan DC, et al. A multicenter, prospective study of a novel nasal EPAP device in the treatment of obstructive sleep apnea: efficacy and 30-day adherence. J Clin Sleep Med 2009;5(6):532–7.

91. Rossi VA, Winter B, Rahman NM, et al. The effects of Provent on moderate to severe obstructive sleep apnoea during continuous positive airway pressure

therapy withdrawal: a randomised controlled trial. Thorax 2013;68(9):854–9.

92. Kaye DM, Mansfield D, Aggarwal A, et al. Acute effects of continuous positive airway pressure on cardiac sympathetic tone in congestive heart failure. Circulation 2001;103(19):2336–8.

93. Barbé F, Duran-Cantolla J, Sanchez-de-la-Torre M, et al. Effect of continuous positive airway pressure on the incidence of hypertension and cardiovascular events in nonsleepy patients with obstructive sleep apnea: a randomized controlled trial. JAMA 2012;307(20):2161–8.

94. Montemurro LT, Floras JS, Millar PJ, et al. Inverse relationship of subjective daytime sleepiness to sympathetic activity in patients with heart failure and obstructive sleep apnea. Chest 2012;142(5):1222–8.

95. Kaneko Y, Floras JS, Usui K, et al. Cardiovascular effects of continuous positive airway pressure in patients with heart failure and obstructive sleep apnea. N Engl J Med 2003;348(13):1233–41.

96. Mansfield DR, Gollogly NC, Kaye DM, et al. Controlled trial of continuous positive airway pressure in obstructive sleep apnea and heart failure. Am J Respir Crit Care Med 2004;169(3):361–6.

97. Kasai T, Narui K, Dohi T, et al. Prognosis of patients with heart failure and obstructive sleep apnea treated with continuous positive airway pressure. Chest 2008;133(3):690–6.

98. Sin DD, Logan AG, Fitzgerald FS, et al. Effects of continuous positive airway pressure on cardiovascular outcomes in heart failure patients with and without Cheyne–Stokes respiration. Circulation 2000;102(1):61–6.

99. Bradley TD, Logan AG, Kimoff RJ, et al. Continuous positive airway pressure for central sleep apnea and heart failure. N Engl J Med 2005;353(19):2025–33.

100. Dohi T, Kasai T, Narui K, et al. Bi-level positive airway pressure ventilation for treating heart failure with central sleep apnea that is unresponsive to continuous positive airway pressure. Circ J 2008;72(7):1100–5.

101. Noda A, Izawa H, Asano H, et al. Beneficial effect of bilevel positive airway pressure on left ventricular function in ambulatory patients with idiopathic dilated cardiomyopathy and central sleep apnea-hypopnea: a preliminary study. Chest 2007;131(6):1694–701.

102. Kasai T, Narui K, Dohi T, et al. Efficacy of nasal bi-level positive airway pressure in congestive heart failure patients with Cheyne-Stokes respiration and central sleep apnea. Circ J 2005;69(8):913–21.

103. Kazimierczak A, Krzesiński P, Krzyżanowski K, et al. Sleep-disordered breathing in patients with

heart failure: new trends in therapy. Biomed Res Int 2013;2013:459613.

104. Philippe C, Stoica-Herman M, Drouot X, et al. Compliance with and effectiveness of adaptive servoventilation versus continuous positive airway pressure in the treatment of Cheyne–Stokes respiration in heart failure over a six month period. Heart 2006;92(3):337–42.

105. Kasai T, Usui Y, Yoshioka T, et al. Effect of flow-triggered adaptive servo-ventilation compared with continuous positive airway pressure in patients with chronic heart failure with coexisting obstructive sleep apnea and Cheyne–Stokes respiration. Circ Heart Fail 2010;3(1):140–8.

106. Randerath WJ, Nothofer G, Priegnitz C, et al. Long-term auto-servoventilation or constant positive pressure in heart failure and coexisting central with obstructive sleep apnea. Chest 2012;142(2):440–7.

107. Fietze I, Blau A, Glos M, et al. Bi-level positive pressure ventilation and adaptive servo ventilation in patients with heart failure and Cheyne–Stokes respiration. Sleep Med 2008;9(6):652–9.

108. Cowie MR, Woehrle H, Wegscheider K, et al. Rationale and design of the SERVE-HF study: treatment of sleep-disordered breathing with predominant central sleep apnoea with adaptive servo-ventilation in patients with chronic heart failure. Eur J Heart Fail 2013;15(8):937–43.

Congenital Central Hypoventilation Syndrome
A Neurocristopathy with Disordered Respiratory Control and Autonomic Regulation

 CrossMark

Casey M. Rand, BS[a], Michael S. Carroll, PhD[a,b],
Debra E. Weese-Mayer, MD[a,b],*

KEYWORDS

- *PHOX2B* • Autonomic • Respiratory • CCHS • Hirschsprung • Neuroblastoma

KEY POINTS

- Congenital central hypoventilation syndrome (CCHS) is a rare neurocristopathy with disordered respiratory control and autonomic nervous system regulation.
- CCHS is caused by mutations in the *PHOX2B* gene, and the *PHOX2B* genotype/mutation anticipates the CCHS phenotype, including the severity of hypoventilation, risk of sinus pauses, and risk of associated disorders including Hirschsprung disease and neural crest tumors.
- It is important to maintain a high index of suspicion in cases of unexplained alveolar hypoventilation, delayed recovery of spontaneous breathing after sedation or anesthesia, or in the event of severe respiratory infection, and unexplained seizures or neurocognitive delay. This will improve identification and diagnosis of milder CCHS cases and later onset/presentation cases, allowing for successful intervention.
- Early intervention and conservative management are key to long-term outcome and neurocognitive development.
- Research is underway to better understand the underlying mechanisms and identify targets for treatment advances and drug interventions.

INTRODUCTION

Congenital central hypoventilation syndrome (CCHS) is a rare disorder of respiratory control with autonomic nervous system dysregulation (ANSD), and a result of maldevelopment of neural crest-derived cells (neurocristopathy). The first reported description of CCHS was in 1970 by

This work was supported in part by the Chicago Community Trust Foundation PHOX2B Patent Fund and Respiratory & Autonomic Disorders of Infancy, Childhood, & Adulthood–Foundation for Research & Education (RADICA-FRE).

[a] Center for Autonomic Medicine in Pediatrics (CAMP), Department of Pediatrics, Ann & Robert H. Lurie Children's Hospital of Chicago, 225 East Chicago Avenue, Chicago, IL 60611-2605, USA; [b] Department of Pediatrics, Northwestern University Feinberg School of Medicine, 303 East Chicago Avenue, Chicago, IL 60611, USA

* Corresponding author.

E-mail addresses: DWeese-Mayer@LurieChildrens.org; D-Weese-Mayer@Northwestern.edu

Clin Chest Med 35 (2014) 535–545
http://dx.doi.org/10.1016/j.ccm.2014.06.010
0272-5231/14/$ – see front matter © 2014 Elsevier Inc. All rights reserved.

Robert Mellins and colleagues.[1] Despite a multitude of case reports, large series were not published until 1992.[2] As of early 2014, laboratories from the United States, France, Italy, Japan, Germany, China, The Netherlands, and Australia have now collectively diagnosed approximately 1200 cases with *PHOX2B* mutation-confirmed CCHS. However, the birth prevalence of CCHS is unknown, because demographically diverse, large, population-based studies have not been reported. Because the milder cases of CCHS and later-onset (LO) CCHS may go unrecognized or misdiagnosed, it is difficult to estimate the true frequency of CCHS in the general population at this time.

CCHS is characteristically diagnosed in the newborn period. However, individuals can also be diagnosed in childhood[3-6] or adulthood,[5,7-13] depending on the severity of symptoms and the inquisivity of the patient, family, and medical team. Impaired breathing regulation (respiratory control) is the hallmark of CCHS. Individuals with CCHS typically present with shallow breathing (alveolar hypoventilation) during sleep and, in more severely affected individuals, during wakefulness and sleep. These breathing complications occur despite the lungs and airways being anatomically and physiologically normal. Conditions associated with CCHS reflecting anatomic ANSD include Hirschsprung disease (HSCR) and tumors of neural crest origin, in addition to a spectrum of symptoms compatible with physiologic ANSD. CCHS is a life-long disease.

PHOX2B Gene Mutations

Individuals with CCHS have a mutation in *PHOX2B*, a gene that plays an important role in the development of the ANS. The normal *PHOX2B* gene has 20 repeats of the amino acid alanine. Approximately 90% of individuals with CCHS are heterozygous for a *PHOX2B* polyalanine repeat expansion mutation (PARM), with expansions to 24 to 33 alanine repeats on the affected allele,[14] genotypes of 20/24 to 20/33 (normal genotype is 20/20; **Fig. 1**). The remaining 9% to 10% of

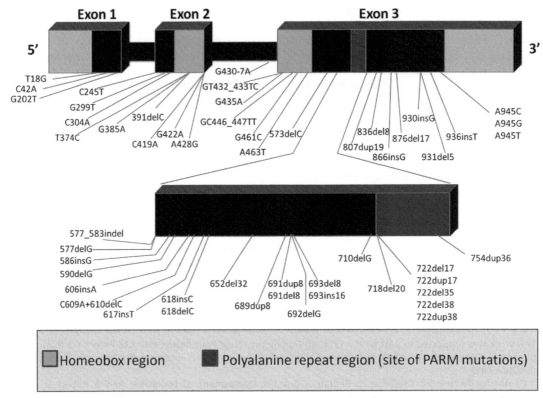

Fig. 1. *PHOX2B* gene with location of all CCHS-associated mutations identified to date. Nearly all polyalanine repeat expansion mutations (PARMs) are located within the second polyalanine expansion region of exon 3 (shown in *red*). Nearly all NPARMs identified thus far have been found at the extreme 3′ end of exon 2 or in exon 3. (*Adapted from* Weese-Mayer DE, Rand CM, Berry-Kravis EM, et al. Congenital central hypoventilation syndrome from past to future: model for translational and transitional autonomic medicine. Pediatr Pulmonol 2009;44:526; with permission.)

individuals with CCHS and LO-CCHS have a different type of alteration in the *PHOX2B* gene, referred to as non-PARM (NPARM). These mutations include missense, nonsense, frameshift, and stop codon mutations, mostly occurring in exon 2 and exon 3 of *PHOX2B*. Fewer than 1% of individuals with CCHS/LO-CCHS or CCHS-like symptoms will have whole gene or exon deletions of *PHOX2B*,[15] and are phenotypically variable. Among PARMS, the 20/25, 20/26, and 20/27 genotypes, and among NPARMs, a 38-bp deletion at the site of the polyalanine repeat, remain the most frequently identified mutations. CCHS-related *PHOX2B* mutations have not been found in thoroughly screened control populations. Although de novo germline mutations cause the majority of CCHS cases, an autosomal-dominant inheritance pattern exists for CCHS. This includes somatic mosaicism, identified in a subset (5%–25%) of parents of CCHS probands,[16–18] as well as inheritance from a fully affected parent (with CCHS).

Mutations in *PHOX2B* result in altered development and regulation of the ANS, primarily by abnormal development in progenitors of early embryonic cells that form the neural crest (hence the term neurocristopathy[19]). Individuals with the NPARMs are typically more severely affected than individuals with the PARMs, and individuals with a greater number of alanine repeats are typically more severely affected than those with fewer (especially among the most common PARMs). The small number of identified cases with whole-gene or exon deletions makes prediction of phenotype difficult in these cases, but thus far disease seems to be less severe in these cases. Typically, dysfunction of *PHOX2B* during development is enough to cause manifestation of disease from the neonatal period; however, the less severe mutations may be "unmasked" by challenges to the respiratory system, such as respiratory infection or exposure to sedation, which can lead to fully manifest disease symptoms.

Genotype–Phenotype Correlations

The symptoms and severity of CCHS vary from one individual to another (**Fig. 2**).[20] This variation is becoming clearer as these patients are studied by *PHOX2B* genotype/mutation, such that repeat length and PARM versus NPARM are related to disease severity. A rapidly expanding understanding of the risks specific to the particular *PHOX2B* mutation is allowing physicians and parents to anticipate risks for continuous ventilation, pauses in the heart rhythm, HSCR, neural crest tumors, and potential factors that influence autonomic regulation in individuals with CCHS.

Ventilatory dependence

In individuals with PARMs, the need for continuous ventilatory dependence has a direct relationship with the length of the alanine expansions.[3,17,21] Specifically, individuals with the 20/25 genotype rarely require 24-hour ventilatory support; individuals with the 20/26 genotype have variable awake needs, depending on the level of activity; and

System		Physiologic Sign/Symptom	Pathologic Condition
	•	decreased/absent pupillary light response	
	•	anisocoria	
	•	esotropia/exotropia	
Ophthalmologic	•	lack of convergent gaze	
Respiratory	•	absent perception of dyspnea	
	•	alveolar hypoventilation	
	•	altered peripheral perfusion	
Cardiovascular	•	decreased heart rate variability	
	•	prolonged sinus pauses	
	•	vasovagal syncope	
	•	esophageal dysmotility	
Gastrointestinal	•	constipation	HSCR
			neural crest tumor
			-sympathetic chain
	•	decreased anxiety	-adrenals
Neuro	•	decreased pain perception	
	•	profuse sweating	
	•	temperature dysregulation	
Sudomotor		(hypothermia)	

Fig. 2. Signs and symptoms of CCHS-related ANS dysregulation. (*From* Weese-Mayer DE, Patwari PP, Rand CM, et al. Congenital central hypoventilation syndrome (CCHS) and *PHOX2B* mutations. Primer on the autonomic nervous system. 3rd edition. Oxford: Elsevier; 2012; with permission.)

individuals with genotypes from 20/27 to 20/33 very often require continuous ventilatory support. LO-CCHS cases with the 20/24 or 20/25 genotype[5,7,8] have the mildest hypoventilation, presenting primarily after exposure to respiratory depressants or severe respiratory infection, and may often be managed with nocturnal ventilatory support only. In contrast with the PARMs, most individuals with NPARMs require continuous ventilatory support (**Fig. 3**).[21]

Hirschsprung disease and tumors of neural crest origin

Some individuals with CCHS have anatomic/structural malformations including HSCR and tumors of neural crest origin. Overall, 16% to 20% of individuals with CCHS have HSCR, with a higher prevalence among individuals with NPARMs than those with PARMs. HSCR is reported in 87% to 100% of NPARMs, in contrast with 13% to 20% of PARMs.[14,16,21] Notably, a high occurrence of HSCR in individuals with the 20/27 genotype has been described[14] and anecdotally in approximately 30% of individuals with the 20/27 to 20/33 genotype. Extracranial solid tumors of neural crest origin have also been reported in CCHS and associated with *PHOX2B* genotype.[14] The tumors include neuroblastomas, ganglioneuromas, and ganglioneuroblastomas. These are found in locations with sympathetic nervous tissue, such as the chest and abdomen in paraspinal ganglia or the adrenal glands. Neural crest tumors in individuals with the NPARMs are typically neuroblastomas, in contrast with the ganglioneuromas and ganglioneuroblastomas in individuals with the longest PARMs (20/30–20/33). However, in 1 case a child with the 20/33 genotype presented with a neuroblastoma.

ANSD

An increased number of symptoms of ANSD has been reported in association with *PHOX2B* genotype in individuals with CCHS.[17] These symptoms can include heart rhythm abnormalities, such as prolonged asystoles (>3 seconds) necessitating a cardiac pacemaker,[22] altered gut motility even in the absence of HSCR (often presenting as severe constipation),[23] altered temperature regulation (as indicated by low body temperatures[24]), decreased pain perception, decreased anxiety, and eye abnormalities that include strabismus, convergence insufficiency, and decreased pupil response to light.[25,26]

LO-CCHS

A growing number of individuals are now being identified who present in later infancy, childhood, or even adulthood and are referred to as LO-CCHS. LO-CCHS seems to reflect the variable penetrance of the *PHOX2B* genotypes 20/24 and 20/25 or rarely an NPARM.[3,5,6,12,27,28] Some of these affected individuals will not be identified until

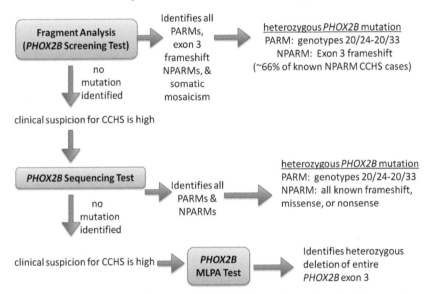

Fig. 3. Algorithm to determine when and what type of *PHOX2B* genetic testing should be performed in various clinical scenarios in which CCHS and LO-CCHS are suspected or confirmed. (*Adapted from* Weese-Mayer DE, Patwari PP, Rand CM, et al. Congenital central hypoventilation syndrome (CCHS) and *PHOX2B* mutations. Primer on the autonomic nervous system. 3rd edition. Oxford: Elsevier; 2012; with permission.)

after receiving sedation, anesthesia, or antiseizure medications.[8] Children with CCHS—both those identified in infancy and those identified later—are now surviving into adulthood, giving new insights into the long-term sequelae of treated and untreated CCHS/ANSD. As more children and adults who were not identified in earlier life are diagnosed with CCHS at an advanced age, and documentation of sinus pauses in individuals with the LO-CCHS 20/25 genotype are reported,[8] a more clear understanding of the importance of aggressive, conservative intervention at the youngest age possible is emerging.

EVALUATION AND PROCEDURE
Diagnosis

The classic presentation of an infant with CCHS includes cyanosis and hypercarbia, resulting from very shallow breathing during sleep (nap and night), but alertness and adequate breathing during wakefulness—and no description of respiratory distress. If on a ventilator, the infant is described as breathing synchronously with the ventilator when asleep but adding extra breaths during wakefulness or in rapid eye movement sleep. These individuals do not properly increase breathing or awaken in response to abnormal oxygen and carbon dioxide levels. This same lack of normal responsivity to low oxygen and elevated

carbon dioxide occurs during wakefulness as well, even when clinical evaluation suggests awake breathing is generally "adequate." LO-CCHS should be considered in the event of centrally mediated alveolar hypoventilation, cyanosis, or seizures after (1) anesthetics or central nervous system depressants, (2) severe pulmonary infection, or (3) obstructive sleep apnea intervention.

Once the diagnosis of CCHS/LO-CCHS is considered, blood should be sent for the clinical *PHOX2B* testing. The American Thoracic Society Statement on CCHS (published in 2010) advises that the *PHOX2B* Screening Test be the first step in making the genetic diagnosis of CCHS (see **Fig. 3**). This test diagnoses all of the PARMs, somatic mosaicism, polyalanine repeat contraction mutations, and the exon frameshift NPARMs. Another name for the *PHOX2B* Screening Test is fragment analysis (see http://www.genetests.org/by-disorder/?disid=217354). If the *PHOX2B* screening test is normal and the subject has the clinical presentation of CCHS, then the sequel *PHOX2B* sequencing test should be performed to identify the subset of patients with small NPARMs. Although the *PHOX2B* sequencing test detects the PARMs and NPARMs, it is typically more costly and it does not detect mosaicism.[29] Because *PHOX2B* mutations can be inherited from a mosaic parent, the sequencing test is rarely useful in parents of children with CCHS (**Fig. 4**).

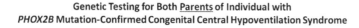

Genetic Testing for Both <u>Parents</u> of Individual with
PHOX2B Mutation-Confirmed Congenital Central Hypoventilation Syndrome

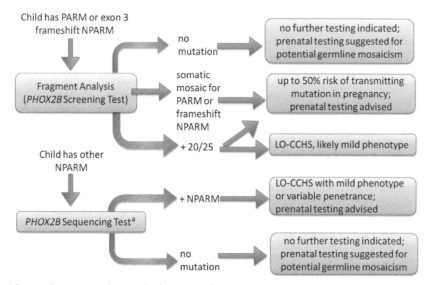

Fig. 4. Algorithm to determine when and what type of *PHOX2B* genetic testing should be performed in parents of CCHS proband. [a] The *PHOX2B* sequencing test does not identify low-level mosaicism.[29] (*Adapted from* Weese-Mayer DE, Patwari PP, Rand CM, et al. Congenital central hypoventilation syndrome (CCHS) and *PHOX2B* mutations. Primer on the autonomic nervous system. 3rd edition. Oxford: Elsevier; 2012; with permission.)

Finally, in cases where both the *PHOX2B* screening and sequel sequencing tests are negative but clinical suspicion remains high, the *PHOX2B* MLPA test for copy number variations should be performed.[15] While awaiting results of the clinically available *PHOX2B* testing, other causes of hypoventilation should be ruled out to expedite proper intervention and facilitate treatment strategies for home care. Primary lung disease, ventilatory muscle weakness, and cardiac disease should be ruled out with the following tests: Chest x-ray and potentially computed tomography of the chest, comprehensive neurologic evaluation and potentially muscle biopsy, and echocardiogram. Causative gross anatomic brain/brainstem lesions should be ruled out with magnetic resonance imaging and/or computed tomography of the brain and brainstem.[30,31] Likewise, inborn errors of metabolism should be considered and a metabolic screen should be performed.

Treatment

Hypoventilation

Alveolar hypoventilation is the hallmark of CCHS, and its most apparent and potentially debilitating phenotypic feature. Characteristically, the diminution of tidal volume with resultant effect on minute ventilation is most apparent in non-rapid eye movement sleep in CCHS, but it is also abnormal during rapid eye movement sleep and wakefulness, although usually to a lesser degree.[2,32,33] The spectrum of sleep-disordered breathing may range in severity from hypoventilation during NREM sleep with adequate ventilation during wakefulness, to complete apnea during sleep and severe hypoventilation during wakefulness. As mentioned, the CCHS phenotype relative to ventilatory needs is in large part *PHOX2B* genotype/mutation dependent. Typically, children with the 20/27 to 20/33 genotype and the NPARMs will require 24-hour mechanical ventilation, especially with exertion and during sleep. Children with the 20/24 and 20/25 genotypes, and a small subset of NPARMs, rarely require 24-hour ventilation, unless they have had suboptimal ventilatory management for prolonged periods in early childhood. The awake ventilatory needs of the children with the 20/26 phenotype varies with activity level. It remains unclear if awake spontaneous breathing improves with puberty, so ventilatory needs should be determined from physiologic testing, not assumptions about developmental stages.

HSCR

For those individuals with constipation symptoms, a barium enema or manometry, and potentially a full-thickness rectal biopsy should be performed to diagnose HSCR.[34] HSCR, a rare gastrointestinal disorder characterized by aganglionosis of the distal hindgut, often presents in individuals with CCHS. Symptoms of HSCR appear soon after birth and may include constipation, abdominal distention, and vomiting. Older infants may have anorexia, failure to thrive, and severe constipation. Short segment HSCR may be diagnosed in older children and adults. Treatment of HSCR usually consists of surgery to remove the nonfunctional segment of aganglionic bowel and relieve obstruction. Typically, a temporary bowel opening of the colon in the abdominal wall (colostomy) is usually performed first. The second operation consists of removing the aganglionic colon and rectum and reconnecting the normal bowel to the anus. In some centers with extensive expertise in HSCR, these procedures can be performed in one operation.

Neuroblastoma

Thus far, tumors of neural crest origin have been identified in children with NPARM (typically neuroblastoma) and in children with 20/30 and 20/33 genotype PARMs (typically ganglioneuroma and ganglioneuroblastoma, though neuroblastoma remains a possibility). The American Thoracic Society Statement on CCHS suggests screening for tumors of neural crest origin in all NPARM cases and in children with the 20/28 to 20/33 *PHOX2B* genotypes. Among infants at greatest risk of a tumor of neural crest origin, chest x-ray/abdominal ultrasonography in infancy and later chest and abdomen magnetic resonance imaging or computed tomography is of value. An iodine meta-iodobenzylguanidine scan, used to find tumors of neural crest-specific origin, might be performed in the patients at greatest risk for neuroblastoma. Neuroblastomas are removed surgically, followed by chemotherapy in some cases. Treatment for other tumors originating from the neural crest depends on the type and location of the tumor.

Neurocognitive function

Suboptimal school performance and/or decreased intellectual function have been observed in CCHS patients.[2,35–37] It is unclear whether this is owing to hypoxemia from inadequate ventilatory support or a direct result of the primary neurologic problem associated with CCHS. As children with CCHS are more consistently identified in the newborn period, and as management for these complex and vulnerable children becomes more standardized, improved neurocognitive performance is anticipated with an increased understanding of the distinction between sequelae of hypoxemia (owing to hypoventilation or asystoles) and innate disease specific to CCHS. There is also new evidence that CCHS patients may have altered cerebral autoregulation, a condition that may contribute to neurocognitive decline related to recurrent hypoxemia/hypercarbia.[38] Comprehensive neurocognitive testing performed annually in a controlled setting assesses the child's progress relative to intervention, management, and compliance and may identify new areas for intervention. Aggressive educational intervention coupled with careful ventilatory and cardiovascular management is essential.[2,35,36,39,40]

Cardiac function

Cardiac rhythm abnormalities include decreased beat-to-beat heart rate variability, reduced respiratory sinus arrhythmia, and transient abrupt asystoles.[22,41,42] Seventy-two–hour Holter monitoring performed annually may identify aberrant cardiac rhythms, typically sinus pauses that necessitate bipolar cardiac pacemaker implantation (ie, any pauses of ≥ 3 seconds),[43] and the frequency of shorter pauses (ie, <3 seconds) that may have physiologic and neurocognitive impact.

Cor pulmonale

Children with CCHS are at risk for progressive pulmonary hypertension and cor pulmonale, as a result of recurrent hypoxemia owing to inadequate ventilator settings or tracheostomy caliber, unrecognized hypoventilation during spontaneous breathing while awake, excessive exercise with resultant physiologic compromise, or suboptimal compliance with artificial ventilation. As a result, echocardiograms, hematocrits, and reticulocyte counts should be performed at least annually to identify potential cor pulmonale and polycythemia.

Ophthalmology

CCHS patients frequently exhibit ophthalmologic abnormalities reflecting the role of PHOX2B in the development of cranial nerves controlling pupillary function.[2,26] Comprehensive ophthalmologic testing and pupillometry determines the nature of the ophthalmologic involvement and allows for intervention strategies to avoid interference with learning.

Other

Anecdotal reports of poor heat tolerance and profuse sweating have been described,[44] although not studied comprehensively. Very limited formal assessment of the ANS has been reported, and none analyzed by PHOX2B genotype. Comprehensive autonomic testing as clinically indicated to assess ANS dysfunction may include head up tilt testing, heart rate–deep breathing, Valsalva maneuver, thermoregulatory chamber sweat testing, quantitative sudomotor sweat testing, pupillometry, and more.

AFTER CARE

Care for individuals with CCHS is ideally provided through centers with extensive expertise in CCHS, working in close partnership with parents and regional pediatric pulmonologists and pediatricians, to provide consistent, state-of-the-art management and guidance, and to provide thorough, up-to-date education regarding CCHS. The concept of centers is based on an understanding that management of children with CCHS is more time intensive and complex than the care of other ventilator-dependent children. Multidisciplinary care must typically be organized to include pediatricians, internists, pulmonologists, cardiologists, intensivists, ENT physicians, surgeons, gastroenterologists, neurologists, ophthalmologists, psychologists, psychiatrists, respiratory therapists, nurses, social workers, speech and language therapists, special education teachers, and more. And because of the nature of the PHOX2B mutations, and the range of phenotype based on these mutations, experience with even 15 to 30 patients does not provide the scope of experience necessary for understanding the needs of children with CCHS. The model of centers with extensive expertise in CCHS working in partnership with regional experts in pediatric pulmonology and pediatricians improves the consistency of management and likely outcome for individuals with CCHS. It also extends education about CCHS in all communities with CCHS patients, thereby improving identification of new patients.

In-hospital, comprehensive, clinical, physiologic testing awake and asleep are essential to assess ventilatory needs during varying levels of activity and concentration and all stages of sleep, with spontaneous breathing and with artificial ventilation. Furthermore, tests of ventilatory responsivity to endogenous and exogenous physiologic challenges awake and asleep ascertain each child's needs for optimal clinical management. This evaluation should be performed annually in CCHS patients 3 years and older, and biannually in the first 3 years of life. These clinical studies performed over the course of a several-day hospitalization in a center with extensive CCHS experience allows for a clear understanding of needs when breathing spontaneously as well as with artificial ventilation, with simulation of activities of daily living. These physiologic studies should include constant supervision by highly trained personnel and continuous audiovisual surveillance with continuous recording (at a minimum) of respiratory inductance plethysmography (chest, abdomen, sum), ECG, hemoglobin saturation, pulse waveform, end-tidal carbon dioxide, sleep state staging, blood pressure, and temperature. Other recommended testing for individuals with CCHS is provided in **Table 1**.

All individuals with CCHS require artificial ventilatory support. In infants, the safest way to deliver this is with a mechanical ventilator via a tracheostomy. Individuals with CCHS require a mechanical ventilator at home (with a backup ventilator, pulse oximeter, end-tidal carbon dioxide monitor, generator and preferably ventilator batteries) as well as experienced registered nursing care 24 hours a day. In select cases, other assistive breathing apparatus and/or techniques may be used, such as diaphragm pacing. Diaphragm pacing may be an option for CCHS patients, who are often ideal candidates (no or mild intrinsic lung disease, not obese with intact phrenic nerve–diaphragm axis integrity, and presence of a tracheostomy at least at the beginning of diaphragm pacing). Diaphragm pacing is an optimal form of ventilatory support during wakefulness because it allows freedom from mechanical ventilator use and participation in age-appropriate activities otherwise not possible.[2,45,46] In general, conservative use of diaphragm pacing is provided in active children, with 12 to 15 hours per day typically recommended. In older children and adults, noninvasive (mask) ventilation may be considered. This technique is discouraged in infants and young children because of the risk of facial deformation from the mask and inadequate stability of mask ventilation at a time of rapidly progressing neurodevelopment. The goal is to optimize oxygenation and ventilation to optimize neurocognitive outcome. Diaphragm pacing is a consideration in older children and adults for support during sleep only, although tracheostomy removal cannot be ensured. CCHS is a life-long disease and affected individuals will, at a minimum, always require artificial ventilation during sleep. Ventilatory needs vary with the specific *PHOX2B* mutation. However, supplemental oxygen alone is not adequate for treating the child with CCHS.

With modern technology for artificial ventilation, most children with CCHS can have prolonged survival with a good quality of life. At present, the oldest neonatally identified patients with CCHS are graduating from college, marrying, and maintaining employment. It behooves the family and medical personnel to provide optimal ventilation and oxygenation to ensure maximization of neurocognitive potential.

COMPLICATIONS
Alcohol and Drug Abuse

With advancing technology and treatment options, CCHS patients are now surviving into adolescence

Table 1
Recommended testing to characterize the CCHS phenotype

PHOX2B Genotype	Annual In-Hospital Comprehensive Physiologic Testing (Awake and Asleep), Exogenous and Endogenous Gas Challenges, Autonomic Testing	Assessment for Hirschsprung Disease	Annual Neurocognitive Assessment	Annual 72-h Holter Recording and Echocardiogram	Annual Imaging to Assess for Tumors of Neural Crest Origin
PARMs					
20/24 and 20/25	X		X	X	
20/26	X	X	X	X	
20/27	X	X	X	X	
20/28–20/33	X	X	X	X	X[a]
NPARMs	X	X	X	X	X[b]

Abbreviations: NPARM, nonpolyalanine repeat expansion mutation (missense, nonsense, frameshift); PARM, polyalanine repeat expansion mutation.
[a] Annual chest and abdominal imaging to identify ganglioneuromas and ganglioneuroblastomas.
[b] Abdominal imaging and urine catecholamines every 3 months in first 2 years, then every 6 months until 7 years of age to identify neuroblastomas.
From Weese-Mayer DE, Berry-Kravis EM, Ceccherini I, et al. An official ATS clinical policy statement: congenital central hypoventilation syndrome: genetic basis, diagnosis, and management. Am J Respir Crit Care Med 2010;181(6):637; with permission.

and adult life. With this advancement comes the normal adolescent temptations of alcohol and drug abuse.[47] The use of drugs and alcohol can further depress ventilatory drive awake and asleep in these patients to the point where continuous assisted ventilation is required; without such support, results can be fatal.[47] Therefore, CCHS patients and families should receive counseling about the special dangers drugs and alcohol present before adolescence, and continuing through adult life.

Pregnancy

CCHS patients are increasingly having children of their own.[48,49] Pregnancy presents potential risks both to the mother with CCHS and the fetus, which may also have a CCHS-associated *PHOX2B* mutation. In the mother with CCHS, the enlarging uterus increases respiratory load; already breathing at a lower minute ventilation and higher P_{CO_2} than other pregnant women,[49] the central respiratory drive to meet these increased ventilatory demands is inadequate. As such, these pregnancies require frequent physiologic monitoring of the mother, evaluating adequacy of gas exchange both during spontaneous awake breathing, and while on assisted ventilation during sleep. Special care must be taken for a caesarian birth occurring in a pregnant woman with CCHS who relies on diaphragm pacing without a tracheostomy. In this situation, the obstetric staff should be prepared to use bilevel positive airway pressure ventilation after delivery, because diaphragm pacing is poorly tolerated after an abdominal incision.[49] For offspring born to individuals with CCHS, prenatal *PHOX2B* testing allows for the anticipated infant with CCHS to be delivered in a tertiary care center with plans for immediate intubation and ventilation in the delivery room. Therefore, prenatal *PHOX2B* testing in any fetus with a CCHS-diagnosed parent (mother or father) or a parent with somatic mosaicism is recommended, even if termination of pregnancy is not anticipated, to optimally plan for the immediate newborn care of a CCHS infant. Plans should also be made to ensure that the mother with CCHS has adequate ventilator support during labor, postpartum, and during and after any general anesthesia which may be required.

SUMMARY

Our understanding of CCHS is expanding rapidly, but it remains a work in progress. Optimal diagnosis and management of CCHS patients requires further advances in our knowledge through research. Owing to the rarity of the disease, these advances require the participation of all CCHS patients and their families and physicians around the world. Because the biology of CCHS is not completely understood, it is hoped that families of the few CCHS patients who die will agree to autopsy, which can provide tissues to further identify and delineate biologic abnormalities. These tissues would include frozen and fixed brain, brainstem, carotid and aortic bodies, adrenal glands, autonomic plexus, sympathetic chain, and the entire intestine. The presentation, symptoms, severity, and relationship of these to *PHOX2B* genotype are complex issues in CCHS. To further our understanding of these issues in the hope of bettering the lives of CCHS patients, and to prepare for possible drug trials in CCHS in the future, an international CCHS registry has been developed. This registry is a secure online interface allowing CCHS families around the world to participate. Further information on this registry can be found on the Center for Autonomic Medicine in Pediatrics at the Ann & Robert H. Lurie Children's Hospital of Chicago website (http://www.luriechildrens.org/en-us/care-services/conditions-treatments/autonomic-medicine/Pages/basics/basics.aspx), or by emailing CRand@LurieChildrens.org.

Recently, the first study in a large cohort of individuals with *PHOX2B* mutation-confirmed CCHS evaluating comprehensive chemosensory function was completed.[38] The study was designed to determine whether residual chemosensory function exists in CCHS patients and if it is associated with *PHOX2B* genotype. The results suggest that CCHS patients maintain a weak residual awake ventilatory response to chemosensory challenge with hypoxia/hypercarbia, independent of *PHOX2B* genotype. However, the *PHOX2B* genotype was found to associate with graded dysfunction in cardiovascular regulation. This contrast in phenotype–genotype association suggests differential effects of *PHOX2B* dysfunction on different autonomic subsystems. Although these results also emphasize the continual risk of physiologic compromise from hypoxemia and hypercarbia to CCHS patients during activities of daily living, they also suggest partial preservation of central nervous system networks that could provide a fulcrum for potential pharmacologic interventions.

A high index of suspicion, early detection, and aggressive, conservative intervention are critical to optimize neurocognitive outcome and quality of life for individuals with CCHS and LO-CCHS of all ages. If inadequately treated, affected individuals will likely suffer neurocognitive compromise and potentially sudden death. If treated conservatively and followed comprehensively, individuals with CCHS can have a good quality of life and an anticipated normal life span. As children with

CCHS are advancing into adulthood, the development of transitional medicine programs in the centers already caring for children with CCHS is essential.

REFERENCES

1. Mellins RB, Balfour HH Jr, Turino GM, et al. Failure of automatic control of ventilation (Ondine's curse). Report of an infant born with this syndrome and review of the literature. Medicine (Baltimore) 1970; 49(6):487–504.
2. Weese-Mayer DE, Silvestri JM, Menzies LJ, et al. Congenital central hypoventilation syndrome: diagnosis, management, and long-term outcome in thirty-two children. J Pediatr 1992;120(3):381–7.
3. Matera I, Bachetti T, Puppo F, et al. PHOX2B mutations and polyalanine expansions correlate with the severity of the respiratory phenotype and associated symptoms in both congenital and late onset central hypoventilation syndrome. J Med Genet 2004;41(5):373–80.
4. Trochet D, Hong SJ, Lim JK, et al. Molecular consequences of PHOX2B missense, frameshift and alanine expansion mutations leading to autonomic dysfunction. Hum Mol Genet 2005;14(23): 3697–708.
5. Repetto GM, Corrales RJ, Abara SG, et al. Later-onset congenital central hypoventilation syndrome due to a heterozygous 24-polyalanine repeat expansion mutation in the PHOX2B gene. Acta Paediatr 2009;98(1):192–5.
6. Trang H, Laudier B, Trochet D, et al. PHOX2B gene mutation in a patient with late-onset central hypoventilation. Pediatr Pulmonol 2004;38(4): 349–51.
7. Weese-Mayer DE, Berry-Kravis EM, Zhou L. Adult identified with congenital central hypoventilation syndrome–mutation in PHOX2b gene and late-onset CHS. Am J Respir Crit Care Med 2005; 171(1):88.
8. Antic NA, Malow BA, Lange N, et al. PHOX2B mutation-confirmed congenital central hypoventilation syndrome: presentation in adulthood. Am J Respir Crit Care Med 2006;174(8):923–7.
9. Diedrich A, Malow BA, Antic NA, et al. Vagal and sympathetic heart rate and blood pressure control in adult onset PHOX2B mutation-confirmed congenital central hypoventilation syndrome. Clin Auton Res 2007;17(3):177–85.
10. Trochet D, de Pontual L, Straus C, et al. PHOX2B germline and somatic mutations in late-onset central hypoventilation syndrome. Am J Respir Crit Care Med 2008;177(8):906–11.
11. Doherty LS, Kiely JL, Deegan PC, et al. Late-onset central hypoventilation syndrome: a family genetic study. Eur Respir J 2007;29(2):312–6.
12. Barratt S, Kendrick AH, Buchanan F, et al. Central hypoventilation with PHOX2B expansion mutation presenting in adulthood. Thorax 2007;62(10): 919–20.
13. Parodi S, Bachetti T, Lantieri F, et al. Parental origin and somatic mosaicism of PHOX2B mutations in congenital central hypoventilation syndrome. Hum Mutat 2008;29(1):206.
14. Weese-Mayer DE, Berry-Kravis EM, Ceccherini I, et al. An official ATS clinical policy statement: congenital central hypoventilation syndrome: genetic basis, diagnosis, and management. Am J Respir Crit Care Med 2010;181(6):626–44.
15. Jennings LJ, Yu M, Rand CM, et al. Variable human phenotype associated with novel deletions of the PHOX2B gene. Pediatr Pulmonol 2012; 47(2):153–61.
16. Trochet D, O'Brien LM, Gozal D, et al. PHOX2B genotype allows for prediction of tumor risk in congenital central hypoventilation syndrome. Am J Hum Genet 2005;76(3):421–6.
17. Weese-Mayer DE, Berry-Kravis EM, Zhou L, et al. Idiopathic congenital central hypoventilation syndrome: analysis of genes pertinent to early autonomic nervous system embryologic development and identification of mutations in PHOX2b. Am J Med Genet A 2003;123A(3):267–78.
18. Bachetti T, Parodi S, Di Duca M, et al. Low amounts of PHOX2B expanded alleles in asymptomatic parents suggest unsuspected recurrence risk in congenital central hypoventilation syndrome. J Mol Med (Berl) 2011;89(5):505–13.
19. Bolande RP. Neurocristopathy: its growth and development in 20 years. Pediatr Pathol Lab Med 1997;17(1):1–25.
20. Weese-Mayer DE, Patwari PP, Rand CM, et al. Congenital central hypoventilation syndrome (CCHS) and PHOX2B mutations. Primer on the autonomic nervous system. 3rd edition. New York: Elsevier; 2012.
21. Berry-Kravis EM, Zhou L, Rand CM, et al. Congenital central hypoventilation syndrome: PHOX2B mutations and phenotype. Am J Respir Crit Care Med 2006;174(10):1139–44.
22. Gronli JO, Santucci BA, Leurgans SE, et al. Congenital central hypoventilation syndrome: PHOX2B genotype determines risk for sudden death. Pediatr Pulmonol 2008;43(1):77–86.
23. Gordon S, Rand C, Vitez S, et al. Ganglion cell presence is only part of the story: gastrointestinal symptoms as a measure of enteric autonomic dysfunction in CCHS (congenital central hypoventilation syndrome). Vancouver (BC): Pediatric Academic Society; 2014. E-PAS2014.
24. Saiyed R, Rand CM, Patwari PP, et al. Altered temperature regulation in respiratory and autonomic disorders of infancy, childhood, and

adulthood (RADICA). Am J Respir Crit Care Med 2011;183A:6394.

25. Patwari PP, Stewart TM, Rand CM, et al. Pupillometry in congenital central hypoventilation syndrome (CCHS): quantitative evidence of autonomic nervous system dysregulation. Pediatr Res 2012;71(3):280–5.

26. Goldberg DS, Ludwig IH. Congenital central hypoventilation syndrome: ocular findings in 37 children. J Pediatr Ophthalmol Strabismus 1996; 33(3):175–80.

27. De Pontual L, Trochet D, Caillat-Zucman S, et al. Delineation of late onset hypoventilation associated with hypothalamic dysfunction syndrome. Pediatr Res 2008;64(6):689–94.

28. Parodi S, Baglietto MP, Pini Prato A, et al. A novel missense mutation in the PHOX2B gene is associated with late onset central hypoventilation syndrome. Pediatr Pulmonol 2008;43(10):1036–9.

29. Jennings LJ, Yu M, Zhou L, et al. Comparison of PHOX2B testing methods in the diagnosis of congenital central hypoventilation syndrome and mosaic carriers. Diagn Mol Pathol 2010;19(4): 224–31.

30. Weese-Mayer DE, Brouillette RT, Naidich TP, et al. Magnetic resonance imaging and computerized tomography in central hypoventilation. Am Rev Respir Dis 1988;137(2):393–8.

31. Bachetti T, Robbiano A, Parodi S, et al. Brainstem anomalies in two patients affected by congenital central hypoventilation syndrome. Am J Respir Crit Care Med 2006;174(6):706–9.

32. Huang J, Colrain IM, Panitch HB, et al. Effect of sleep stage on breathing in children with central hypoventilation. J Appl Phys 2008;105(1):44–53.

33. Fleming PJ, Cade D, Bryan MH, et al. Congenital central hypoventilation and sleep state. Pediatrics 1980;66(3):425–8.

34. Amiel J, Sproat-Emison E, Garcia-Barcelo M, et al. Hirschsprung disease, associated syndromes and genetics: a review. J Med Genet 2008;45(1):1–14.

35. Oren J, Kelly DH, Shannon DC. Long-term follow-up of children with congenital central hypoventilation syndrome. Pediatrics 1987;80(3):375–80.

36. Marcus CL, Jansen MT, Poulsen MK, et al. Medical and psychosocial outcome of children with congenital central hypoventilation syndrome. J Pediatr 1991;119(6):888–95.

37. Zelko FA, Nelson MN, Leurgans SE, et al. Congenital central hypoventilation syndrome: Neurocognitive functioning in school age children. Pediatr Pulmonol 2010;45(1):92–8.

38. Carroll MS, Patwari PP, Kenny AS, et al. Residual chemosensitivity to ventilatory challenges in genotyped congenital central hypoventilation syndrome. J Appl Phys 2014;116(4):439–50.

39. DeMarchi GA, NM, Wuu J, et al. Cognitive phenotype of PHOX2B mutation-confirmed congenital central hypoventilation syndrome. Am J Respir Crit Care Med 2007;175A:810.

40. Charnay A, Antisdel J, Zelko F, et al. Congenital central hypoventilation syndrome: neurodevelopmental performance in preschool children. Mclean (VA): Pediatric Academic Society; 2014. E-PAS2014.

41. Woo MS, Woo MA, Gozal D, et al. Heart rate variability in congenital central hypoventilation syndrome. Pediatr Res 1992;31(3):291–6.

42. Silvestri JM, Hanna BD, Volgman AS, et al. Cardiac rhythm disturbances among children with idiopathic congenital central hypoventilation syndrome. Pediatr Pulmonol 2000;29(5):351–8.

43. Epstein AE, DiMarco JP, Ellenbogen KA, et al. ACC/AHA/HRS 2008 guidelines for device-based therapy of cardiac rhythm abnormalities: a report of the American College of Cardiology/American Heart Association Task Force on practice guidelines (writing committee to revise the ACC/AHA/NASPE 2002 guideline update for implantation of cardiac pacemakers and antiarrhythmia devices) developed in collaboration with the American Association for Thoracic Surgery and Society of Thoracic Surgeons. J Am Coll Cardiol 2008;51(21):e1–62.

44. Weese-Mayer DE, Shannon DC, Keens TG, et al. Idiopathic congenital central hypoventilation syndrome: diagnosis and management. American Thoracic Society. Am J Respir Crit Care Med 1999;160(1):368–73.

45. Weese-Mayer DE, Hunt CE, Brouillette RT, et al. Diaphragm pacing in infants and children. J Pediatr 1992;120(1):1–8.

46. Chin AC, Shaul DB, Patwari PP, et al. Diaphragmatic pacing in infants and children with congenital central hypoventilation syndrome (CCHS). In: Kheirandish-Gozal L, Gozal D, editors. Sleep disordered breathing in children: a clinical guide. New York: Springer; 2012. p. 553–73.

47. Chen ML, Turkel SB, Jacobson JR, et al. Alcohol use in congenital central hypoventilation syndrome. Pediatr Pulmonol 2006;41(3):283–5.

48. Silvestri JM, Chen ML, Weese-Mayer DE, et al. Idiopathic congenital central hypoventilation syndrome: the next generation. Am J Med Genet 2002;112(1):46–50.

49. Sritippayawan S, Hamutcu R, Kun SS, et al. Mother-daughter transmission of congenital central hypoventilation syndrome. Am J Respir Crit Care Med 2002;166(3):367–9.

Sleep-Disordered Breathing in Neurologic Conditions

Maryann C. Deak, MD[a,b],*, Douglas B. Kirsch, MD[a,b]

KEYWORDS

- Sleep-disordered breathing • Neurologic disorders • Obstructive sleep apnea

KEY POINTS

- Sleep-disordered breathing (SDB) is common in neurologic disorders.
- Obstructive sleep apnea, central sleep apnea, and sleep-related hypoventilation can all be seen in neurologic conditions, with certain sleep-related breathing disorders being more common in specific neurologic conditions.
- The underlying cause of SDB is complex and often multifactorial.
- Identification and treatment of SDB is an important aspect of treating patients with neurologic disease.

INTRODUCTION

Sleep-related breathing disorder or sleep-disordered breathing (SDB) encompasses a range of conditions, including central sleep apnea (CSA), obstructive sleep apnea (OSA), and sleep-related hypoventilation or hypoxemic syndromes.[1] For a list of possible presentations of SDB in neurologic disease, see **Box 1**. SDB is common in neurologic conditions that impact the central and/or peripheral nervous systems. Patients with neurologic conditions are at risk for SDB due to a combination of factors such as muscular weakness, damage to areas of the brain that control respiration, use of sedating medications, and, in some cases, weight gain from limited physical activity (**Box 2**). Recognition and treatment of SDB is an important aspect of treating patients with neurologic disease.

NEUROMUSCULAR DISEASES AND BREATHING DURING SLEEP

Disordered breathing during sleep and neuromuscular diseases are intimately linked. Breakdowns in nerves, muscles, and the connections between them may lead to severe compromises in respiratory function. However, each neuromuscular disorder may have a different impact on breathing, given the variance in the location of the dysfunction. This section discusses some of the common neuromuscular conditions and their resultant SDB.

Amyotrophic Lateral Sclerosis

Amyotrophic lateral sclerosis (ALS), also known as Lou Gehrig disease for the well-known New York Yankee first baseman who suffered from the disorder, is a disease of neuron degeneration in the brain, brainstem, and ventral horn of the spinal cord. Symptoms of this often rapidly progressive disorder include weakness, muscle atrophy and fasciculation, spasticity, dysarthria, dysphagia, and respiratory compromise. Dysfunction of the respiratory system occurs on multiple levels, including pharynx, larynx, intercostal muscles, and diaphragm. Thus, neurons supplying the inspiratory, expiratory, and upper-airway muscles are all affected. A variety of causes have been

Disclosures: None.
[a] Division of Sleep and Circadian Disorders, Departments of Neurology and Medicine, Brigham and Women's Hospital, Boston, MA, USA; [b] Department of Neurology, Harvard Medical School, Boston, MA, USA
* Corresponding author. 1153 Centre Street, Suite 47, Boston, MA 02138.
E-mail address: MDEAK@partners.org

http://dx.doi.org/10.1016/j.ccm.2014.06.009
0272-5231/14/$ – see front matter © 2014 Elsevier Inc. All rights reserved.

chestmed.theclinics.com

Box 1
Possible presentations of SDB in neurologic conditions

OSA

Nocturnal stridor

CSA, Cheyne-Stokes

Sleep-related hypoventilation

Mixed OSA and CSA

Acquired central alveolar hypoventilation

proposed for this disease, including toxic exposure, genetic disorders, and autoimmune conditions, although no single cause for the disease has been identified.[2] Approximately 15 new cases are diagnosed per day (5600 per year) with an estimate of 30,000 patients currently diagnosed with the disease in the United States at any given time.[3]

Sleep complaints are common in ALS. In one study, 59% of subjects with ALS had sleep complaints compared with 36% of controls. Common sleep complaints include nocturia, sleep fragmentation, and nocturnal cramping.[4] Although not all of the sleep complaints are likely related to underlying SDB, it seems likely that at least some of the symptoms have a respiratory-related underpinning.

In late stages of ALS, patients will have daytime respiratory problems; however, patients will often have nocturnal breathing disturbance much earlier due to the vulnerability of the respiratory system during sleep. In particular, diaphragmatic dysfunction leads to reduced ventilation during sleep, particularly rapid eye movement (REM) sleep, when other accessory muscles do not lend support to breathing. Early intervention with noninvasive ventilation in patients suffering from ALS has improved their quality of life and may also prolong survival.[5,6] Several types of abnormal sleep-related breathing disorders have been discovered in ALS, including OSA, CSA, and hypoventilation, with the frequency of reporting widely variable.

Box 2
Potential contributors to SDB in neurologic conditions

Muscular weakness, including muscles of respiration

Damage to respiratory control areas of brainstem

Sedating medications

Obesity

Most common of the sleep-related breathing disturbances in ALS is hypoventilation. Because the disease affects the diaphragm, intercostal muscles, and accessory muscles of respiration, the patient moves less air in and out of the lungs (reduced tidal volume). REM sleep is a period of particularly notable hypoventilation. Human REM-related respiration is nearly completely dependent on diaphragmatic movement, which is limited by motor neuron disease. Nocturnal hypoventilation may be difficult to unmask initially, with subtle symptoms that might include restless sleep, insomnia, and morning headaches. As the hypoventilation worsens, it causes frequent arousals from sleep, leading to both nocturnal symptoms of insomnia and daytime symptoms of sleepiness. For a more complete list of symptoms of hypoventilation, see **Box 3**.

Myasthenia Gravis and Lambert Eaton Myasthenic Syndrome

Myasthenia gravis (MG) is characterized by episodic weakness related to the fatigability of voluntary muscles. This autoimmune disorder is defined by prevention of neuromuscular transmission due to blockage of postsynaptic acetylcholine receptors. Repetitive use of the voluntary muscles will cause weakness; rest restores normal function.[7] There are approximately 36,000 to 60,000 cases of MG in the United States, with an estimated prevalence of 14 to 20 cases per 100,000

Box 3
Symptoms of nocturnal hypoventilation

Air hunger

Snoring

Choking

Orthopnea

Cyanosis

Restlessness

Insomnia

Daytime hypersomnolence

Morning headaches

Drowsiness

Fatigue

Depression

Impaired cognition

Adapted from Perrin C, Unterborn JN, Ambrosio CD, et al. Pulmonary complications of chronic neuromuscular diseases and their management. Muscle Nerve 2004;29(1):5–27; with permission.

people.[8] Approximately 30% of patients with MG develop a degree of respiratory muscle weakness. Limited correlation exists between the severity of the respiratory muscle weakness and that of other skeletal muscles; thus, a mild case of MG can be associated with a clinically relevant reduction of the ability to appropriately ventilate.[9]

According to available research, 40% to 60% of patients with diurnally stable MG have SDB, of which a large portion is central, rather than obstructive. Interestingly, these studies suggest that a large fraction of the SDB in patients with MG is of central origin and more commonly observed during REM sleep. The presence of disrupted breathing during the night may be relevant, given reports that patients with MG die of early morning respiratory failure. However, not all research confirms the relationship between SDB and MG; much of the research variability with subjects with MG is likely related to the instability of the disease.[9]

Lambert Eaton myasthenic syndrome is a less common disorder of the neuromuscular junction, which most commonly occurs in association with small cell lung cancer. This disorder affects the presynaptic portion of the neuromuscular junction. Though the effect on respiratory function is similar, there are several clinical differences, including areflexia and more significant autonomic dysfunction.[10]

Inherited Myopathies

Myotonic dystrophy

Myotonic dystrophy type I (MD1) is the most common adult-onset form of muscular dystrophy. The worldwide prevalence of MD1 ranges from 2.1 to 14.3 per 100 000 people. Also referred to as Steinert disease, MD1 is a progressive disorder caused by an abnormality on chromosome 19; an expansion of a CTG repeat of the myotonic dystrophy protein kinase gene is the cause. Symptoms of this disease may include limb, facial and respiratory muscle weakness, myotonia, cardiomyopathy, endocrinopathy, and, neuropsychological deficit. There are three different forms of MD1: congenital, childhood onset, and adult onset. Both the timing of onset (earlier is worse) and the muscles affected (proximal is worse) impacts the life expectancy of patients with this disorder.[4]

Multiple sleep symptoms occur in patients with MD1, including prominent excessive daytime sleepiness (EDS) in the absence of other abnormal symptoms. This sleepiness appears central in etiology and occurs prominently in most patients with MD1.[11] Some reports suggest up to 70% to 80% of patients have a complaint of EDS, which may be the most common nonmuscular symptom.

EDS may predate the diagnosis of MD1 in some cases.[12]

Sleep studies on patients with MD1 may demonstrate SDB, including nocturnal desaturations and hypercapnia. There are multiple possible reasons for the SDB, including the direct effects of the disease on the respiratory muscles and abnormalities of central control of ventilation. Diaphragmatic weakness is common in MD1, contributing to the observed hypoventilation; in some cases it is observed even during the daytime. Central ventilatory dysfunction in patients with MD1 may be related to neuronal loss in several medullary nuclei linked to respiratory function.[13]

Myotonic dystrophy type 2 (MD2), also known as proximal myotonic myopathy, is a less common disorder stemming from an autosomal dominant CCTG expansion on chromosome 3. Limited studies of sleep in patients with MD2 have been performed; however, the data suggest that several different sleep disorders may occur, including OSA, insomnia, and REM sleep behavior disorder (RBD). Hypersomnolence is also present in some patients with MD2, although it may not be as common a symptom as in MD1.[4] Pilot data suggest that OSA was common in a group of 12 consecutive MD2 subjects when compared with matched controls.[14] Conjectures about the source of the sleep disorders include the peripheral effect of the muscular weakness (OSA) as well as a central nervous system process to explain sleepiness and the other sleep symptoms.[15]

Duchenne muscular dystrophy and Becker muscular dystrophy

Duchenne muscular dystrophy (DMD) is a progressive disorder of muscular weakness, beginning in the legs and pelvis but, over time, affecting all skeletal muscles. This disorder, as well as its milder variant, Becker muscular dystrophy (BMD), occurs due to an X-linked recessive mutation of the dystrophin gene. In DMD, dystrophin is absent, whereas, in BMD, dystrophin is reduced. The Center for Disease Control estimates 1 of every 5600 to 7700 male patients 5 through 24 years of age had either DMD or BMD.[16] Typically, as the disease progresses, alveolar hypoventilation occurs in all sleep stages due to restricted pulmonary function (from both respiratory muscle weakness and scoliosis), although the hypoventilation is typically worst during REM sleep. In addition, due to loss of tone in the upper airway muscles, obstructive SDB is also common in patients with muscular dystrophy.[4]

Neuropathies

Most neuropathies do not have a dramatic impact on breathing during sleep. A notable exception is acute inflammatory demyelinating polyradiculo-neuropathy, also known as Guillain-Barre syndrome. Often a post-infectious condition, this disorder has worldwide incidence of 0.6 to 4 cases per 100,000, more commonly occurring in men than women, and in older people compared with younger people.[17] Sleep disturbance is common in this disorder. One study suggested than more than half of subjects had difficulty with sleep.[18] Dysfunction of the diaphragm is commonly observed in this disorder; mechanical ventilation may be necessary both during wake and sleep.[4]

Assessment of SDB in Neuromuscular Disease

SDB is common in patients with neuromuscular disorders. In one neuromuscular clinic, 60 consecutive patients were evaluated for SDB. Of these patients, 80% had an apnea-hypopnea index (AHI) greater than 5 per hour and 42% had an AHI greater than 15 per hour. SDB is often seen before the onset of respiratory insufficiency in this patient population and may be more easily identified by symptoms of EDS or fatigue than direct muscle function testing or spirometery.[19] Other symptoms that may be helpful to identify SDB include snoring, gasping or choking during sleep, morning headache, poor concentration, and issues with memory.[20]

History taking, questionnaires such as the Sleep-Disordered Breathing in Neuromuscular Disease Questionnaire (SiNQ-5),[21] and physical examination are useful first steps in assessment of a neuromuscular condition. Even a single-breath counting task may be useful assessment of respiratory function. A score of up to 50 is common in normal patients; scores of less than 15 demonstrate significant impairment of vital capacity. Other physical signs suggesting respiratory dysfunction may include use of accessory muscles for breathing, paradoxic breathing, and rapid, shallow breathing.

Early in the assessment of patients with neuromuscular conditions, pulmonary function testing and arterial blood gases help gauge the current respiratory status of a patient. Nocturnal polysomnography is the gold standard for assessment of abnormal breathing during sleep. In particular, patients with suspected hypoventilation should have polysomnography that includes monitoring of carbon dioxide levels, either via end-tidal or transcutaneous carbon dioxide monitoring. An example of a polysomnogram with end-tidal carbon dioxide demonstrating hypoventilation is observed in **Fig. 1**. Overnight oximetry and limited channel home sleep testing may provide limited information about SDB; however, in-laboratory polysomnography is generally felt to be the test of choice for diagnosis of hypoventilation.

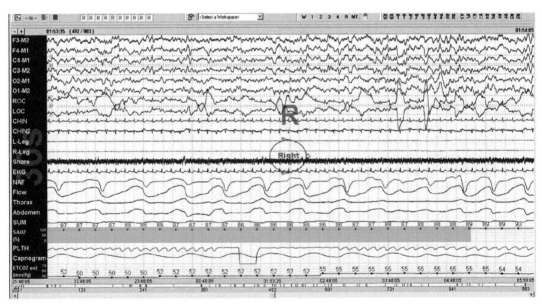

Fig. 1. A 30-second epoch of polysomnography from Nihon Kohden software demonstrating hypoventilation. The leads from the top include six electroencephalogram leads: left and right pairs of frontal (F3 and F4), central (C3 and C4), and occipital (O1 and O2); right and left eye (ROC, LOC); chin, left, and right leg electromyography (CHIN, L-Leg, R-Leg), snore microphone channel, electrocardiogram (EKG); nasal pressure transducer (NAF); oro-nasal thermistor (Flow); thorax and abdominal effort bands (Thorax and Abdomen) with a summation channel (SUM); oxygen saturation (SAO2); plethysmography (PLTH); capnogram, and end-tidal carbon dioxide signal (Capnogram and ETCO2-ext).

Treatment of SDB in Neuromuscular Disease

Positive pressure therapy is a common treatment of SDB. When OSA is the sole condition, continuous positive airway pressure (CPAP) is the gold standard for treatment. However, when hypoventilation is present, noninvasive positive pressure ventilation (NPPV) is a superior option. Best practices for titration of NPPV during a sleep study have been described by the American Academy of Sleep Medicine.[22] Use of supplemental oxygen as sole therapy in hypoventilation is controversial; although it can be used adjunctively with bilevel positive pressure therapy.

In some cases, such as in patients with ALS, patients may be placed on NPPV without a diagnostic sleep study, based on daytime respiratory findings such as a low functional ventilatory capacity (less than 50% of predicted), maximal inspiratory pressure less than −60 cm of water, sniff nasal inspiratory pressure less than 40 cm of water, or sleep evaluation showing desaturation at nighttime.[10]

In some cases, NPPV may not be a good option for the patient. These situations include facial weakness, such as in myotonic dystrophy, causing difficulty in fitting NPPV or when oral secretions are poorly managed and place the patient at risk for aspiration, such as in late stage ALS. Depending on the clinical scenario, tracheostomy is an alternative option to ventilate and bypass the airway. However, patients and family should always be involved early when considering this therapy mechanism to ensure all risks and potential benefits are reviewed and discussed. Also, the Food and Drug Administration has approved diaphragmatic pacing in patients with ALS; however, not all patients may be candidates for this treatment.

NEURODEGENERATIVE DISEASE

Neurodegenerative diseases such as multiple system atrophy (MSA), Alzheimer dementia, and multiple sclerosis (MS) are commonly associated with sleep disruption. SDB is a frequent cause of sleep disruption in these patient populations. Treatment of SDB may lead to improvements in quality of life, neurologic symptoms, or survival in some patient populations with neurodegenerative disease.

MSA

MSA is a sporadic progressive neurodegenerative disorder characterized by parkinsonism, cerebellar ataxia, and autonomic failure. MSA is grouped into two subtypes based on the predominant motor feature: MSA-parkinsonian (MSA-P) and MSA- cerebellar (MSA-C). Life expectancy is approximately 6 to 9 years from the time of diagnosis, with pneumonia and sudden death being the most common causes of death.[23] Sleep disturbance in MSA is common and may present as sleep fragmentation, EDS, RBD, or SDB.[24] SDB in MSA may manifest as nocturnal stridor, CSA, OSA, or as a combination of these disorders.[24]

Stridor

Stridor is caused by obstruction of the larynx due to partial or complete vocal cord palsy. It is characterized by an inspiratory high-pitched sound, which may be mixed with snoring in patients with comorbid OSA.[24] It can be diagnosed by polysomnography with synchronized audiovisual recording or by daytime laryngoscopy. Between 13% and 42% of MSA patients experience nocturnal stridor.[24] Nocturnal stridor precedes the development of stridor during wakefulness, which can develop with disease progression.[23] Stridor is associated with sudden death, and nocturnal sudden death is the most common cause of death in patients with MSA.[25] Median survival is decreased by 1 year in MSA patients with stridor compared with those without stridor.[26]

Treatment options for stridor include CPAP and tracheostomy.[23,24] Stridor can often be effectively treated with CPAP, which improves subjective sleep quality and survival time.[27,28] A CPAP titration study should be performed to confirm the resolution of stridor. Tracheostomy is indicated in patients with stridor during wakefulness or in whom CPAP is ineffective or poorly tolerated.[23] The degree of motor impairment at the time of CPAP therapy initiation plays an important role in determining CPAP acceptance in patients with MSA.[29] Tracheostomy has also been shown to increase survival.[24,26]

CSA and OSA

CSA, Cheyne-Stokes respiration (CSR), irregular and apneustic breathing, and OSA have all been described in MSA.[23,30] Although prevalence estimates are limited, OSA is more common than CSA, with up to 37% of patients meeting criteria for OSA (defined as a respiratory disturbance index >10).[23,31] CSA may result from damage to centers of automatic breathing control in the brainstem such as chemosensitive neurons in the ventral medulla.[32] CSA is typically found in late stages of MSA, although it is rarely a feature of initial presentation.[30] The long-term effects of CSA in MSA are unclear. Polysomnography is used to diagnose SDB in MSA and can determine if CSA, OSA, or both are present. CPAP is the treatment of choice for OSA, and may be effective in CSA. In some cases, adaptive servoventilation or oxygen therapy are warranted for the treatment CSA.[33] CPAP may be contraindicated in MSA patients with floppy epiglottis, which is obstruction of the laryngeal inlet by the epiglottis.[34]

Alzheimer Disease

Alzheimer disease (AD) is the most common form of dementia.[35] AD causes progressive cognitive decline, characterized by memory impairment as well as disturbance in one or more other domains, including apraxia, aphasia, or executive function. Sleep disturbance, common in AD, is a significant factor contributing to institutionalization of patients and reduces both patient and caregiver quality of life.[36]

The cause of sleep disturbance in AD is multifactorial. Patients may experience insomnia, circadian rhythm disturbance, nocturnal agitation, and nocturnal wandering. Estimates of the prevalence of SDB in dementia are high. More than 70% of institutionalized patients with dementia are estimated to have OSA, defined as 5 five or more apnea or hypopneas per hour of sleep based on portable monitoring.[37] More than 38% are estimated to have 20 or more apneas or hypopneas per hour.[37] The apolipoprotein E4 genotype is a risk factor for both AD and OSA and may play a pathophysiological role in these disorders.[23] OSA may worsen or cause cognitive impairment.[38,39] OSA has been associated with a significantly higher likelihood of developing cognitive impairment or dementia over 5 years of follow-up, with the risk increasing with more sleep apnea events or a lower oxygen nadir.[39]

The frequency of CSA in AD is unclear but it is likely significantly less common than OSA.[36] Dysfunction of brainstem respiratory regulation networks may predispose patients with AD to CSA.[36] There is a paucity of data on the potential impact of CSA in AD.

CPAP is the treatment of choice for OSA, and patients with AD have been shown to tolerate CPAP.[40] CPAP reduces subjective daytime sleepiness in patients with AD.[41] Preliminary data suggest that CPAP improves cognition in AD and may also improve sleep quality and mood.[42,43] The presence of comorbid depression is a potential barrier to CPAP use in AD.[40] The presence of caregivers invested in treatment likely improves compliance with CPAP therapy in dementia.[44] CSA is often treated with CPAP, adaptive servo-ventilation, or oxygen.[33]

MS

MS, which causes T-cell–mediated demyelination of focal areas of the brain and spinal cord, is a leading cause of disability in young adults. Sleep-related problems are common in MS, reported by approximately 50% of patients.[45] Sleep disorders are often under-recognized in the MS population.

SDB including OSA, CSA, and respiratory death during sleep (Ondine curse) have been described in MS.[45] Prevalence of SDB in MS is unclear due to lack of large-scale studies. Available data are conflicted regarding prevalence of SDB in MS. Some studies have found that SDB is not more common in MS than the general population.[46,47] A recent study suggests a higher prevalence, with 12% of patients with MS having polysomnography-confirmed SDB.[48] MS patients with fatigue are more likely to have comorbid sleep-related breathing disorders.[48] SDB is more severe in MS, and patients with MS have been found to have an AHI and central apnea index (CAI) compared with two control groups matched for age, gender, and body mass index.[49]

Several factors may contribute to the development of SDB in patients with MS. Demyelinating lesions in the brainstem, particularly in the medullary reticular formation may contribute directly the development of SDB.[47] Patients with MS who have clinical or radiographic evidence of brainstem involvements have a higher AHI and CAI compared with patients with MS who do not have brainstem involvement. Sedating medications for pain or spasticity may contribute to the development of SDB.[47] Obesity related to lack of activity may also contribute.[47] Positive airway pressure is the mainstay of treatment of SDB, although controlled treatment trials in MS subjects are lacking.

OTHER NEUROLOGIC CONDITIONS
Stroke

Stroke, which is one of the most common neurologic disorders, is an acute vascular event that results in focal neurologic impairment. Estimates of the prevalence of SDB in stroke are high, with approximately 50% to 70% of patients with stroke having an AHI greater than or equal to 10 events per hour.[50,51] Although OSA is the most common form of SDB in stroke, CSR and CSA may also been seen in stroke, at times in combination with OSA. **Fig. 2** demonstrates mixed apneas in a patient with stroke. OSA increases the risk of stroke, with prospective cohort or cross-sectional cohort studies demonstrating odds or hazard ratios ranging between 1.6 and 3.8.[50] OSA also adversely affects outcomes after stroke, resulting in worse functional outcome, longer hospitalization, and increased mortality.[50]

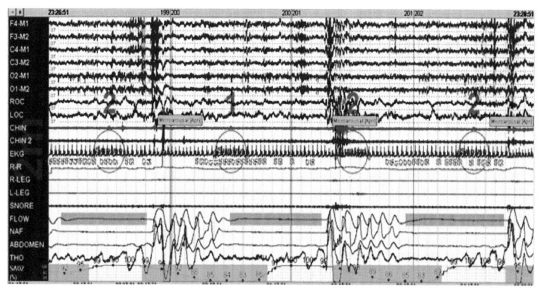

Fig. 2. A 2-minute segment of a polysomnography from Nihon Khoden software demonstrating mixed apneas in a patient with a history of stroke. The leads from the top include six electroencephalogram leads: left and right pairs of frontal (F3 and F4), central (C3 and C4), and occipital (O1 and O2); right and left eye (ROC, LOC); chin electromyography (CHIN); electrocardiogram (EKG); right and left leg electromyography (R-LEG, L-LEG); snore microphone channel; oronasal thermistor (FLOW); nasal pressure transducer (NAF); abdominal and thoracic effort bands (ABDOMEN and THO); oxygen saturation (SAO2).

CSR is most prevalent in the initial days following stroke. Estimates of the prevalence of CSR respirations in the acute poststroke period are 10% to 40%.[52–54] CSR is associated with higher age and stroke severity.[52] In addition, cardiac abnormalities are more likely to be present in patients with stroke who have CSR, including ECG abnormalities on hospital admission and lower ejection fraction on echocardiography.[52] However, patients may not have clinically apparent congestive heart failure.[52] Unlike OSA, CSR commonly resolves, at least in part, within 1 to 3 months of acute stroke.[53,54] The effect of CSR on stroke risk is unclear and CSR may be a consequence of stroke, rather than a clear contributor to stroke risk. Central hypoventilation is rare in stroke and typically occurs in brainstem or spinal cord stroke.[51]

CPAP is the treatment of choice for OSA. CSA is often treated with CPAP, oxygen, or adaptive servoventilation.[51] Randomized controlled clinical trials examining treatment of OSA or CSA in stroke subjects are lacking. CPAP adherence may be limited in patients with stroke by neurologic impairment, mask discomfort, and claustrophobia. Available data suggest that patients with stroke on CPAP long-term for treatment of OSA likely have a reduced risk or a delayed recurrence of vascular events after stroke.[55] Treatment of SDB in stroke has been associated with improvement in subjective wellbeing, nocturnal blood pressure, and mood.[51]

Epilepsy

Patients with epilepsy experience recurrent unprovoked seizures, which are characterized by abnormal electrical activity in the brain. Sleep disturbance is common in epilepsy and is related to several factors, including nocturnal seizures, antiepileptic medications, comorbid psychiatric disorders, and comorbid sleep disorders such as OSA.[56]

OSA is common in epilepsy, with a prevalence of approximately 10% in unselected adults with epilepsy and up to 30% in patients with refractory epilepsy.[57] Predictors of a diagnosis of OSA in epilepsy include male sex, older age, obesity, and higher seizure frequency.[58,59] Both seizures and epilepsy treatments, including antiepileptic drugs and vagus nerve stimulators, contribute to the increased incidence of OSA in epilepsy.[60]

OSA likely increases seizure frequency in patients with epilepsy.[60] In addition, OSA adversely affects mood, cognitive function, and quality of life in epilepsy patients.[57] Treatment of OSA in epilepsy with CPAP likely improves seizure control, particularly in the setting of medically refractory epilepsy.[58,61,62] Patients with epilepsy on stable antiepileptic drug regimens who are compliant with CPAP have better seizure control compared with pre-CPAP baseline, whereas noncompliant CPAP-users do not experience any change in seizure control.[63]

CSA is less common than OSA, although the prevalence of CSA in epilepsy is uncertain. A recent retrospective study of epilepsy patients referred for polysomnography found that 75% had OSA, 3.7% had CSA, and 7.9% had mixed CSA and OSA.[64] Focal seizures were more prevalent in patients with CSA compared with patients with OSA alone or with mixed CSA and OSA. Ictal or postictal central apneas during sleep have been described in case reports and are considered a possible risk factor for sudden unexplained death in epilepsy.[65–67] Further research is needed regarding the prevalence of CSA in epilepsy.

SDB of Other Neurologic Causes

There are many other neurologic conditions that have been associated with SDB. Both disturbed sleep and SDB are common in spinal cord injury.[68] Patients with spinal cord injury are susceptible to SDB due to muscle weakness, including muscles of respiration, as well as use of sedating medications for pain or spasticity.[68] Patients with spinal cord injury are at risk of OSA and hypoventilation in sleep particularly during REM sleep.[68,69] SDB is more likely with higher levels of spinal cord lesion. Treatment options include positive airway pressure, noninvasive ventilation, or mechanical ventilation via tracheostomy depending on the severity and type of SDB. Chiari malformations, which are acquired or congenital herniations of the cerebellum through the foramen magnum with the potential to cause brainstem compression, have been associated with CSA and OSA.[70] SDB may be reversible with surgical decompression. Posterior fossa tumors have also been associated with SDB.[71] SDB can occur with involvement of the cerebellar peduncles, even in the absence of brainstem involvement.[71]

Acquired central alveolar hypoventilation

Acquired central alveolar hypoventilation (CAH) (previously known as Ondine curse) is a condition characterized by loss of automatic breathing during sleep. CAH is very rare and is described in case reports in the literature.[72,73] CAH can be caused by brainstem damage resulting from tumors, anoxic ischemic damage or infection. It can also be caused by brainstem ischemia or demyelination (see above discussion). Treatment options include mechanical ventilatory support at night or diaphragmatic pacing.[74]

SUMMARY

SDB is common in neurologic disorders that affect the central and/or peripheral nervous system. SDB and neurologic disorders have an important bidirectional impact. Identification and treatment of SDB is an important aspect of treating patients with neurologic disease. More research is needed to clarify the prevalence and optimal treatment of SDB.

REFERENCES

1. AASM. The International classification of sleep disorders, 2nd edition: diagnostic and coding manual. Westchester (IL): American Academy of Sleep Medicine; 2005.
2. Perrin C, Unterborn JN, Ambrosio CD, et al. Pulmonary complications of chronic neuromuscular diseases and their management. Muscle Nerve 2004;29(1):5–27.
3. Available at: www.alsa.org/about-als/who-gets-als.html. Accessed October 20, 2013.
4. Bhat S, Gupta D, Chokroverty S. Sleep disorders in neuromuscular diseases. Neurol Clin 2012;30(4):1359–87.
5. Miller RG, Jackson CE, Kasarskis EJ, et al. Practice parameter update: the care of the patient with amyotrophic lateral sclerosis: multidisciplinary care, symptom management, and cognitive/behavioral impairment (an evidence-based review): report of the Quality Standards Subcommittee of the American Academy of Neurology. Neurology 2009; 73(15):1227–33.
6. Miller RG, Jackson CE, Kasarskis EJ, et al. Practice parameter update: the care of the patient with amyotrophic lateral sclerosis: drug, nutritional, and respiratory therapies (an evidence-based review): report of the Quality Standards Subcommittee of the American Academy of Neurology. Neurology 2009;73(15):1218–26.
7. Quera-Salva MA, Guilleminault C, Chevret S, et al. Breathing disorders during sleep in myasthenia gravis. Ann Neurol 1992;31(1):86–92.
8. Available at: www.myasthena.org/healthprofessionals/clinicaloverviewofMG.aspx. Accessed October 20, 2013.
9. Prudlo J, Koenig J, Ermert S, et al. Sleep disordered breathing in medically stable patients with myasthenia gravis. Eur J Neurol 2007;14(3):321–6.
10. Benditt JO, Boitano LJ. Pulmonary issues in patients with chronic neuromuscular disease. Am J Respir Crit Care Med 2013;187(10):1046–55.
11. Laberge L, Gagnon C, Dauvilliers Y. Daytime sleepiness and myotonic dystrophy. Curr Neurol Neurosci Rep 2013;13(4):340.
12. Dauvilliers YA, Laberge L. Myotonic dystrophy type 1, daytime sleepiness and REM sleep dysregulation. Sleep Med Rev 2012;16(6):539–45.
13. Ono S, Kanda F, Takahashi K, et al. Neuronal loss in the medullary reticular formation in myotonic

dystrophy: a clinicopathological study. Neurology 1996;46(1):228–31.

14. Romigi A, Albanese M, Placidi F, et al. Sleep disorders in myotonic dystrophy type 2: a controlled polysomnographic study and self-reported questionnaires. Eur J Neurol 2014;1(6):929–34.

15. Bhat S, Sander HW, Grewal RP, et al. Sleep disordered breathing and other sleep dysfunction in myotonic dystrophy type 2. Sleep Med 2012; 13(9):1207–8.

16. Available at: http://www.cdc.gov/ncbddd/muscular dystrophy/data.html. Accessed October 30, 2013.

17. Pithadia AB, Kakadia N. Guillain-Barre syndrome (GBS). Pharmacol Rep 2010;62(2):220–32.

18. Karkare K, Sinha S, Taly AB, et al. Prevalence and profile of sleep disturbances in Guillain-Barre syndrome: a prospective questionnaire-based study during 10 days of hospitalization. Acta Neurol Scand 2013;127(2):116–23.

19. Bassetti CL, Gugger M. Sleep disordered breathing in neurologic disorders. Swiss Med Wkly 2002;132(9–10):109–15.

20. Panossian L, Daley J. Sleep-disordered breathing. Continuum (Minneap Minn) 2013;19(1 Sleep Disorders):86–103.

21. Steier J, Jolley CJ, Seymour J, et al. Screening for sleep-disordered breathing in neuromuscular disease using a questionnaire for symptoms associated with diaphragm paralysis. Eur Respir J 2011;37(2):400–5.

22. Berry RB, Chediak A, Brown LK, et al. Best clinical practices for the sleep center adjustment of noninvasive positive pressure ventilation (NPPV) in stable chronic alveolar hypoventilation syndromes. J Clin Sleep Med 2010;6(5):491–509.

23. Gaig C, Iranzo A. Sleep-disordered breathing in neurodegenerative diseases. Curr Neurol Neurosci Rep 2012;12(2):205–17.

24. Ferini-Strambi L, Marelli S. Sleep dysfunction in multiple system atrophy. Curr Treat Options Neurol 2012;14(5):464–73.

25. Shimohata T, Ozawa T, Nakayama H, et al. Frequency of nocturnal sudden death in patients with multiple system atrophy. J Neurol 2008; 255(10):1483–5.

26. Yamaguchi M, Arai K, Asahina M, et al. Laryngeal stridor in multiple system atrophy. Eur Neurol 2003;49(3):154–9.

27. Iranzo A, Santamaria J, Tolosa E, et al. Long-term effect of CPAP in the treatment of nocturnal stridor in multiple system atrophy. Neurology 2004;63(5): 930–2.

28. Iranzo A, Santamaria J, Tolosa E. Continuous positive air pressure eliminates nocturnal stridor in multiple system atrophy. Barcelona Multiple System Atrophy Study Group. Lancet 2000;356(9238): 1329–30.

29. Ghorayeb I, Yekhlef F, Bioulac B, et al. Continuous positive airway pressure for sleep-related breathing disorders in multiple system atrophy: long-term acceptance. Sleep Med 2005;6(4):359–62.

30. Iranzo A. Sleep and breathing in multiple system atrophy. Curr Treat Options Neurol 2007;9(5):347–53.

31. Vetrugno R, Provini F, Cortelli P, et al. Sleep disorders in multiple system atrophy: a correlative video-polysomnographic study. Sleep Med 2004; 5(1):21–30.

32. Benarroch EE, Schmeichel AM, Low PA, et al. Depletion of putative chemosensitive respiratory neurons in the ventral medullary surface in multiple system atrophy. Brain 2007;130(Pt 2):469–75.

33. Aurora RN, Chowdhuri S, Ramar K, et al. The treatment of central sleep apnea syndromes in adults: practice parameters with an evidence-based literature review and meta-analyses. Sleep 2012;35(1): 17–40.

34. Shimohata T, Tomita M, Nakayama H, et al. Floppy epiglottis as a contraindication of CPAP in patients with multiple system atrophy. Neurology 2011; 76(21):1841–2.

35. Matthews BR. Alzheimer disease update. Continuum (Minneap Minn) 2010;16(2 Dementia):15–30.

36. Boeve BF. Update on the diagnosis and management of sleep disturbances in dementia. Sleep Med Clin 2008;3(3):347–60.

37. Ancoli-Israel S, Klauber MR, Butters N, et al. Dementia in institutionalized elderly: relation to sleep apnea. J Am Geriatr Soc 1991;39(3):258–63.

38. Bliwise DL. Is sleep apnea a cause of reversible dementia in old age? J Am Geriatr Soc 1996; 44(11):1407–9.

39. Yaffe K, Laffan AM, Harrison SL, et al. Sleep-disordered breathing, hypoxia, and risk of mild cognitive impairment and dementia in older women. JAMA 2011;306(6):613–9.

40. Ayalon L, Ancoli-Israel S, Stepnowsky C, et al. Adherence to continuous positive airway pressure treatment in patients with Alzheimer's disease and obstructive sleep apnea. Am J Geriatr Psychiatry 2006;14(2):176–80.

41. Chong MS, Ayalon L, Marler M, et al. Continuous positive airway pressure reduces subjective daytime sleepiness in patients with mild to moderate Alzheimer's disease with sleep disordered breathing. J Am Geriatr Soc 2006;54(5):777–81.

42. Ancoli-Israel S, Palmer BW, Cooke JR, et al. Cognitive effects of treating obstructive sleep apnea in Alzheimer's disease: a randomized controlled study. J Am Geriatr Soc 2008;56(11):2076–81.

43. Cooke JR, Ayalon L, Palmer BW, et al. Sustained use of CPAP slows deterioration of cognition, sleep, and mood in patients with Alzheimer's disease and obstructive sleep apnea: a preliminary study. J Clin Sleep Med 2009;5(4):305–9.

44. Bliwise DL. Alzheimer's disease, sleep apnea, and positive pressure therapy. Curr Treat Options Neurol 2013;15(6):669–76.

45. Fleming WE, Pollak CP. Sleep disorders in multiple sclerosis. Semin Neurol 2005;25(1):64–8.

46. Ferini-Strambi L. Sleep disorders in multiple sclerosis. Handb Clin Neurol 2011;99:1139–46.

47. Caminero A, Bartolome M. Sleep disturbances in multiple sclerosis. J Neurol Sci 2011;309(1–2): 86–91.

48. Veauthier C, Radbruch H, Gaede G, et al. Fatigue in multiple sclerosis is closely related to sleep disorders: a polysomnographic cross-sectional study. Mult Scler 2011;17(5):613–22.

49. Braley TJ, Segal BM, Chervin RD. Sleep-disordered breathing in multiple sclerosis. Neurology 2012;79(9):929–36.

50. Hermann DM, Bassetti CL. Sleep-related breathing and sleep-wake disturbances in ischemic stroke. Neurology 2009;73(16):1313–22.

51. Bassetti CL, Hermann DM. Sleep and stroke. Handb Clin Neurol 2011;99:1051–72.

52. Siccoli MM, Valko PO, Hermann DM, et al. Central periodic breathing during sleep in 74 patients with acute ischemic stroke - neurogenic and cardiogenic factors. J Neurol 2008;255(11):1687–92.

53. Hermann DM, Siccoli M, Kirov P, et al. Central periodic breathing during sleep in acute ischemic stroke. Stroke 2007;38(3):1082–4.

54. Parra O, Arboix A, Bechich S, et al. Time course of sleep-related breathing disorders in first-ever stroke or transient ischemic attack. Am J Respir Crit Care Med 2000;161(2 Pt 1):375–80.

55. Tomfohr LM, Hemmen T, Natarajan L, et al. Continuous positive airway pressure for treatment of obstructive sleep apnea in stroke survivors: what do we really know? Stroke 2012;43(11):3118–23.

56. van Golde EG, Gutter T, de Weerd AW. Sleep disturbances in people with epilepsy; prevalence, impact and treatment. Sleep Med Rev 2011;15(6): 357–68.

57. Manni R, Terzaghi M. Comorbidity between epilepsy and sleep disorders. Epilepsy Res 2010; 90(3):171–7.

58. Li P, Ghadersohi S, Jafari B, et al. Characteristics of refractory vs. medically controlled epilepsy patients with obstructive sleep apnea and their response to CPAP treatment. Seizure 2012;21(9): 717–21.

59. Manni R, Terzaghi M, Arbasino C, et al. Obstructive sleep apnea in a clinical series of adult epilepsy patients: frequency and features of the comorbidity. Epilepsia 2003;44(6):836–40.

60. Eriksson SH. Epilepsy and sleep. Curr Opin Neurol 2011;24(2):171–6.

61. Vaughn BV, D'Cruz OF, Beach R, et al. Improvement of epileptic seizure control with treatment of obstructive sleep apnoea. Seizure 1996;5(1):73–8.

62. Malow BA, Foldvary-Schaefer N, Vaughn BV, et al. Treating obstructive sleep apnea in adults with epilepsy: a randomized pilot trial. Neurology 2008; 71(8):572–7.

63. Vendrame M, Auerbach S, Loddenkemper T, et al. Effect of continuous positive airway pressure treatment on seizure control in patients with obstructive sleep apnea and epilepsy. Epilepsia 2011;52(11): e168–71.

64. Vendrame M, Jackson S, Syed S, et al. Central sleep apnea and complex sleep apnea in patients with epilepsy. Sleep Breath 2014;18(1):119–24.

65. So EL, Sam MC, Lagerlund TL. Postictal central apnea as a cause of SUDEP: evidence from near-SUDEP incident. Epilepsia 2000;41(11):1494–7.

66. Nadkarni MA, Friedman D, Devinsky O. Central apnea at complex partial seizure onset. Seizure 2012; 21(7):555–8.

67. Schuele SU, Afshari M, Afshari ZS, et al. Ictal central apnea as a predictor for sudden unexpected death in epilepsy. Epilepsy Behav 2011;22(2):401–3.

68. Biering-Sorensen F, Jennum P, Laub M. Sleep disordered breathing following spinal cord injury. Respir Physiol Neurobiol 2009;169(2):165–70.

69. Castriotta RJ, Murthy JN. Hypoventilation after spinal cord injury. Semin Respir Crit Care Med 2009; 30(3):330–8.

70. Zolty P, Sanders MH, Pollack IF. Chiari malformation and sleep-disordered breathing: a review of diagnostic and management issues. Sleep 2000; 23(5):637–43.

71. Lee A, Chen ML, Abeshaus S, et al. Posterior fossa tumors and their impact on sleep and ventilatory control: a clinical perspective. Respir Physiol Neurobiol 2013;189(2):261–71.

72. Kuhn M, Lutolf M, Reinhart WH. The eye catcher. Ondine's curse. Respiration 1999;66(3):265.

73. Heckmann JG, Ernst S. Central alveolar hypoventilation (Ondine's Curse) caused by megadolichobasilar artery. J Stroke Cerebrovasc Dis 2014;23(2): 390–2.

74. Mendoza M, Latorre JG. Pearls and oy-sters: reversible Ondine's curse in a case of lateral medullary infarction. Neurology 2013;80(2):e13–6.

Medication Effects on Sleep and Breathing

Gilbert Seda, MD, PhD[a],*, Sheila Tsai, MD[b], Teofilo Lee-Chiong, MD[c]

KEYWORDS

- Obstructive sleep apnea • Central sleep apnea • Hypnotics • Benzodiazepines • Antipsychotics
- Estrogen • Progesterone • Testosterone

KEY POINTS

- Benzodiazepines are generally safe in low doses but in higher doses and in select patients they may be associated with respiratory depression, hypoventilation, hypoxemia, and obstructive sleep apnea (OSA).
- Narcotics can be associated with apneas and hypoventilation with increased risk with higher doses and use of other central nervous system depressants.
- Nonbenzodiazepine hypnotics, acetazolamide, and theophylline promote stable respirations at high altitude.
- Antidepressants may partially improve OSA by suppressing stage rapid eye movement and increasing upper airway tone but do not completely treat OSA.
- Hormonal therapy may effect sleep-disordered breathing and hypoventilation.
- Nasal steroids and leukotriene antagonists improve OSA by improving nasal airway resistance.

INTRODUCTION

Respiration during sleep is regulated by circadian, endocrine, mechanical, and chemical factors. The volitional control of breathing during wakefulness is abolished during sleep and the hypercapnic threshold is increased.[1] Furthermore, the diminished hypoxic and hypercapnic ventilatory responses are more pronounced in rapid eye movement (REM) sleep compared with non-REM (NREM) sleep.[2] Sleep stage also affects the respiratory pattern. Periodic breathing can be observed in stages N1 or N2 of NREM sleep. In contrast, respiration is stable and regular during stage N3 sleep.[3] Stage REM is characterized by an irregular respiratory pattern. Additionally, REM-associated atonia in which the diaphragm remains the sole primary muscle of respiration may be associated with severe respiratory events.[4] Tidal volume and minute ventilation decrease during sleep and functional residual capacity is reduced.[5] Finally, upper airway (UA) dilator muscle tone decreases during sleep; this may increase the risk of sleep-disordered breathing (SDB).[6]

Medications can alter respiration during sleep through a variety of mechanisms. During sleep, medications can suppress the chemical or neural control of respiration resulting in central or obstructive apneas, hypopneas, hypoxemia, or hypoventilation. Medications can also alter sleep architecture by decreasing arousals, reducing the distribution of stage REM, or increasing the

Disclosure: No conflicts of interest to declare.
Disclaimer: The opinions expressed herein are those of the authors and do not necessarily reflect those of the Department of the Navy, Department of Defense, the US government, or any of its agencies.
[a] Department of Pulmonary and Sleep Medicine, Naval Medical Center San Diego, 34730 Bob Wilson Drive, Building 3-3, Suite 301, San Diego, CA 92134, USA; [b] Division of Pulmonary, Critical Care and Sleep Medicine, National Jewish Health, 1400 Jackson Street, Denver, CO 80206, USA; [c] Division of Pulmonary and Critical Care Medicine, National Jewish Health, University of Colorado, 1400 Jackson Street, Denver, CO 80206, USA
* Corresponding author.
E-mail address: gilbert.seda@gmail.com

Clin Chest Med 35 (2014) 557–569
http://dx.doi.org/10.1016/j.ccm.2014.06.011
0272-5231/14/$ – see front matter Published by Elsevier Inc.

duration of N2 or N3 sleep stages with secondary consequences on respiratory patterns. Medications can also improve respiration during sleep by functioning as respiratory stimulants or by increasing UA tone. Patient factors such as obesity, medical disorder such as chronic obstructive pulmonary disease (COPD) or asthma, psychiatric disorders, sleep disorders, and concomitant medication use can also influence a specific-agent effect on breathing during sleep.

SEDATIVE HYPNOTIC AGENTS
Benzodiazepines

Gamma-amino butyric acid (GABA) is the principle inhibitory neurotransmitter in the central nervous system (CNS). Benzodiazepines are widely used hypnotics and bind nonselectively to the pentameric $GABA_A$ receptor resulting in CNS inhibition.[7] Benzodiazepine hypnotics differ in duration of action, absorption, and potency. As a class, they reduce sleep latency (SOL), increase total sleep time (TST), decrease wake after sleep onset (WASO), and improve sleep quality. They increase N2 sleep and suppress N3 sleep. They increase REM latency and increase the number of spindles known as pseudospindles.[8]

Benzodiazepines can affect respiration during sleep through their sedative effects, suppression of arousals, and myorelaxation properties, or by increasing N2 sleep. Although considered respiratory depressants, they are generally safe in low doses. Stege and colleagues[9] investigated breathing and gas exchange during sleep in subjects with severe COPD but no baseline hypercapnia. Compared with placebo, temazepam was not associated with worsening hypoxemia, hypercapnia, or apnea-hypopnea index (AHI). A limitation of the study was the low doses of temazepam tested. Triazolam, a short-acting hypnotic, was also shown to have no adverse effects on respiration in subjects with COPD.[10] However, in another trial of subjects with mild-to-moderate OSA, temazepam (10 mg) was associated with greater respiratory impairment in subjects with a higher chemosensitivity in wakefulness.[11] Hypoxemia worsened during sleep but SDB did not.

Benzodiazepines can improve periodic breathing that develops at high altitude. These agents reduce wakefulness and augment stage N3 during the period of acclimatization after ascent. Dubowitz[12] studied the effects of temazepam 10 mg at 5300 m after acclimatization. Subjects taking temazepam versus placebo had fewer arousals, reduced periodic breathing, and a decreased frequency and severity of nocturnal oxygen desaturation. In another high-altitude study, temazepam reduced periodic breathing but was associated with a small decrease in mean nocturnal oxygen saturation (SaO_2).[13]

Other investigators have demonstrated that benzodiazepine administration resulted in adverse effects during early ascent to high altitude. Röggla and colleagues[14] performed a crossover trial comparing temazepam (10 mg) and placebo in 7 healthy men at 171 m and 3000 m. Measuring arterial blood gas at the two different elevations, they noted that temazepam use increased hypoxemia and hypercapnia at the moderate altitude.

Benzodiazepines can worsen SDB, hypoventilation, hypoxemia, and hypercapnia, and can increase UA collapsibility during sleep. Elderly patients taking higher doses of benzodiazepines, patients using agents with longer half-lives or agents with active metabolites, patients with underlying lung disease such as COPD, and those concomitantly using other sedative medications or substances such as narcotics or alcohol are more susceptible to adverse effects.[15] Flurazepam has been associated with increased apnea frequency, longer apnea duration, and worse oxygen desaturation during sleep.[16] In another study, flurazepam at high doses (30 mg) but not at lower doses (15 mg) increased SDB events in subjects with COPD.[17,18] Genta and colleagues[19] demonstrated the critical closing pressure (Pcrit) of the UA during midazolam-induced sleep is similar to the Pcrit during natural sleep.

Overall, the data suggest that low-dose benzodiazepines are relatively safe for patients with underlying lung disease or SDB and may improve periodic breathing associated with ascent to high altitude.

Nonbenzodiazepine Hypnotics

Nonbenzodiazepine sedative hypnotics include zolpidem, eszopiclone, and zaleplon. They promote sleep by acting on a subset of the $GABA_A$ receptors. These agents have no significant adverse effects on respiratory patterns or SaO_2. The nonbenzodiazepine hypnotics have been investigated for treatment of high altitude periodic breathing, central apnea, and obstructive apnea. They have also been shown to enhance short-term adherence to continuous positive airway pressure (CPAP) therapy compliance.[20]

Eckert and colleagues[21] investigated the effect of eszopiclone on OSA. Seventeen subjects with OSA without significant nocturnal hypoxemia received eszopiclone (3 mg) or placebo. Eszopiclone increased arousal threshold and sleep duration, improved sleep quality, and lowered AHI without prolonging respiratory events or worsening hypoxemia. The subgroup of subjects with a lower arousal threshold from stage N1 to N2 sleep had greater opportunity to enable sufficient UA dilator muscle recruitment, thereby increasing airway patency and improving respiration.

Rosenberg and colleagues[22] reported that, in subjects with mild-to-moderate OSA, eszopiclone improved sleep maintenance and efficiency and did not worsen AHI, SaO_2, or duration of apneas and hypopneas. In a prospective, double-blind, placebo-controlled trial, pretreatment with eszopiclone 3 mg improved the quality of CPAP titration by reducing SOL, improving sleep efficiency (SE), reducing WASO and prolonging TST, which collectively resulted in fewer poor quality studies.[23]

Coyle and colleagues[24] also observed that short-acting, nonbenzodiazepine hypnotic agents are safe in middle-aged subjects with mild-to-moderate OSA, who are receiving CPAP therapy in the home environment. Using home monitoring, they studied 15 mild-to-moderate subjects with OSA for the presence of worsening apnea during zaleplon use. There were no statistically significant treatment differences between zaleplon and placebo in AHI, apneas, hypopneas, or mean SaO_2. The zaleplon group, however, had a lower SaO_2 nadir. Steens and colleagues[25] compared zolpidem with triazolam to determine the effects on respiration in subjects with mild-to-moderate COPD; neither agent had adverse effects on respiration during sleep.

Zolpidem may also be useful in the treatment of central sleep apnea (CSA). In a case series, 20 subjects with idiopathic CSA received zolpidem (20 mg) for an average of 9 weeks. Zolpidem use was associated with reduced arousals, improved SE, and decreased central apnea hypopnea index but not with worse hypoxemia.[26]

Nonbenzodiazepine hypnotics have also been used for periodic breathing at high altitude. Beaumont and colleagues[27] studied the effects of zolpidem 10 mg and zaleplon 10 mg on sleep and respiration at high altitude (4000 m). Both zolpidem and zaleplon improved slow wave sleep; changes were more marked with zolpidem. Nocturnal respiration and daytime cognitive and physical performance were not adversely affected. In another double-blind, placebo-controlled, crossover trial, this research team noted that zolpidem and zaleplon had positive effects on sleep at altitude without adversely affecting respiration, attention, alertness, or mood.[28] Both hypnotic agents increased SE, WASO, and increased stage N3 sleep without adverse effects on nocturnal SaO_2.

Girault and colleagues[29] investigated the effects of zolpidem on nocturnal respiratory function in 10 subjects with stable COPD. Zolpidem had no significant effect on apnea index, mean SaO_2, or duration of SaO_2 less than 90%. Thus, use of zolpidem in COPD patients does not alter nocturnal respiration, sleep architecture, pulmonary function tests, central control of breathing, and physical performance.

Melatonin Agonist

Ramelteon is a hypnotic with a unique mechanism of action. It functions as a melatonin agonist binding to melatonin-1 and melatonin-2 receptors. It is used to treat insomnia and has a short half-life. It has no CNS depressant effects and, therefore, does not affect respiration during sleep. Several studies report that ramelteon is safe and effective in patients with mild-to-moderate OSA and mild-to-severe COPD.[30–32] Ramelteon has not been associated with respiratory depression, abnormal respiratory patterns, or nocturnal oxygen desaturation even when the recommended dose was doubled.

NARCOTICS

A substantial number of patients receive narcotics for management of pain. Narcotics can induce respiratory depression by actions on the brainstem respiratory center, central and peripheral chemoreceptors, and actions on decreasing respiratory effort in response to airway resistance.[33,34] Narcotics reduce the hypoxic and hypercapnic ventilatory drive during sleep.[35] Besides hypoxemia and hypoventilation, narcotics are associated with central and obstructive apneas. There is an increased risk of adverse reactions with narcotics in the elderly, in patients on higher doses of medication, in those with medical comorbidities such as morbid obesity and COPD in which respiration is altered, and concurrent use of other CNS depressants. Abnormal respiratory patterns such as ataxic breathing during NREM sleep and Biot breathing patterns are associated with the use of narcotics.[36]

Sharkey and colleagues[37] investigated obstructive and CSA in subjects on methadone maintenance therapy. OSA was observed in 35% of subjects and CSA was noted in 14% of subjects. OSA was associated with higher body mass index (BMI) and longer duration on methadone maintenance therapy. Risk factors for CSA included prior structural damage from drugs of abuse, disrupted hypoxic or hypercapnic respiratory responses, and concurrent use of antidepressants and benzodiazepines. Teichtahl and colleagues[38] found subjects on methadone maintenance therapy had a diminished ventilatory response to hypercapnia, but an increased ventilatory response to hypoxemia. In a case series, three subjects on opiates developed irregular breathing patterns characteristic of Biot or ataxic breathing.[36] This pattern of breathing is related to a morphine equivalent dose of greater than 200 mg daily.[33]

Although endogenous opioids are postulated to have a central depressive effect on the stability of the UA resulting in suppression of the hypercapnic drive, opioid antagonists may increase respiratory drive. Naloxone is a short-acting opiate antagonist and naltrexone is a long-acting opiate antagonist. Both have been investigated for treatment of OSA. Meurice and colleagues[39] showed that an infusion of naloxone reduced UA collapsibility following sleep fragmentation. Atkinson and colleagues[40] gave a naloxone infusion to 10 obese subjects with OSA and found that 9 out of 10 subjects had a lower desaturation index with naloxone; however, REM sleep decreased by 80% in subjects with stage REM. Naltrexone also reduces the number and magnitude of hypoxemia and hypercapnic events during sleep in patients with OSA; however, this is not considered the standard of care for treating OSA.[41]

ANTIHISTAMINES

Antihistamines are widely used medications in allergic diseases and asthma and insomnia. First-generation antihistamines are nonselective histamine antagonists, cross the blood brain barrier, and may have antimuscarinic, anti–α-adrenergic, and sedative effects.[42] Few studies have investigated the effects of antihistamines on respiratory function but respiratory depression has not been reported.[43–46] They are generally effective for insomnia in the elderly without respiratory complications.[47]

Because antihistamines in infants are implicated in apparent life-threatening events and sudden infant death syndrome, McKelvey and colleagues[48] investigated the effects of promethazine on airway protective mechanisms and cardiorespiratory function in 42 neonatal piglets. Promethazine significantly decreased the spontaneous occurrence of swallowing and arousal, and increased the occurrence of both CSA and OSA. Low-dose promethazine profoundly altered sleep characteristics, airway protective mechanisms, and cardiorespiratory responses in normal healthy sleeping piglets.

Antihistamines are not associated with respiratory depression. Alexander and colleagues[49] evaluated the effects of diphenhydramine on hypercapnic and hypoxic ventilatory control in healthy volunteers. Diphenhydramine did not affect the ventilatory response to carbon dioxide (CO_2) during hyperoxia or the ventilatory response to hypoxia at an end-tidal CO_2 tension ($PetCO_2$) of 46 mm Hg. Diphenhydramine augmented the hypoxic response under conditions of hypercapnia in young healthy volunteers.

In patients receiving narcotics, antihistamines are often used as antiemetics and antipruritics. In patients receiving alfentanil infusion, diphenhydramine counteracted the alfentanil-induced decrease in the slope of the ventilatory response to CO_2.[50] However, at $PetCO_2$ of 46 mm Hg, it did not significantly alter the alfentanil-induced shift in the CO_2 response curve. In addition, diphenhydramine does not exacerbate the opioid-induced depression of the hypoxic ventilatory response during moderate hypercarbia.

GABAPENTIN AND PREGABALIN

Gabapentin is used for treatment of partial seizures, neuropathic pain, restless legs syndrome, and behavioral agitation.[51–53] It is a reversible inhibitor of GABA transaminase and can have an inhibitory effect on the medullary respiratory center. There are two case reports of hypoventilation with use of gabapentin. In one an elderly man with COPD taking clonazepam and zolpidem developed hypercapnic respiratory failure with the addition of gabapentin.[54] In the other, central hypoventilation occurred with insomnia.[55]

Pregabalin is used for neuropathic pain, postoperative pain management, and restless legs syndrome (RLS). Eipe and Penning[56] report three cases of subjects receiving pregabalin in the postoperative period that developed respiratory depression. The first involved an elderly subject with borderline renal dysfunction. The second subject presented with severe respiratory depression 12 hours after receiving a spinal anesthetic for joint replacement, and was later found to have clinically significant OSA. The third subject was a healthy elderly individual on benzodiazepines for anxiety, who experienced respiratory arrest in the postanesthesia care unit after an uneventful surgery for lumbar spine decompression.

SODIUM OXYBATE

Sodium oxybate is a CNS sedative used to treat hypersomnia and cataplexy associated with narcolepsy. Its mechanism of action is CNS inhibition via actions at the $GABA_B$ and gamma hydroxylbutyrate receptors. Although generally safe with proper administration, it has an increased risk of CSA and worsening nocturnal hypoxemia in patients with OSA. Overdose can result in respiratory depression, coma, and death. Oxybate-induced obstructive apneas have been reported.[57] Sodium oxybate-induced central apneas were reported in a 39-year-old woman with narcolepsy.[58] Zvosec and colleagues[59] report three deaths associated with the use of sodium oxybate that are presumed secondary to respiratory depression.

STIMULANTS

Stimulant agents include over-the-counter agents such as caffeine, which antagonizes adenosine and inhibits phosphodiesterase; medications for attention deficit hyperactivity disorder (ADHD) such as methylphenidate, which increase the synaptic availability of monoamines such as dopamine, norepinephrine, and serotonin; substances such as nicotine, which increase central cholinergic neurons; and wake-promoting agents including modafinil and armodafinil. These medications generally have no effects on respiration during sleep. They may indirectly improve OSA by promoting weight loss.

Modafinil and armodafinil are approved by the Food and Drug Administration for treatment of narcolepsy, shift work sleep disorder, and residual sleepiness despite treatment of OSA. They do not alter respiration during sleep. Modafinil has been shown to be effective and well-tolerated in the adjunctive treatment of OSA.[60] Armodafinil use in patients with residual daytime sleepiness on CPAP demonstrated no significant effects on nighttime sleep, as assessed by polysomnogram.[61]

Winslow and colleagues[62] conducted a randomized, double-blind, placebo-controlled trial involving 45 individuals with moderate-to-severe OSA with a BMI of 30 to 40 kg/m² not receiving positive pressure therapy. Subjects received a combination of phentermine and extended-release topiramate. There was a significant decline in AHI, and improvement in nocturnal oxygenation that was attributed to drug-associated weight loss.

PSYCHIATRIC MEDICATIONS
Antidepressants

Antidepressants may benefit patients with OSA by suppressing stage REM sleep, increasing UA patency, and by central respiratory stimulant effects. Protriptyline improves oxygenation by reducing REM-associated apneas.[63] Smith and colleagues[64] studied protriptyline in 12 subjects with moderate-to-severe OSA. Treatment with protriptyline resulted in a reduction in the amount of stage REM sleep, and improvement in apnea

severity and nocturnal oxygenation. Hanzel and colleagues[65] compared the effect of fluoxetine with protriptyline in 12 subjects with OSA. Although there was variability in the response to each antidepressant, 6 of the 12 subjects had favorable responses, including improvement in oxygenation, to either fluoxetine or protriptyline; however, fluoxetine was better tolerated.

Atomoxetine is a norepinephrine reuptake inhibitor used for ADHD. Bart Sangal and colleagues[66] investigated whether atomoxetine would improve respiration in subjects with OSA similar to protriptyline. Subjects with a respiratory disturbance index (RDI) greater than 5 demonstrated improvement in daytime sleepiness but had no significant change in RDI.

Decreased serotonergic activity of UA neurons has been postulated as a risk factor for UA collapse. Mirtazapine is a 5HT2 and 5HT3 receptor antagonist. In animal studies, 5HT3 antagonists have been shown to reduce apneas in stages REM and NREM sleep.[67] Two studies investigate mirtazapine in OSA. In seven subjects with OSA, mirtazapine reduced the AHI by 50%.[68] In another trial investigating the effectiveness of mirtazapine for OSA, there was no improvement in OSA and the drug increased weight that might, in turn, further worsen OSA.[69]

Paroxetine, a selective serotonin reuptake inhibitor, has been investigated for treatment of OSA. The postulated mechanism is increased genioglossus muscle activity during sleep to maintain UA patency. In one study of male OSA subjects, paroxetine reduced the apnea index during NREM but not REM sleep.[70] There was no significant effect on hypopnea indices. Berry and colleagues[71] studied paroxetine (40 mg) in 8 men with OSA. Although paroxetine increased genioglossus activity during NREM sleep it had no significant effect on the frequency of OSA.

Atypical Antipsychotics

Atypical antipsychotics are prescribed for mood and psychotic disorders. They antagonize postsynaptic serotonin receptors and dopamine receptors, have sedative effects, and can worsen OSA independent of their weight-promoting effects. Winkelman[72] used logistical regression to investigate the risk factors for OSA in psychiatric patients. These included obesity, male gender, and chronic neuroleptic administration. In a retrospective study, subjects receiving atypical antipsychotics had more severe AHIs compared with subjects not taking atypical antipsychotics, despite similar BMI and neck circumference.[73] In a retrospective review of polysomnogram data in

200 subjects with a depressive disorder compared with 331 healthy controls, the use of atypical antipsychotics increased the risk of OSA independent of age, sex, BMI, and neck circumference.[74]

There are case reports associating atypical antipsychotics with respiratory complications during sleep, particularly in the elderly, patients with medical comorbidities, and those using concomitant CNS depressants. Kohen and Sarcevic[75] report a case of a geriatric patient developing CSA with aripiprazole. CSA resolved when the medication was withdrawn. There are two case reports of hyperventilation associated with quetiapine.[76,77] Jabeen and colleagues[78] report a case of acute respiratory failure in a 92-year-old man with COPD after a single dose of quetiapine 50 mg. Freudenmann and colleagues[79] report two adverse respiratory events with quetiapine in obese subjects with OSA. In one case, acute respiratory failure and coma occurred after a single normal dose of quetiapine when combined with lorazepam. In the second case, quetiapine was associated with nocturnal respiratory dysfunction and delirium in a subject who received operative treatment with OSA.

RESPIRATORY AGENTS
Nasal Steroids

Nasal airflow resistance can contribute to UA obstruction during sleep. Fluticasone has been shown to lower the AHI in snorers and patients with OSA.[80] Furthermore, a 6-week treatment with intranasal budesonide decreased the severity OSA syndrome and the magnitude of adenoidal hypertrophy.[81] The budesonide effect persisted up to 8 weeks after cessation of therapy. A combination of intranasal budesonide and montelukast, a leukotriene antagonist, effectively treated children with residual OSA after adeonotonsillectomy.[82]

Acetazolamide

Acetazolamide is the most studied medication for sleep disturbances at altitude as well as for treating acute mountain sickness (AMS).[83] Its primary action is the enzymatic inhibition of CO_2 to carbonic acid in a wide array of sites, including kidney, peripheral chemoreceptors, red blood cells, and brain.[84] Antagonism of carbonic anhydrase results in the accumulation of CO_2, which may increase cerebral blood flow and stimulate central chemoreceptors. Administration of acetazolamide at altitude stabilizes ventilator control by stimulating ventilation, improving oxygenation and increasing hypocapnia. Acetazolamide acts primarily on the kidney to produce a metabolic acidosis, and not by affecting chemoreceptor sensitivity. It decreases periodic breathing during sleep via metabolic acidosis-mediated chemical stimulation of respiration. Acetazolamide has been shown to eliminate central apneas at both low and high altitudes.[85]

Nussbaumer-Ochsner and colleagues[86] conducted a randomized controlled trial to determine the effectiveness of acetazolamide in subjects with OSA at altitude. Subjects discontinued use of CPAP and took acetazolamide (250 mg twice a day). Acetazolamide improved oxygenation, decreased breathing disturbances, and enhanced sleep quality. Latshang and colleagues[87] investigated the combined effects of autotitrating CPAP and acetazolamide in subjects with OSA who traveled to altitude. Subject with OSA undergoing 3 days at moderate altitude benefitted from autotitrating CPAP combined with acetazolamide compared with autotitrating CPAP alone. Combination treatment was associated with higher nocturnal saturation and better control of OSA.

Theophylline

Theophylline is a methylxanthine that antagonizes adenosine receptors and is an inhibitor of phosphodiesterase. Adenosine is a respiratory depressant. Theophylline is used for COPD and asthma. It may improve respiration during sleep by blocking adenosine receptors and stimulating respiration.

Theophylline has been used to treat Cheyne-Stokes respiration (CSR) in patients with heart failure. Short-term oral theophylline reduced the number of apneas and hypopneas and decreased the duration of nocturnal desaturation in subjects with compensated heart failure and CSR.[88] Oberndorfer and colleagues[89] investigated the effects of theophylline in snoring, obstructive snorers, and OSA. Subjects with moderate OSA had significant improvement in nocturnal respiration, obstructive snorers showed a tendency to improvement, and snorers were unchanged. A small but clinically insignificant improvement in AHI with theophylline has also been shown in subjects with mild OSA.[90]

Theophylline decreases symptoms of acute mountain sickness and improves sleep acutely after ascent to moderate altitude (3454 m) with improvement in SDB, desaturation index, and arousals.[91] Low-dose, slow-release theophylline reduced AMS and periodic breathing associated with ascent to altitude.[92] Theophylline is a viable alternative to acetazolamide in patients with sulfonamide hypersensitivity. A potential limitation of theophylline is an increased risk of arrhythmias.

Oxygen Therapy

Long-term oxygen therapy has been shown to improve survival and quality of life in patients with COPD.[93] With respect to respiration during sleep, oxygen is an effective treatment of CSA. It also improves SaO_2 in patients with OSA but it may increase the duration of apnea-hypopnea events. Mehta and colleagues[94] conducted a systematic review on the effects of oxygen therapy on OSA. When CPAP was compared with oxygen therapy, all but one subject showed a significant improvement in AHI. Ten studies demonstrated that oxygen therapy improved SaO_2 compared with placebo but the average duration of apnea and hypopnea episodes were longer in subjects receiving oxygen therapy than in those receiving placebo. Chowdhuri and colleagues[95] showed the supplemental oxygen added to positive pressure therapy in veterans taking narcotics reduced CSA.

In infants with Prader-Willi syndrome, oxygen therapy has been shown to significantly reduce the central apnea index.[96]

HORMONAL THERAPY
Estrogen and Progesterone

The prevalence of sleep apnea in women is estimated to be half of that in men.[97] In addition, women seem to have fewer episodes of complete airway occlusion as well as shorter duration of apneas than men.[98] Thus, female gender is thought to be protective from OSA. This protection has been attributed at least partially to estrogen and progesterone. It has been observed that lower levels of progesterone are seen in woman with AHI greater than 10 versus less than 10 events per hour.[99] The benefit of female gender in sleep apnea wanes postmenopause. Although premenopausal women have a decreased incidence of sleep apnea compared with age-matched men, this effect diminishes postmenopause with SDB in postmenopausal women resembling that of SDB in men.[17,100]

Exogenous estrogen and progesterone use may have some beneficial effects on SDB. Studies have shown variable results. One study noted a slight benefit on sleepiness as well as a decrease in the duration, but not number, of events.[101] Another study revealed a decrease in the number of obstructive apneas during sleep and improvement in daytime sleepiness but no significant improvement in the overall AHI.[102] Discontinuing hormonal therapy led to a recurrence of obstructive apneas. Shahar and colleagues[103] looked at the relationship between SDB and replacement hormones in more than 2800 postmenopausal women. There was an inverse relationship between hormone use and SDB, especially in the 50 to 59 age group. This benefit of estrogen and

progestin treatment in decreasing SDB may be seen in as little as 1 week of hormonal therapy.[104]

Estrogen and progesterone therapy in men is less clearly beneficial for management of sleep apnea. In one study with 9 subjects with sleep apnea, 7 days of progesterone therapy led to a statistically significant decrease in the AHI from around 51.1 to 43.6; however, the clinical significance of this decrease is less notable.[105] In 10 men receiving medroxyprogesterone acetate (MPA) versus placebo, no changes in apneas were noted but there was associated decrease in testosterone.[106] In nonhypercapnic men, it seems that MPA does not improve SDB.[107]

Progesterone has also been shown to be a respiratory stimulant. It was administered to 10 subjects resulting in increase in Pao_2 and decrease in $Paco_2$, which reverted to previous values on discontinuation of the therapy. When administered to healthy men, MPA was associated with a decrease in the arterial $Paco_2$.[108] As such, it is considered a respiratory stimulant associated with hyperventilation and hypocapnia; therefore, it may be useful in patients with obesity hypoventilation syndrome.[109]

Although surgically induced menopause has been associated with risk of SDB similar to natural menopause,[101] sex hormone suppression, such as with the gonadotropin releasing hormone leuprolide acetate, has not been associated with a change in SDB.[110]

Testosterone

The gender differences in sleep apnea have also lead to the suspicion of the role of testosterone in SDB. In men, sleep apnea has been associated with low testosterone levels[111] and there seems to be a negative correlation between serum testosterone levels and BMI and testosterone levels and severity of OSA.[112] When CPAP therapy is administered for OSA, serum testosterone levels have been shown to improve.[113]

It has been suspected that testosterone administration worsens sleep apnea. There are significant data that support this hypothesis. In a published case report, a woman with a testosterone-producing tumor had concurrent OSA. When the tumor was resected, her testosterone level normalized and her OSA resolved.[114] Obese women with polycystic ovarian syndrome (PCOS), a condition associated with high testosterone levels and insulin resistance, seem to be at increased risk of OSA.[115] However, this risk seems more closely associated with obesity than with PCOS itself.[116] In another published case report, a 13-year-old male subject received testosterone, which was associated with an increase in UA collapsibility during sleep.[117] With this case in mind, it is proposed that testosterone affects neuromuscular control of UA patency during sleep. Also testosterone administration has been associated with an increase in neck size and tongue thickness.[118] It has been further proposed that it is supraphysiologic rather than physiologic replacement doses that contribute to sleep apnea.[119] High-dose, short-term testosterone worsens OSA. However, when evaluating low-dose testosterone in obese men with OSA, the effects are time-limited. The oxygen desaturation index and nocturnal hypoxemia worsened at 7 weeks but not at 18 weeks.[120] However, androgen blockers do not seem to have an effect on OSA.[121]

Thyroid Hormone

Hypothyroidism is associated with an increased risk of OSA. This may result from a combination of decreased ventilatory responses, UA narrowing from deposition of mucopolysaccharides in UA tissues, hypothyroid myopathy, macroglossia, and obesity.[118] This seems to improve after treatment with thyroxine.[118] There is also some suggestion that apneas disappear in patients with hypothyroidism when they are treated with medroxyprogesterone.[118]

However, this effect is not reproduced when supraphysiologic doses of levothyroxine have been administered to euthyroid study subjects. It resulted in an increase in the heart rate and respiratory rate but did not affect the sleep architecture.[122]

Somatostatin

Acromegaly is associated with OSA, which is thought to be related to changes in UA tissue such as macroglossia. The prevalence of OSA in the acromegalic population is about 50%. Patients with acromegaly controlled with surgery, radiotherapy, and/or somatostatin analogues have a decrease in the prevalence of sleep apnea and an improvement in the AHI when compared with active acromegalic patients. However, the treatments do not often resolve sleep apnea.[123] Somatostatin therapy has been associated with a decrease in UA soft tissue, RDI, and total apnea time. Patients also notice improvements in subjective sleepiness.

Melatonin

Melatonin is a hormone secreted by the pineal gland, which helps regulate the sleep-wake cycle. Elevated melatonin levels have been noted in patients with nocturnal asthma,[124] suggesting a role in this disease state. However, after oral melatonin administration, pulmonary function testing demonstrated a decrease in diffusing capacity but no significant change in forced expiratory volume in 1 second, forced vital capacity, peak expiratory flow, or minute volume.[125] In addition, studies have demonstrated improved sleep in subjects with COPD who have received melatonin or ramelteon, a melatonin receptor antagonist.[32,126] Similarly, improved sleep has been noted in asthma subjects who have been given melatonin.[127]

SUBSTANCES
Nicotine

Nicotine has been studied for treatment of OSA. Nicotine is hypothesized to increase UA tone through central cholinergic effects. However, no significant benefit in SDB has been demonstrated.[128–130]

Alcohol

Alcohol has CNS-depressant effects. Its use is associated with SDB in healthy men who snore and do not have sleep apnea.[131] Alcohol use is associated with increased nocturnal oxygen desaturation in men more than in women, and with exacerbation of SDB.[132] Bedtime use of alcohol is associated with increased UA resistance particularly after the first 2 hours of ingestion.[133] Even moderate doses of alcohol worsen respiratory events in patients with mild-to-moderate OSA.[134] Alcohol suppresses the arousal response during airway occlusion in sleep as well as the magnitude of inspiratory effort.[135] Alcohol-related SDB is also associated with reduced processing of sensory respiratory neural information and nasal congestion.[136]

EMERGING DRUGS

AVE0118 is a nasal topically administered potassium channel blocker to the UA.[137] It is a proposed treatment of OSA and works by maintaining UA patency. AVE0118 shifts the mechanoreceptor response threshold for the genioglossus muscle to more positive pressures. Given as a slow-release formulation it showed a complete inhibition of UA collapsibility at 10 mg per nostril for more than 4 hours, supporting its potential for the treatment of OSA. In animals, it showed greater efficacy for maintaining UA airway patency better than fluoxetine, mirtazapine, and paroxetine, whereas no benefit was seen with naloxone or acetazolamide.

SUMMARY

Medications during sleep can stabilize respiration and reduce periodic breathing. Studies have primarily examined subjects with SDB, COPD, and periodic breathing at high altitude. Narcotics, sodium oxybate, and benzodiazepines are the classes of medications with the greatest risk of respiratory complications and should be used judiciously. Certain medications can result in partial improvement in respiratory events but none are superior to positive pressure therapy.

REFERENCES

1. Pever JH, Sessle BJ. Sensory and motor processes during sleep and wakefulness. In: Kryger MH, Roth T, Dement WC, editors. Principles and Practice of Sleep Medicine. Missouri: Saunders; 2010. p. 348–59.

2. Douglas NJ, White DP, Weil JV, et al. Hypercapnic ventilatory response in sleeping adults. Am Rev Respir Dis 1982;126(5):758–62.

3. San T, Polat S, Cingi C, et al. Effects of high altitude on sleep and respiratory system and theirs adaptations. ScientificWorldJournal 2013;2013:241569.

4. Stradling JR, Chadwick GA, Frew AJ. Changes in ventilation and its components in normal subjects during sleep. Thorax 1985;40(5):364–70.

5. Douglas NJ, White DP, Pickett CK, et al. Respiration during sleep in normal man. Thorax 1982;37:840–4.

6. Ioachimescu OC, Collop NA. Sleep-disordered breathing. Neurol Clin 2012;30:1095–136.

7. Lee-Chiong T. Somnology 2: Learn sleep medicine in one weekend. CreateSpace Independent Publishing Platform; 2011. p. 17.

8. Roux FJ, Kryger MH. Medication effects on sleep. Clin Chest Med 2010;31(2):397–405.

9. Stege G, Heijdra YF, van den Elshout FJ, et al. Temazepam 10mg does not affect breathing and gas exchange in patients with severe normocapnic COPD. Respir Med 2010;104(4):518–24.

10. Timms RM, Dawson A, Hajdukovic RM, et al. Effect of triazolam on sleep and arterial oxygen saturation in patients with chronic obstructive pulmonary disease. Arch Intern Med 1988;148(10):2159–63.

11. Wang D, Marshall NS, Duffin J, et al. Phenotyping interindividual variability in obstructive sleep apnoea response to temazepam using ventilatory chemoreflexes during wakefulness. J Sleep Res 2011;20(4):526–32.

12. Dubowitz G. Effect of temazepam on oxygen saturation and sleep quality at high altitude: randomised placebo controlled crossover trial. BMJ 1998;316(7131):587–9.

13. Nickol AH, Leverment J, Richards P, et al. Temazepam at high altitude reduces periodic breathing without impairing next-day performance: a randomized cross-over double-blind study. J Sleep Res 2006;15(4):445–54.

14. Röggla G, Moser B, Röggla M. Effect of temazepam on ventilatory response at moderate altitude. BMJ 2000;320(7226):56.

15. Guilleminault C. Benzodiazepines, breathing, and sleep. Am J Med 1990;88(3A):25S–8S.

16. Dolly FR, Block AJ. Effect of flurazepam on sleep-disordered breathing and nocturnal oxygen desaturation in asymptomatic subjects. Am J Med 1982;73(2):239–43.

17. Block AJ, Wynne JW, Boysen PG. Sleep-disordered breathing and nocturnal oxygen desaturation in postmenopausal women. Am J Med 1980;69(1):75–9.

18. Cummiskey J, Guilleminault C, Del Rio G, et al. The effects of flurazepam on sleep studies in patients with chronic obstructive pulmonary disease. Chest 1983;84(2):143–7.

19. Genta PR, Eckert DJ, Gregorio MG, et al. Critical closing pressure during midazolam-induced sleep. J Appl Physiol (1985) 2011;111(5):1315–22.

20. Collen J, Lettieri C, Kelly W, et al. Clinical and polysomnographic predictors of short-term continuous positive airway pressure compliance. Chest 2009;135(3):704–9.

21. Eckert DJ, Owens RL, Kehlmann GB, et al. Eszopiclone increases the respiratory arousal threshold and lowers the apnoea/hypopnoea index in obstructive sleep apnoea patients with a low arousal threshold. Clin Sci (Lond) 2011;120(12):505–14.

22. Rosenberg R, Roach JM, Scharf M, et al. A pilot study evaluating acute use of eszopiclone in patients with mild to moderate obstructive sleep apnea syndrome. Sleep Med 2007;8(5):464–70.

23. Lettieri CJ, Quast TN, Eliasson AH, et al. Eszopiclone improves overnight polysomnography and continuous positive airway pressure titration: a prospective, randomized, placebo-controlled trial. Sleep 2008;31(9):1310–6.

24. Coyle MA, Mendelson WB, Derchak PA, et al. Ventilatory safety of zaleplon during sleep in patients with obstructive sleep apnea on continuous positive airway pressure. J Clin Sleep Med 2005;1(1):97.

25. Steens RD, Pouliot Z, Millar TW, et al. Effects of zolpidem and triazolam on sleep and respiration in mild to moderate chronic obstructive pulmonary disease. Sleep 1993;16(4):318–26.

26. Quadri S, Drake C, Hudgel DW. Improvement of idiopathic central sleep apnea with zolpidem. J Clin Sleep Med 2009;5(2):122–9.

27. Beaumont M, Batéjat D, Coste O, et al. Effects of zolpidem and zaleplon on sleep, respiratory patterns and performance at a simulated altitude of 4,000 m. Neuropsychobiology 2004;49(3):154–62.

28. Beaumont M, Batéjat D, Piérard C, et al. Zaleplon and zolpidem objectively alleviate sleep disturbances in mountaineers at a 3,613 meter altitude. Sleep 2007;30(11):1527–33.

29. Girault C, Muir JF, Mihaltan F, et al. Effects of repeated administration of zolpidem on sleep, diurnal and nocturnal respiratory function, vigilance, and physical performance in patients with COPD. Chest 1996;110(5):1203–11.

30. Kryger M, Wang-Weigand S, Roth T. Safety of ramelteon in individuals with mild to moderate obstructive sleep apnea. Sleep Breath 2007; 11(3):159–64.

31. Kryger M, Wang-Weigand S, Zhang J, et al. Effect of ramelteon, a selective MT(1)/MT (2)-receptor agonist, on respiration during sleep in mild to moderate COPD. Sleep Breath 2008;12(3):243–50.

32. Kryger M, Roth T, Wang-Weigand S, et al. The effects of ramelteon on respiration during sleep in subjects with moderate to severe chronic obstructive pulmonary disease. Sleep Breath 2009;13(1): 79–84.

33. Yue HJ, Guilleminault C. Opioid medication and sleep-disordered breathing. Med Clin North Am 2010;94(3):435–46.

34. Drummond GB. Comparison of decreases in ventilation caused by enflurane and fentanyl during anaesthesia. Br J Anaesth 1984;55:825–35.

35. Weil JV, McCullough RE, Kline JS, et al. Diminished ventilatory response to hypoxia and hypercapnia after morphine in normal man. N Engl J Med 1975;292:1103–6.

36. Farney RJ, Walker JM, Cloward TV, et al. Sleep-disordered breathing associated with long-term opioid therapy. Chest 2003;123(2):632–9.

37. Sharkey KM, Kurth ME, Anderson BJ, et al. Obstructive sleep apnea is more common than central sleep apnea in methadone maintenance patients with subjective sleep complaints. Drug Alcohol Depend 2010;108(1–2):77–83.

38. Teichtahl H, Wang D, Cunnington D, et al. Ventilatory responses to hypoxia and hypercapnia in stable methadone maintenance treatment patients. Chest 2005;128(3):1339–47.

39. Meurice JC, Marc I, Sériès F. Effects of naloxone on upper airway collapsibility in normal sleeping subjects. Thorax 1996;51(8):851–2.

40. Atkinson RL, Suratt PM, Wilhoit SC, et al. Naloxone improves sleep apnea in obese humans. Int J Obes 1985;9(4):233–9.

41. Ferber C, Duclaux R, Mouret J. Naltrexone improves blood gas patterns in obstructive sleep apnoea syndrome through its influence on sleep. J Sleep Res 1993;2(3):149–55.

42. Kalpaklioglu F, Baccioglu A. Efficacy and safety of H1-antihistamines: an update. Antiinflamm Antiallergy Agents Med Chem 2012;11(3):230–7.

43. Krystal AD, Durrence HH, Scharf M, et al. Efficacy and safety of Doxepin 1 mg and 3 mg in a 12-week sleep laboratory and outpatient trial of elderly subjects with chronic primary insomnia. Sleep 2010; 33(11):1553–61.

44. Krystal AD, Lankford A, Durrence HH, et al. Efficacy and safety of doxepin 3 and 6 mg in a 35-day sleep laboratory trial in adults with chronic primary insomnia. Sleep 2011;34(10):1433–42.

45. Roth T, Rogowski R, Hull S, et al. Efficacy and safety of doxepin 1 mg, 3 mg, and 6 mg in adults with primary insomnia. Sleep 2007;30(11): 1555–61.

46. Roth T, Heith Durrence H, Jochelson P, et al. Efficacy and safety of doxepin 6 mg in a model of transient insomnia. Sleep Med 2010;11(9):843–7.

47. Lankford A, Rogowski R, Essink B, et al. Efficacy and safety of doxepin 6 mg in a four-week outpatient trial of elderly adults with chronic primary insomnia. Sleep Med 2012;13(2):133–8.

48. McKelvey GM, Post EJ, Jeffery HE, et al. Sedation with promethazine profoundly affects spontaneous airway protection in sleeping neonatal piglets. Clin Exp Pharmacol Physiol 1999;26(11):920–6.

49. Alexander CM, Seifert HA, Blouin RT, et al. Diphenhydramine enhances the interaction of hypercapnic and hypoxic ventilatory drive. Anesthesiology 1994;80(4):789–95.

50. Babenco HD, Blouin RT, Conard PF, et al. Diphenylhydramine increases ventilatory drive during alfentanil infusion. Anesthesiology 1998;89(3): 642–7.

51. Regan WM, Gordon SM. Gabapentin for behavioral agitation in Alzheimer's disease. J Clin Psychopharmacol 1997;17:59–60.

52. Rowbotham M, Harden N, Stacey B, et al. Gabapentin for the management of postherpetic neuralgia: a randomized controlled trial. JAMA 1998;280: 1837–42.

53. Garcia-Borreguero D, Kohnen R, Silber MH, et al. The long-term treatment of restless legs syndrome/Willis-Ekbom disease: evidence-based guidelines and clinical consensus best practice guidance: a report from the International Restless Legs Syndrome Study Group. Sleep Med 2013; 14(7):675–84.

54. Batoon SB, Vela AT, Dave D, et al. Recurrent hypoventilation and respiratory failure during gabapentin therapy. J Am Geriatr Soc 2001;49(4):498.

55. Català Pérez R, Gámez Lechuga M, Martínez-Lage Alvarez M, et al. Gabapentin-induced central hypoventilation. Med Clin (Barc) 2007;128(13):519 [in Spanish].

56. Eipe N, Penning J. Postoperative respiratory depression with pregabalin: a case series and a preoperative decision algorithm. Pain Res Manag 2011;16(5):353–6.

57. Hartley S, Quera-Salva MA, Machou M. Sodium oxybate and sleep apnea: a clinical case. J Clin Sleep Med 2011;7(6):667–8.

58. Frase L, Schupp J, Sorichter S, et al. Sodium oxybate-induced central sleep apneas. Sleep Med 2013;14(9):922–4.

59. Zvosec DL, Smith SW, Hall BJ. Three deaths associated with use of Xyrem. Sleep Med 2009;10(4): 490–3.

60. Inoue Y, Takasaki Y, Yamashiro Y. Efficacy and safety of adjunctive modafinil treatment on residual excessive daytime sleepiness among nasal continuous positive airway pressure-treated japanese patients with obstructive sleep apnea syndrome: a double-blind placebo-controlled study. J Clin Sleep Med 2013;9(8):751–7.

61. Roth T, White D, Schmidt-Nowara W, et al. Effects of armodafinil in the treatment of residual excessive sleepiness associated with obstructive sleep apnea/hypopnea syndrome: a 12-week, multicenter, double-blind, randomized, placebo-controlled study in nCPAP-adherent adults. Clin Ther 2006; 28(5):689–706.

62. Winslow DH, Bowden CH, DiDonato KP, et al. A randomized, double-blind, placebo-controlled study of an oral, extended-release formulation of phentermine/topiramate for the treatment of obstructive sleep apnea in obese adults. Sleep 2012;35(11):1529–39.

63. Brownell LG, Perez-Padilla R, West P, et al. The role of protriptyline in obstructive sleep apnea. Bull Eur Physiopathol Respir 1983;19(6):621–4.

64. Smith PL, Haponik EF, Allen RP, et al. The effects of protriptyline in sleep-disordered breathing. Am Rev Respir Dis 1983;127(1):8–13.

65. Hanzel DA, Proia NG, Hudgel DW. Response of obstructive sleep apnea to fluoxetine and protriptyline. Chest 1991;100(2):416–21.

66. Bart Sangal R, Sangal JM, Thorp K. Atomoxetine improves sleepiness and global severity of illness but not the respiratory disturbance index in mild to moderate obstructive sleep apnea with sleepiness. Sleep Med 2008;9(5):506–10.

67. Carley DW, Radulovacki M. Mirtazapine, a mixed-profile serotonin agonist/antagonist, suppresses sleep apnea in the rat. Am J Respir Crit Care Med 1999;160(6):1824–9.

68. Carley DW, Olopade C, Ruigt GS, et al. Efficacy of mirtazapine in obstructive sleep apnea syndrome. Sleep 2007;30(1):35–41.

69. Marshall NS, Yee BJ, Desai AV, et al. Two randomized placebo-controlled trials to evaluate the efficacy and tolerability of mirtazapine for the treatment of obstructive sleep apnea. Sleep 2008; 31(6):824–31.

70. Kraiczi H, Hedner J, Dahlöf P, et al. Effect of serotonin uptake inhibition on breathing during sleep and daytime symptoms in obstructive sleep apnea. Sleep 1999;22(1):61–7.

71. Berry RB, Yamaura EM, Gill K, et al. Acute effects of paroxetine on genioglossus activity in obstructive sleep apnea. Sleep 1999;22(8):1087–92.

72. Winkelman JW. Schizophrenia, obesity, and obstructive sleep apnea. J Clin Psychiatry 2001; 62(1):8–11.

73. Rishi MA, Shetty M, Wolff A, et al. Atypical antipsychotic medications are independently associated with severe obstructive sleep apnea. Clin Neuropharmacol 2010;33(3):109–13.

74. Shirani A, Paradiso S, Dyken ME. The impact of atypical antipsychotic use on obstructive sleep apnea: a pilot study and literature review. Sleep Med 2011;12(6):591–7.

75. Kohen I, Sarcevic A. Central sleep apnea in a geriatric patient treated with aripiprazole. Am J Ther 2009;16(2):197–8.

76. Mutschler J, Obermann C, Grosshans M. Quetiapine-induced hyperventilation and dyspnea. Clin Neuropharmacol 2010;33(4):214.

77. Shelton PS, Barnett FL, Krick SE. Hyperventilation associated with quetiapine. Ann Pharmacother 2000;34(3):335–7.

78. Jabeen S, Polli SI, Gerber DR. Acute respiratory failure with a single dose of quetiapine fumarate. Ann Pharmacother 2006;40(3):559–62.

79. Freudenmann RW, Süssmuth SD, Wolf RC, et al. Respiratory dysfunction in sleep apnea associated with quetiapine. Pharmacopsychiatry 2008;41(3): 119–21.

80. Kiely JL, Nolan P, McNicholas WT. Intranasal corticosteroid therapy for obstructive sleep apnoea in patients with co-existing rhinitis. Thorax 2004; 59(1):50–5.

81. Kheirandish-Gozal L, Gozal D. Intranasal budesonide treatment for children with mild obstructive sleep apnea syndrome. Pediatrics 2008;122(1):e149–55.

82. Kheirandish L, Goldbart AD, Gozal D. Intranasal steroids and oral leukotriene modifier therapy in residual sleep-disordered breathing after tonsillectomy and adenoidectomy in children. Pediatrics 2006;117(1):e61–6.

83. Forwand SA, Landowne M, Follansbee JN, et al. Effect of acetazolamide on acute mountain sickness. N Engl J Med 1968;279:839–45.

84. Leaf DE, Goldfarb DS. Mechanisms of action of acetazolamide in the prophylaxis and treatment of acute mountain sickness. J Appl Physiol (1985) 2007;102:1313–22.

85. DeBacker WA, Verbraecken J, Willemen M, et al. Central apnea index decreases after prolonged treatment with acetazolamide. Am J Respir Crit Care Med 1995;151:87–91.

86. Nussbaumer-Ochsner Y, Latshang TD, Ulrich S, et al. Patients with obstructive sleep apnea

syndrome benefit from acetazolamide during an altitude sojourn: a randomized, placebo-controlled, double-blind trial. Chest 2012;141(1):131–8.

87. Latshang TD, Nussbaumer-Ochsner Y, Henn RM, et al. Effect of acetazolamide and autoCPAP therapy on breathing disturbances among patients with obstructive sleep apnea syndrome who travel to altitude: a randomized controlled trial. JAMA 2012;308(22):2390–8.

88. Javaheri S, Parker TJ, Wexler L, et al. Effect of theophylline on sleep-disordered breathing in heart failure. N Engl J Med 1996;335(8):562–7.

89. Oberndorfer S, Saletu B, Gruber G, et al. Theophylline in snoring and sleep-related breathing disorders: sleep laboratory investigations on subjective and objective sleep and awakening quality. Methods Find Exp Clin Pharmacol 2000;22(4):237–45.

90. Hein H, Behnke G, Jörres RA, et al. The therapeutic effect of theophylline in mild obstructive sleep Apnea/Hypopnea syndrome: results of repeated measurements with portable recording devices at home. Eur J Med Res 2000;5(9):391–9.

91. Fischer R, Lang SM, Leitl M, et al. Theophylline and acetazolamide reduce sleep-disordered breathing at high altitude. Eur Respir J 2004;23(1):47–52.

92. Küpper TE, Strohl KP, Hoefer M, et al. Low-dose theophylline reduces symptoms of acute mountain sickness. J Travel Med 2008;15(5):307–14.

93. Cranston JM, Crockett AJ, Moss JR, et al. Domiciliary oxygen for chronic obstructive pulmonary disease. Cochrane Database Syst Rev 2005;(4):CD001744.

94. Mehta V, Vasu TS, Phillips B, et al. Obstructive sleep apnea and oxygen therapy: a systematic review of the literature and meta-analysis. J Clin Sleep Med 2013;9(3):271–9.

95. Chowdhuri S, Ghabsha A, Sinha P, et al. Treatment of central sleep apnea in U.S. veterans. J Clin Sleep Med 2012;8(5):555–63.

96. Urquhart DS, Gulliver T, Williams G, et al. Central sleep-disordered breathing and the effects of oxygen therapy in infants with Prader-Willi syndrome. Arch Dis Child 2013;98(8):592–5.

97. Young T, Palta M, Dempsey J, et al. The occurrence of sleep-disordered breathing among middle-aged adults. N Engl J Med 1993;328(17):1230–5.

98. Leech JA, Onal E, Dulberg C, et al. A comparison of men and women with occlusive sleep apnea syndrome. Chest 1988;94(5):983–8.

99. Netzer NC, Eliasson AH, Strohl KP. Women with sleep apnea have lower levels of sex hormones. Sleep Breath 2003;7(1):25–9.

100. Kapsimalis F, Kryger MH. Gender and obstructive sleep apnea syndrome, part 1: clinical features. Sleep 2002;25(4):412–9.

101. Block AJ, Wynne JW, Boysen PG, et al. Menopause, medroxyprogesterone and breathing during sleep. Am J Med 1981;70(3):506–10.

102. Strohl KP, Hensley MJ, Saunders NA, et al. Progesteron administration and progressive sleep apneas. JAMA 1981;145(12):1230–2.

103. Shahar E, Redline S, Young T, et al. Hormone replacement therapy and sleep-disordered breathing. Am J Respir Crit Care Med 2003;167(9):1186–92.

104. Pickett CK, Regensteiner JG, Woodard WD, et al. Progestin and estrogen reduce sleep-disordered breathing in postmenopausal women. J Appl Physiol (1985) 1989;66(4):1656–61.

105. Kimura H, Tatsumi K, Kunitomo F, et al. Progesterone therapy for sleep apnea syndrome evaluated by occlusion pressure responses to exogenous loading. Am Rev Respir Dis 1989;139(5):1198–206.

106. Cook WR, Benich JJ, Wooten SA. Indices of severity of obstructive sleep apnea syndrome do not change during medroxyprogesterone acetate therapy. Chest 1989;96(2):262–6.

107. Rajagopal KR, Abbrecht PH, Jabbari B. Effects of medroxyprogesterone acetate in obstructive sleep apnea. Chest 1986;90(6):815–21.

108. Skatrud JB, Dempsey JA, Kaiser DG. Ventilatory response to medroxyprogesterone acetate in normal subjects: time course and mechanism. J Appl Physiol Respir Environ Exerc Physiol 1978;44(6):939–44.

109. Zwillich CW, Sutton FD, Pierson DJ, et al. Decreased hypoxic ventilatory drive in the obesity-hypoventilation syndrome. Am J Med 1975;59(3):343–8.

110. D'Ambrosio C, Stachenfeld NS, Pisani M, et al. Sleep, breathing, and menopause: the effect of fluctuating estrogen and progesterone on sleep and breathing in women. Gend Med 2005;2(4):238–45.

111. Santamaria JD, Prior JC, Fleetham JA. Reversible reproductive dysfunction in men with obstructive sleep apnoea. Clin Endocrinol (Oxf) 1988;28(5):461–70.

112. Canguven O, Salepci B, Albayrak S, et al. Is there a correlation between testosterone levels and the severity of the disease in male patients with obstructive sleep apnea? Arch Ital Urol Androl 2010;82(4):143–7.

113. Meston N, Davies RJ, Mullins R, et al. Endocrine effects of nasal continuous positive airway pressure in male patients with obstructive sleep apnoea. J Intern Med 2003;254(5):447–54.

114. Dexter DD, Dovre EJ. Obstructive sleep apnea due to endogenous testosterone production in a woman. Mayo Clin Proc 1998;73(3):246–8.

115. Fogel RB, Malhotra A, Pillar G, et al. Increased prevalence of obstructive sleep apnea syndrome in obese women with polycystic ovary syndrome. J Clin Endocrinol Metab 2001;86(3):1175–80.

116. Mokhlesi B, Scoccia B, Mazzone T, et al. Risk of obstructive sleep apnea in obese and nonobese women with polycystic ovary syndrome and healthy reproductively normal women. Fertil Steril 2012;97(3):786–91.

117. Cistulli PA, Grunstein RR, Sullivan CE. Effect of testosterone administration on upper airway collapsibility during sleep. Am J Respir Crit Care Med 1994;149(2 Pt 1):530–2.

118. Robinson RW, Zwillich CW. The effect of drugs on breathing during sleep. Symposium on Sleep Disorders. Clin Chest Med 1985;6:603–14.

119. Hanafy HM. Testosterone therapy and obstructive sleep apnea: is there a real connection? J Sex Med 2007;4(5):1241–6.

120. Hoyos CM, Killick R, Yee BJ, et al. Effects of testosterone therapy on sleep and breathing in obese men with severe obstructive sleep apnoea: a randomized placebo-controlled trial. Clin Endocrinol (Oxf) 2012;77(4):599–607.

121. Stewart DA, Grunstein RR, Berthon-Jones M, et al. Androgen blockade does not affect sleep-disordered breathing or chemosensitivity in men with obstructive sleep apnea. Am Rev Respir Dis 1992;146(6):1389–93.

122. Kraemer S, Danker-Hopfe H, Pilhatsch M, et al. Effects of supraphysiological doses of levothyroxine on sleep in healthy subjects: a prospective polysomnography study. J Thyroid Res 2011;2011:420580.

123. Davi' MV, Dalle Carbonare L, Giustina A, et al. Sleep apnoea syndrome is highly prevalent in acromegaly and only partially reversible after biochemical control of the disease. Eur J Endocrinol 2008; 159(5):533–40.

124. Sutherland ER, Ellison MC, Kraft M, et al. Elevated serum melatonin is associated with the nocturnal worsening of asthma. J Allergy Clin Immunol 2003;112(3):513–7.

125. Vardar SA, Altun GD, Günerbuyuk C, et al. Melatonin administration acutely decreases the diffusing capacity of carbon monoxide in human lungs. Respiration 2006;73(4):509–13.

126. Nunes DM, Mota RM, Machado MO, et al. Effect of melatonin administration on subjective sleep quality in chronic obstructive pulmonary disease. Braz J Med Biol Res 2008;41(10):926–31.

127. Campos FL, da Silve-Junior FP, de Bruin VM, et al. Melatonin improves sleep in asthma: a randomized, double-blind, placebo-controlled study. Am J Respir Crit Care Med 2004;170(9):947–51.

128. Davila DG, Hurt RD, Offord KP, et al. Acute effects of transdermal nicotine on sleep architecture, snoring, and sleep-disordered breathing in nonsmokers. Am J Respir Crit Care Med 1994;150(2): 469–74.

129. Hein H, Kirsten D, Jugert C, et al. Nicotine as therapy of obstructive sleep apnea? Pneumologie 1995;49(Suppl 1):185–6.

130. Zevin S, Swed E, Cahan C. Clinical effects of locally delivered nicotine in obstructive sleep apnea syndrome. Am J Ther 2003;10(3):170–5.

131. Taasan VC, Block AJ, Boysen PG, et al. Alcohol increases sleep apnea and oxygen desaturation in asymptomatic men. Am J Med 1981;71(2):240–5.

132. Peppard PE, Austin D, Brown RL. Association of alcohol consumption and sleep disordered breathing in men and women. J Clin Sleep Med 2007; 3(3):265–70.

133. Mitler MM, Dawson A, Henriksen SJ, et al. Bedtime ethanol increases resistance of upper airways and produces sleep apneas in asymptomatic snorers. Alcohol Clin Exp Res 1988;12(6):801–5.

134. Scanlan MF, Roebuck T, Little PJ, et al. Effect of moderate alcohol upon obstructive sleep apnoea. Eur Respir J 2000;16(5):909–13.

135. Berry RB, Bonnet MH, Light RW. Effect of ethanol on the arousal response to airway occlusion during sleep in normal subjects. Am Rev Respir Dis 1992; 145(2 Pt 1):445–52.

136. Eckert DJ, Elgar NJ, McEvoy RD, et al. Alcohol alters sensory processing to respiratory stimuli in healthy men and women during wakefulness. Sleep 2010;33(10):1389–95.

137. Wirth KJ, Steinmeyer K, Ruetten H. Sensitization of upper airway mechanoreceptors as a new pharmacologic principle to treat obstructive sleep apnea: investigations with AVE0118 in anesthetized pigs. Sleep 2013;36(5):699–708.

Sleep Disorders in Pregnancy

Dennis Oyiengo, MD[a], Mariam Louis, MD[b], Beth Hott, BA[c], Ghada Bourjeily, MD[d],*

KEYWORDS

- Pregnancy • Restless legs syndrome • Narcolepsy • Insomnia • Circadian rhythm
- Sleep-disordered breathing

KEY POINTS

- Pregnancy is associated with physiologic changes that may disrupt sleep, cause sleep disorders, or worsen underlying sleep conditions.
- Restless legs syndrome may occur de novo in pregnancy or could potentially be exacerbated by increased iron or folate requirements.
- Sleep-disordered breathing may be exacerbated or caused by pregnancy; the disorder is associated with adverse pregnancy outcomes.

Sleep disturbances in pregnancy have been well recognized since Hippocrates. In 2000, the American Academy of Sleep Medicine officially recognized sleep disorders associated with pregnancy as a separate entity defined as the occurrence of insomnia or excessive daytime sleepiness in the course of pregnancy.[1] The past decade has witnessed the emergence of numerous publications on various sleep disorders associated with pregnancy.

Pregnancy is a unique, short-lived state that is associated with profound physiologic changes that may predispose individuals to the development of sleep disturbances; these changes also may exacerbate preexisting conditions. Many pregnancy-related factors may result in sleep disruption.[2] Heartburn is significantly more common in pregnancy and has been reported in up to 75% of pregnancies in one study.[3] Oxytocin, the hormone that is responsible for uterine contractions, is known to peak at night, possibly causing sleep fragmentation in late pregnancy. Nocturia is a common occurrence in the first and third trimesters. Nocturia is related to an increase in the overnight sodium secretion, leading to a higher overnight urine flow. In late pregnancy, nocturia is worsened by the effect of the growing uterus on bladder capacity.[4] Fetal movements can disrupt sleep, and musculoskeletal discomfort related to musculoskeletal changes of pregnancy also can result in sleep fragmentation. In the postpartum period, sleep is naturally disrupted and restricted by the needs of the newborn. Some pathologic respiratory conditions, such as asthma, may be exacerbated by physiologic changes of pregnancy, such as nasal congestion, heartburn, and immune changes, resulting in disrupted sleep.

Management of the various conditions in the pregnant population is complicated by concern for fetal well-being and the impact of treatment on the safety of the unborn child. Nonetheless, management decisions should also take into

a Pulmonary and Critical Care Fellowship Program, The Warren Alpert Medical School of Brown University, 593 Eddy Street, Providence, RI 02903, USA; b Department of Medicine, University of Florida, 655 West 8th Street, Jacksonville, FL 32209, USA; c Department of Medicine, Women's Medicine Collaborative, The Miriam Hospital, 146 West River Street, Suite 11C, Providence, RI 02904, USA; d Department of Medicine, The Miriam Hospital, The Warren Alpert Medical School of Brown University, 146 West River Street, Suite 11C, Providence, RI 02904, USA
* Corresponding author. The Miriam Hospital, 146 West River Street, Suite 11C, Providence, RI 02904.
E-mail address: Ghada_Bourjeily@brown.edu

Clin Chest Med 35 (2014) 571–587
http://dx.doi.org/10.1016/j.ccm.2014.06.012

consideration the effect of the untreated conditions on the health of the pregnancy and the fetus. This review focuses on nonbreathing-related sleep disorders, with a brief mention of sleep-disordered breathing. A detailed discussion of physiologic changes of pregnancy resulting in sleep disruption is outside the scope of this article.

SLEEP-DISORDERED BREATHING

Many of the physiologic changes of pregnancy predispose to sleep-disordered breathing. Upper airway edema,[5] increased Mallampati score,[6] nasal congestion,[7] and reduction in functional residual capacity[8] are all predisposing factors, as they contribute to decreased airway patency and increased collapsibility. Despite protective factors, the balance tips toward a higher incidence of sleep-disordered breathing in this population compared with the nonpregnant population. Sleep-disordered breathing has been repeatedly associated with negative pregnancy outcomes, such as gestational hypertensive disorders,[9,10] gestational diabetes,[9,11–14] and cesarean deliveries.[9,10] Adverse fetal outcomes also have been described, but are less consistent. Growth restriction has been described in some studies,[15,16] but not others.[9,17–20] Preterm birth has been described in women who snore or have obstructive sleep apnea,[9,10] but this complication is likely mediated by preeclampsia. Fetal heart rate decelerations were described in clinical studies[21,22]; however, recent polysomnographic data do not show decelerations following apneic episodes.[23]

One recent retrospective study has shown that the risk of a composite set of adverse outcomes increases with the severity of sleep-disordered breathing.[24] These data suggest that, like the nonpregnant population, pregnant women with more severe disease need to be offered treatment. It remains unclear, however, whether continuous positive airway pressure (CPAP) alters pregnancy outcomes. Small studies and case series of women with obstructive sleep apnea[25,26] show an improvement in daytime somnolence, quality of life, and other symptoms, such as morning headaches. However, the impact of CPAP on the prevention of gestational hypertension, gestational diabetes, or fetal outcomes in the setting of obstructive sleep apnea remains unclear. Minimal data have assessed sleep-disordered breathing outside the setting of obstructive sleep apnea and snoring. Central sleep apnea appears to be quite uncommon in pregnant women with sleep-disordered breathing.[27] Treatment of these conditions is usually extrapolated from the nonpregnant population.

In summary, sleep-disordered breathing is prevalent in pregnancy and is associated with adverse outcomes. Optimal management of pregnant women with obstructive sleep apnea is unclear and should follow nonpregnant guidelines until evidence suggesting that CPAP modifies pregnancy-specific outcomes exists.

RESTLESS LEGS SYNDROME

Restless legs syndrome (RLS), now known as Willis Ekbom disease (WED), is a sensorimotor phenomenon characterized by an urge to move the legs because of an unpleasant sensation; the urge is worse during periods of rest or inactivity and is partially or totally relieved by movement, and the sensation is worse during the evening or at night. Although a sleep study is not required to make the diagnosis of RLS/WED, the vast majority of patients with RLS/WED have evidence of periodic limb movements and arousals on polysomnography.[28]

Depending on methodology in community-based surveys in the nonpregnant population, RLS/WED estimates fall between 1.9% and 15.0%[29] and appear to have a female predominance.[30] RLS/WED has a higher prevalence in pregnancy, with more than a quarter of pregnant women reported to have the syndrome in some studies.[31,32] However, the methodology and the gestational age at the time of administration of questionnaires in these epidemiologic studies varied significantly. Although some used self-administered questionnaires,[33,34] others used interview-based information.[35–37] Timing of data collection also varied significantly, with some studies performing the assessment longitudinally throughout pregnancy,[38,39] while others performed a cross-sectional analysis at various points during pregnancy.[31,40] Importantly, the number of criteria met for the diagnosis of RLS also differed between studies.

In a study that performed face-to-face interviews with pregnant women conducted at delivery, nearly a quarter of pregnant women met criteria for RLS according to the International Restless Legs Syndrome Study Group criteria.[35] Almost two-thirds of these women had new-onset symptoms, whereas about one-third had symptoms predating pregnancy. The prevalence of RLS appears to increase with gestational age,[33,38,39] suggesting de novo symptoms. For most women, symptoms resolve shortly after delivery.[36,40] Lower prevalence was reported in other studies[33] and the discrepancy may be related to methodology and the diagnostic criteria used.

Pathophysiology

RLS has been linked to dopamine metabolism in the brain, and it is thought that the disorder arises from dysfunction of hypothalamic dopaminergic cells that are the source of spinal dopamine. By impeding the production of tyrosine hydroxylase in the central nervous system, reduced serum iron hinders the production of dopamine. A potential mechanism for the higher prevalence of RLS in pregnancy may be the threefold to fourfold increase in iron requirements in pregnancy.[32] As the mother is the sole source of nutrients to the fetus, the placenta upregulates its iron transfer systems to maintain adequate supply to the fetus, which often occurs at the expense of the mother's stores.[41] This upregulation is more pronounced under conditions of maternal iron deficiency.[42] As many as 30% of women have limited iron stores in wealthy cities in developed countries[43] and up to 90% of pregnant American women have suboptimal iron intake.[44] Serum iron follows a circadian pattern and levels are 50% to 60% lower at night than in the daytime, and nadir levels appear to correlate with the highest severity of symptoms. Although serum iron and iron saturation are decreased in 62% and 77% of patients with RLS, respectively, serum ferritin levels and markers of anemia based on hemoglobin and red blood cell mass were decreased in fewer than a quarter of patients in one study.[45] Ferritin levels less than 50 ng/mL correlate well with poor sleep quality and higher symptom severity scores.[46] As attractive as this theory of iron deficiency is in explaining the higher prevalence of RLS in pregnancy, it does not explain the rapid improvement that occurs postpartum, as blood loss at delivery and fluid shifts postpartum would likely worsen anemia.

Furthermore, folate deficiency also may play a role in the pathogenesis of RLS in pregnancy. Folate requirements increase 8-fold to 10-fold in pregnancy because of the increased demands of the fetus. The incidence of RLS is significantly lower in women who use vitamin supplementation throughout pregnancy compared with those who do not,[37,47] and resolution of symptoms correlates with normalization of levels.[48]

Female hormones may be culprits as well. Through interactions with the dopaminergic system, namely the nigrostriatal dopaminergic neurons, estradiol may play a role in RLS.[49] In a small study of 10 pregnant women with RLS and pregnant controls without RLS, estradiol levels were significantly higher in women with RLS, irrespective of whether estradiol predated the pregnancy or occurred de novo in pregnancy.[50] A more recent study that excluded pregnant women being treated with intravenous iron for iron deficiency, reported a lower prevalence of the disorder than previously described (12%) and showed similar levels of third-trimester estradiol levels in pregnant women with RLS compared with controls.[51] Prolactin also influences the dopaminergic system, has the same circadian rhythmicity as RLS, and may play a role in RLS in pregnancy. However, the drastic improvement in symptoms in the postpartum period, even in lactating women,[52] argues against a prominent role of this hormone. Progesterone increases several-fold in pregnancy. Although progesterone increases neuronal excitability and may theoretically manifest this excitability as RLS, progesterone levels in pregnant women with RLS were not found to be higher than those without the syndrome.[37,50]

Management

Certain conditions should be excluded before diagnosing a patient with RLS, such as electrolyte imbalance and peripheral vasculopathy, but some conditions need to be specifically considered in the pregnant population. Leg cramps are quite common in pregnancy and may mimic RLS symptoms. Musculoskeletal discomfort is common, and nerve impingement should be considered, especially if symptoms are unilateral.

RLS has been linked to hypertension in some general population studies,[53,54] but only one recent study has evaluated a link between RLS and pregnancy outcomes.[55] Until this association is confirmed in additional studies, it is premature to think that treatment of RLS could modify any pregnancy outcomes.

Similar to nonpregnant patients, known triggers to RLS, such as caffeine, smoking, and certain drugs, should be eliminated if possible. RLS has been described in association with the use of some antidepressants in some studies[56–58] but not in others.[59,60] As untreated mood disorders are associated with adverse pregnancy outcomes, the safety of withholding or switching antidepressants should be carefully assessed, preferably by a perinatal psychiatrist, and the risk and benefit of such a decision carefully weighed.

In 2012, American Academy of Sleep Medicine practice parameters summarized available options for the treatment of RLS in the general population and in some special populations, but provided no recommendations for the pregnant population.[61] Although moderate and high-quality evidence supports the use of some drugs in the treatment of RLS, first-line therapy varies in pregnancy because of the scarcity of safety data in this population. **Table 1** summarizes the safety

Table 1
Pharmacotherapy and drug safety in restless legs syndrome

Medications Restless Leg Syndrome (RLS)	Pregnancy Safety	Lactation
Pramipexole (Approved for indication)	Based on studies in rats and rabbits, an increase in malformations is not anticipated in women treated with pramipexole during pregnancy.[62] Human safety data are limited to case reports and case series but do not show evidence of malformations.	No human studies assessing levels in breast milk are available. Pramipexole is known to reduce the secretion of prolactin, and it is possible that it could significantly reduce milk synthesis in breastfeeding mothers. This product should probably not be used in breastfeeding mothers.[63]
Ropinirole (Approved for indication)	There are no human data. Based on experimental animal studies, ropinirole is not expected to increase the risk of congenital anomalies. One case report has been identified on use of Ropinirole in pregnancy.[135]	No human studies are available concerning levels in milk. Medication might inhibit lactation because of its prolactin-lowering effects. This product should probably not be used in breastfeeding mothers.[63]
Levodopa (Approved, but off-label use)	Levodopa produces adverse pregnancy and fetal outcomes[136–138] in experimental animals after high-dose treatment. Case reports in humans have not identified abnormal embryo or fetal development. Theoretic concern about placental perfusion with levodopa.[139] Current data do not support the safety of this drug in pregnancy.	No pediatric concerns reported. However, reduced prolactin levels by dopamine may reduce milk production.[63]
Opioids (Approved, but off-label use)	Neonatal withdrawal after maternal use has occurred with opioid medications. Oxycodone use in the first trimester was associated with an increase in pulmonary valve stenosis in one retrospective study.[140] Study limited by maternal recall and findings confounded by indication for use. These findings were not confirmed in other studies.[141–143]	Small amounts are secreted in breast milk. Sedation of the newborn may be observed.[63]
Gabapentin (Approved for indication)	Gabapentin has been reported to interfere with embryo development in some but not all experimental studies. There are case reports of normal pregnancy outcomes after gabapentin therapy, but there are also reports of malformations. It is not known if the risk of malformations in increased with this medication.	Data reveal that the infant plasma levels following exposure to gabapentin through breastfeeding are probably too low to cause untoward effects in the breastfed infant. Weigh the potential benefits of drug treatment against potential risks before prescribing this drug during breastfeeding.
Carbamazepine (Approved, but off-label use)	Carbamazepine use during early pregnancy has been associated with an increased risk of neural tube defects and possibly an increased risk of craniofacial abnormalities and developmental delay. In spite of these risks, this drug has been used for optimal seizure control as benefit likely outweighs the risk in most cases. However, until RLS is clearly linked to adverse pregnancy outcomes, the use of carbamazepine for the treatment of RLS may not outweigh the risk of fetal malformations.	The amount of carbamazepine transferred to the infant is apparently quite low. Medication usually compatible with breastfeeding according to the American Academy of Pediatrics (AAP) and World Health Organization (WHO).

Drug	Pregnancy	Lactation
Clonidine (Approved, but off-label use)	Based on experimental animal studies, clonidine use during pregnancy is not expected to increase the risk of structural malformations. Possible behavioral effects, such as hyperactivity and sleep disturbances, were reported in children exposed prenatally compared with a control population.[144] Similar behavioral effects of prenatal clonidine exposure have been reported in experimental animals.	Clonidine is minimally excreted in human milk. No pediatric concerns reported, but newborns may need to be observed for hypotension. Clonidine may reduce milk production by reducing prolactin secretion.
Pregabalin (Approved, but off-label use)	Pregabalin has adverse effects on embryo development and viability in rats at plasma levels about twice those achieved in humans on therapy. Human data are limited.	There are no data available on the transfer of pregabalin into human milk. However, due to the kinetics of the drug, its passage into the milk compartment is probable, and its oral bioavailability to the infant would be high. Therefore, infant risk cannot be ruled out.
Rotigotine (Withdrawn from US market because of drug crystallization affecting absorption)	Magnitude of potential teratogenic effect is undetermined. No animal teratology studies have been published.	No data are available on the transfer of rotigotine into human milk. It is possible that this medication could significantly decrease prolactin release and in turn, decrease milk production.
Bromocriptine	Based on experimental animal studies and limited human experience, bromocriptine use during pregnancy is not believed to increase the risk of congenital anomalies. Risk and benefit of the use of this drug should be carefully weighed in women with RLS.	No reports of direct toxicity to infant via milk, but use with caution. May inhibit lactation.
Cabergoline	Human studies of more than 500 pregnancies exposed to cabergoline suggest that the drug does not increase the risk of congenital malformations. Cabergoline has been used to increase fertility in women with prolactinomas.	Drug used to treat prolactinomas and is known to decrease prolactin levels. If lactation can be maintained, watch infant for ergot effects, if any.
Valproic acid	Maternal use of valproic acid alone or in combination with other antiepileptic drugs has been found to cause valproic acid syndrome in infants. Facial dysmorphology, congenital heart defects, spina bifida, cleft lip and palate, and developmental delays are some of the teratogenic effects seen. The use of this drug for the treatment of RLS in pregnancy cannot be justified.	No adverse events have been associated with breastfeeding. Maternal medication usually compatible with breastfeeding according to the AAP and WHO. Monitor infant for side effects.
Clonazepam	Maternal use is not thought to increase the risk of congenital malformations. Risk of transient respiratory distress and hypotonia in women taking clonazepam in combination with paroxetine.	One case report of apnea, cyanosis, and hypotonia in a newborn exposed to clonazepam via breast milk.[145] Other reports (11 newborns) showed no side effects.[146]

data available both in pregnancy and lactation. Reprotox.org and Thomas Hale's Medications and Mothers' Milk[62,63] are excellent sources of updated information on drug safety during pregnancy and lactation. Briefly, iron supplementation starting at ferritin less than 50 ng/mL or hemoglobin less than 11 g/dL may result in symptomatic improvement in women with low iron stores or iron deficiency. Preliminary data describing the use of intravenous iron supplementation appear to be promising. Data published in an abstract form on 11 women with moderate to severe iron deficiency–associated RLS and treated with intravenous iron in the third trimester showed a significant improvement in RLS severity score from 25 ± 5 to 7 ± 6, P = .01, 4 weeks after administration.[64] The effect of the mild reduction in blood pressure associated with iron infusion on placental perfusion remains unclear and more data are needed to assess the exact role of this therapy in pregnancy. Although case reports of intravenous magnesium were associated with significant improvement in RLS symptom score, the Food and Drug Administration recently issued a warning against the use of intravenous magnesium for more than 5 to 7 days because of the effect of this mineral on calcium metabolism and fetal bone development. In addition to oral or intravenous iron supplementation in women with iron deficiency, clonidine, opioids, and clonazepam are potential therapeutic options in pregnancy, although none is standard therapy based on the recent practice parameters classification.[61] Newborns exposed to opioids in utero should be observed closely for respiratory depression, or the drugs discontinued close to term. Although bromocriptine and cabergoline have been used to improve fertility and in pregnancy in women with prolactinomas, the risk-benefit ratio of the use of these drugs in RLS in pregnancy is less clear. In our opinion, these medications should be reserved for more severe cases in which symptoms are significantly disrupting sleep and are not responding to other therapy.

In summary, RLS/WED is a common disorder in pregnancy that adversely affects sleep. Iron, folate, and hormones may each play a role in the pathogenesis of this disorder; however, the exact mechanism underlying this higher prevalence is unclear. Drugs with lower quality of evidence in the nonpregnant population than first-line therapy may be options for therapy in pregnancy.

INSOMNIA

The National Sleep Foundation recommends 7 to 9 hours of sleep per 24 hours for adults[65]; however, sleep needs and duration vary by age and gender and are likely different in pregnancy. Although self-reported sleep duration does not correlate well with subjective measurements, such as actigraphy, in pregnancy,[66,67] most epidemiologic studies evaluating sleep duration rely on self-reports.[68,69] Based on these studies, it appears that sleep duration increases starting in the first trimester and is then reduced late in pregnancy.[70–72] These reports suggest that sleep needs are likely increased in pregnancy, or that longer sleep duration is related to rising levels of hormones necessary for maintaining pregnancy, such as human chorionic gonadotropin and progesterone.[2] However, the emerging literature suggesting an association of sleep deficiency with some adverse outcomes in pregnancy may indicate that the longer sleep duration may be a necessary phenomenon rather than a mere side effect of hormonal changes.

Sleep disruption is a common occurrence in pregnancy, and in many cases, sleep fragmentation may be related to physiologic changes of pregnancy. Many factors, such as musculoskeletal discomfort, heartburn, nocturia, uterine contractions, and fetal movement, may all disrupt sleep.[2,73] Disrupted sleep is more prevalent in the third trimester and more than half of women report poor sleep in the last 8 weeks of gestation.[74] As a result of fragmented nocturnal sleep, daytime napping increases in late pregnancy. Factors that have been associated with shorter sleep duration[75] and worse insomnia severity scores in pregnancy[76] include nulliparity, younger age,[75] smoking, advanced gestational age, and higher blood pressure.[76] Postpartum sleep is usually disrupted by the newborn's nocturnal needs and potential postpartum discomfort, with more frequent complaints of insomnia in women with operative deliveries.[77]

Higher Epworth Sleepiness Scale (ESS) scores also have been described in pregnancy, with up to 24% of women reporting excessive sleepiness.[76,78,79] Although daytime sleepiness may relate to physiologic sleep disruption, ESS scores appear to correlate with sleep-disordered breathing[80] and may add to the risk of some adverse pregnancy outcomes related to snoring.[8]

Sleep Deficiency and Pregnancy Outcomes

Although poor sleep in the antepartum period is related to normal physiologic changes of pregnancy in many, differentiating between normal and abnormal sleep in pregnancy may be challenging but an important task nonetheless, as poor sleep has been linked to adverse pregnancy outcomes. Sleep disruption or deficiency during pregnancy is considered a significant risk factor for the occurrence of mood disturbances,[81–85] as well as the recurrence of depression.[86] More so, a recent placebo-controlled randomized clinical trial with diphenhydramine, trazodone, or placebo has shown a significant improvement in the sleep profile of women treated with any of the active drugs during pregnancy compared with placebo, and a significant reduction in depressive symptoms 2 and 6 weeks after delivery.[87] Another pilot open intervention tested the effect of cognitive behavioral therapy for insomnia on mood, sleep, and fatigue in women with depression and insomnia.[88] This study has shown significant improvement in sleep efficiency and total wake time on sleep diary, in addition to significant enhancement of subjective mood and insomnia severity, sleep quality, and fatigue. These studies do suggest that there may be a causal link between sleep duration and quality and insomnia in peripartum women.

Other outcomes that have been linked to short sleep duration include labor duration and delivery mode. In a study by Lee and Gay,[89] the investigators showed that short sleep duration (less than 6 hours) in the last month of pregnancy was associated with longer labor duration and a higher risk of cesarean deliveries in nulliparous women. Similar studies have demonstrated the association of nocturnal and diurnal total sleep time with these outcomes.[75,90,91] It is possible that abnormal sleep may lead to fatigue, which may then predispose to longer labor. However, factors that may lead to both poor sleep and longer labor, such as emotional stressors, also may explain these findings but have not yet been elucidated.

Preterm birth, defined as birth occurring before 37 completed weeks of gestation, is a major health burden and a source of significant infant morbidity. Studies from more than 2 decades ago suggested a connection between sleep disruption and preterm labor. Nearly half of women residents who spent at least 1 night a week without any sleep or worked long hours were more likely to experience preterm labor than male residents' partners.[92,93] More recently, poor sleep quality measured by the Pittsburgh Sleep Quality Index (PSQI) was shown to be associated with preterm birth.[94] Despite of these findings, little has been done to investigate the link between sleep deprivation and preterm labor. It is possible that inflammation and hypothalamic pituitary axis (HPA) dysfunction, which are believed to be potential underlying mechanisms for preterm labor, are negatively influenced by poor sleep. Sleep disturbances measured by the PSQI and sleep diaries were shown to be associated with increased levels

of interleukin 6[95] and C-reactive protein[96] in pregnancy. As sleep, mood disturbances, and stress may be associated with HPA dysfunction, which has been linked to preterm birth, preliminary data are evaluating the interactions among these disturbances.[97]

Treatment

Cognitive behavioral therapy (CBT) is recommended for the treatment of insomnia in the nonpregnant population. Data on the use of CBT in pregnancy are lacking. One recent study has reported an improvement in sleep measures and mood in women with insomnia and depression who were treated with CBT for insomnia.[88] Because of fears of teratogenicity, many drugs are avoided in pregnancy. A recent study[98] showed no increase in the risk of congenital anomalies in women treated with nonbenzodiazepines zaleplon (n = 32), zolpidem (n = 603), and zopiclone (n = 692). **Table 2** summarizes the safety data of drugs commonly used for the treatment of insomnia.

In summary, sleep disruption is common in pregnancy and may be due to physiologic factors. As poor sleep has been associated with adverse pregnancy outcomes, testing whether interventions to improve sleep quality would have a positive effect on pregnancy outcomes is needed.

NARCOLEPSY

Narcolepsy is an uncommon clinical syndrome of daytime sleepiness and may be accompanied by cataplexy, hypnagogic hallucinations, and sleep paralysis. Narcolepsy can occur with or without cataplexy. According to the US population estimates, it afflicts approximately 1 in 3000 individuals.[99] As narcolepsy peaks in the adolescent years to early 20s, it is likely that women who carry the diagnosis will have a pregnancy complicated by the disorder.

Pathophysiology

The symptoms of narcolepsy largely reflect a dysregulation of the transition between wakefulness, non–rapid eye movement (REM), and REM sleep.[100–102] The normal sleep-wake cycle is regulated by a complex interaction of neurohormones and chemicals. Hypocretin 1 and 2 (Orexin A and B) are neuropeptides synthesized in the lateral hypothalamus and are implicated in the pathogenesis of narcolepsy.[103,104] Hypocretins/orexins, peptides produced by the lateral hypothalamus, orchestrate the interaction of the monoaminergic and cholinergic systems in the regulation of sleep

Table 2
Pharmacotherapy and drug safety in insomnia

	Pregnancy Safety	Lactation
Zaleplon	Study of 32 pregnant women suggests no increased risk of teratogenicity; however, numbers too small to be conclusive.[98]	Estimated infant dose <0.02% the maternal dose.[147] Unlikely to adversely affect the neonate, but no available studies evaluating consequences of such exposure.
Zolpidem	Study of 603 pregnancies with zolpidem exposure showed no increased risk of congenital anomalies.[98] However, population-based study in Taiwan (n = 2497 exposed women and 12,485 unexposed) showed an increased risk of low birth weight and preterm deliveries in women but no increased risk of congenital anomalies.[148]	Estimated infant dose <0.02% the maternal dose.[149] The American Academy of Pediatrics (AAP) classifies the drug as safe for lactation.[150]
Zopiclone	Study of 692 pregnancies showed no increased risk of malformations.[98] Other smaller studies showed similar results.[151,152] Crosses placental barrier and withdrawal reported at birth.[153]	Estimated infant dose about 3.2%.[153] Unlikely toxicity but effects of chronic exposure unknown.
Ramelteon	Animal studies suggest dose-dependent incidence of diaphragmatic hernia and scapular shape abnormalities.[154] Human data are lacking.	No human data on lactation are available.
Amytriptyline	Large-scale studies and case-control data fail to show an association with congenital malformations.[155,156]	Distributed in milk at concentrations similar to mothers. AAP considers the effect unknown.[150]
Trazodone	Not likely to result in major congenital malformations based on human reports.[157–159]	Distributed in milk but in small amounts.[160]
Doxepin	Based on animal and human reports, the drug is not expected to increase the risk of congenital malformations but human reports are scarce.	Despite only 2.5% of dose is found in breast milk, reports of muscle hypotonia exist. The World Health Organization deems the drug incompatible with breastfeeding.[161]
Diphenhydramine	Based on animal and human studies, the drug is not expected to increase the risk of congenital malformations.[162] There is some suggestion in the literature that first-trimester use may be associated with various (rather than a single) anomalies.[163,164]	Manufacturer advises against the use in lactating mothers, especially in premature newborns; however, no major adverse effects have been reported.
Temazepam	Early data on diazepam and chlordiazepoxide use in first trimester suggesting increased risk of cleft palate were not supported by later studies. Concern about neonatal withdrawal with late third-trimester use. Concomitant use with diphenhydramine has been associated with fetal death.[165]	Occasional use of benzodiazepines in breastfeeding mothers is acceptable.[161]

and wakefulness.[100–102] In persons with narcolepsy, there is an up to 90% selective reduction in orexin-producing neurons that is associated with an absence of orexin A in the spinal fluid.[105] Loss of orexin neurons may allow breakthrough REM phenomena, such as hypnagogic hallucinations, sleep paralysis, cataplexy, or sleep attacks to occur during periods of wakefulness.[100–102] The interaction of pregnancy with the orexin system is unclear. Recent preliminary data have shown immunohistochemical presence of orexin A and orexin 1 and 2 receptors in the feline placenta.[106] It is unclear if the human placenta expresses the same and whether such expression may result in any extraplacental and systemic effects of orexin.

As the age at diagnosis occurs mostly before the reproductive peak, most women will be diagnosed before pregnancy.[107] It is not clear whether the physiologic and pathologic sleep disruption in pregnancy[52,65,80] may precipitate or worsen symptoms of narcolepsy. As in the nonpregnant population, diagnosis is established by full nocturnal polysomnography followed by a multiple sleep latency test.[108]

Pregnancy and Neonatal Outcomes

Studies evaluating pregnancy and fetal outcomes are scarce and most of the literature on narcolepsy in pregnancy is based on case reports and reviews of the literature. In 2013, a European multinational cohort study of 249 mothers (414 pregnancies) with narcolepsy reported anemia and glucose intolerance more frequently in women with narcolepsy than in the general population.[107] In this study, nearly 40% of women had worsening in their symptoms of narcolepsy.[107] The average body mass index was, however, higher in the narcolepsy group and could have confounded the findings of glucose intolerance. Mean birth weight and gestational age at birth were within the normal range, suggesting that the effect of this disorder on intrauterine growth and preterm delivery is likely minimal.[107] In a previous study published by the same investigators, women with symptoms of narcolepsy during pregnancy had a higher percentage of a composite set of complications, including edema, anemia, and gestational diabetes compared with the group who developed narcolepsy symptoms after the index pregnancy.[109] This difference was no longer significant when the individual complications were compared.

In the multinational European study,[107] fewer than 1% of mothers with a history of cataplexy reported cataplexy during delivery, but there was an increased rate of cesarean deliveries in the overall sample. Pain may be a trigger for cataplexy, and so is interrupted sleep from prolonged labor. Thus, it is possible that labor may be a trigger for cataplexy. In addition, a case report describes status cataplecticus during labor in a woman with a history of cataplexy triggered by sexual intercourse, suggesting that genital stimulation during labor or intercourse may be a potential stimulant as well.[110]

Treatment

Management of narcolepsy in pregnancy is quite challenging due to the dearth of data evaluating medication safety. However, the implications of untreated disease in pregnancy and the postpartum period can be quite dramatic in some symptomatic patients. Unpredictable sleep attacks and cataplexy can have some devastating consequences for the mother and the fetus, such as car accidents, falls, or trauma. In the postpartum period, narcolepsy may be exacerbated by newborn-induced sleep restrictions, and the lack of treatment may have the same consequences but certainly have some additional repercussions on child care. There are currently no standardized guidelines to guide the treatment of narcolepsy in pregnancy. A recent survey of 34 sleep physicians who treat 5 patients with narcolepsy per week on average showed that opinions differed significantly regarding the use or discontinuation of drugs at the time of conception, pregnancy, or lactation.[111,112] The decision to withdraw or continue stimulant or anticataplectic medications should essentially be individualized, and the risk of untreated disease weighed against that of exposure of the fetus to these medications. Women with minimal symptoms that are unlikely to affect their safety or that their unborn child will likely do well with scheduled naps and the avoidance of sleep loss. For those with more significant symptoms that may lead to falls for instance, or excessive sleepiness that may affect driving or being in public places, the decision is more challenging. **Table 3** summarizes the data available on stimulants and REM suppressants. Essentially some of the medications are not associated with a teratogenic risk but are associated with poor growth, the clinical relevance of which is unclear given the quality of the available data. Reproductive-age women should be counseled before pregnancy of the risk of the disorder and the drugs and a plan decided on early, when possible.

As in the nonpregnant population, optimization of nonpharmacological and behavioral measures is important. Patients should be educated on good sleep hygiene, with regular sleep-wake cycles;

Table 3
Pharmacotherapy and drug safety in narcolepsy

	Pregnancy Safety	Lactation
Modafinil	Based on experimental animal studies and limited human data, the drug is not expected to increase the risk of congenital abnormalities.[62] Ongoing registry by the manufacturer.	No human data available on transfer to breast milk. Small molecular weight makes it likely that the drug is transferred. By stimulating dopamine, the drug may inhibit breast milk production.
Armodafinil	Experimental animal studies suggest resorption and skeletal variations. Very limited human data. Ongoing pregnancy exposure registry by manufacturer.	No human data available.
Amphetamines	Reduced pup and litter size in animal studies. Limited human data show an effect on growth and neonatal behavior. Despite case reports associating amphetamines with various congenital anomalies, case-control and prospective studies fail to show such associations.[142,166–168] However, reports of minor malformations continue to exist.[167]	Not compatible with breastfeeding.[150,169]
Methylphenidate	The drug is not expected to increase the risk of congenital anomalies[170]; however, possible increase in risk of prematurity, growth restriction, and neonatal withdrawal.	Small amounts transfer into breast milk. Limited reports of no adverse effects on the nursling.
Sodium oxybate	Report of 150 cesarean deliveries performed with sodium hydroxybutyrate has identified maternal seizure, arterial hypertension, and excessive blood loss as possibly being associated with the use of the drug. Poor fetal condition reported in 12% of subjects.[171] There are no available studies to support safe use of this drug to date.	No available data on breastfeeding.
Venlafaxine	Animal studies and some human studies suggest reduction in birth weight of the offspring. The drug is not anticipated to cause congenital anomalies.[172] Transient neonatal complications have been reported.	Transfer in milk has been documented but found to be variable.
Fluoxetine	No significant association with birth defects. Transient neonatal complications with third-trimester use. Risk of social-behavioral abnormalities in childhood.	Small amount found in breast milk.
Clomipramine	Possible increase in the risk of cardiac malformations.[173] Increased risk of transient neonatal complications as selective serotonin reuptake inhibitors.	Small amount found in breast milk. May be a concern in breastfeeding.[174]
Protriptyline	The drug is not anticipated to increase the risk of congenital malformations. Withdrawal symptoms in the newborn have been reported.[175]	There are no available data on the transfer of this drug into breast milk.
Selegiline	Limited animal and human data. Vasoconstrictive effect is concerning in pregnancy.	No safety data available.

avoidance of potentially hazardous situations, especially when alone; and avoiding driving, cooking, or operating machinery. Scheduled naps in the late morning or early afternoon, along with regular exercise may be beneficial.

Recommending a mode of delivery is another step in the management of pregnant women with narcolepsy. Because of the increased risk of medical and obstetric complications associated with cesarean deliveries compared with vaginal deliveries, it is hard to recommend cesarean delivery in women with cataplexy if the risk of cataplexy during labor is only 1%.[107] Good pain control, careful history to investigate individual triggers, and avoiding sleep loss when possible may minimize the risk of cataplexy during labor. In the postpartum period, partner education may be necessary to enlist help with nocturnal chores to help minimize maternal sleep deprivation.

In summary, women with narcolepsy may have worsening symptoms with pregnancy but cataplexy during labor is rare. Although most responders to a survey would opt to stop medications at the onset of pregnancy and many would do so for the duration of pregnancy, we would recommend making individualized decisions based on the drug in question and the risk of untreated disease.

CIRCADIAN RHYTHM DISTURBANCES

The circadian system is the main pacemaker in mammals and regulates many physiologic and behavioral functions. It is located in the suprachiasmatic nucleus, within the anterior hypothalamus, and is controlled by several factors, with the most significant and potent being light. Causes for desynchronization of the circadian patterns may be spontaneous and due to intrinsic dysfunction of the circadian clock, but desynchronization is much more likely to be due to exogenous factors such as jet lag or shift work. Desynchronization of circadian patterns in conditions, such as night-shift work, have been associated with adverse outcomes in the general population. These include increased risk of cancer,[113] metabolic syndrome,[114] and adverse cardiovascular outcomes.[115]

Circadian rhythm likely plays an important role in pregnancy. In the first trimester, rapid rises in estrogen and progesterone occur to promote implantation and gestation and their levels continue to rise throughout pregnancy. There also are increases in the levels of prolactin, cortisol, and thyroid hormones. These hormones are all regulated via the circadian system and have circadian variations. Hence, it is possible that misalignment of the circadian pattern may lead to dysregulation of these hormones, and potentially impact fertility

and pregnancy. Indeed, in reproductive-age women, shift work has been repeatedly shown to be associated with irregular menses and infertility.[116,117] Labyak and colleagues[118] found that among women who worked the overnight shift, 53% reported irregularities in their menstrual cycle, leading to potential subfertility.

In the animal model, circadian disturbances during pregnancy have detrimental effects on both maternal and pup outcomes. Rats exposed to circadian desynchrony during pregnancy had a higher incidence of embryo resorption and poor pup survival.[119] Furthermore, rats that underwent chronic jet lag during pregnancy produced pups with metabolic derangements, including obesity, hyperleptinemia, and modulation of glucose tolerance/insulin insensitivity.[120] Data linking circadian desynchrony with adverse outcomes in human pregnancies are scarce, but some evidence exists that shift work during pregnancy may contribute to poor outcomes. Evidence from the National Birth Cohort in Denmark suggests that shift work leads to early fetal loss.[121] Another study by Lin and colleagues[122] demonstrated that factory employees working rotating shifts had infants with lower birth weights. A recent meta-analysis by Bonzini and colleagues[123] showed that nurses exposed to shift work had a higher, albeit small, risk of having small for gestational age and low birth weight infants along with preterm delivery. Although these results are interesting, it should be noted that these studies did not assess the influence of sleep duration on this association. Shift workers have been shown to be sleep deprived by virtue of their circadian misalignment, and there is a growing body of literature to suggest that short sleep duration is associated with increased adverse health outcomes.[124] These adverse outcomes may be mediated via increased proinflammatory markers and reactive species, and altered immunity.[125–128] As discussed previously, short sleep duration may be associated with some perinatal adverse outcomes.

There are no convincing data to date to suggest an association between circadian desynchrony and preeclampsia. Haelterman and colleagues[129] did not find any correlation between work schedule and preeclampsia. This result was similar to a study by Chang and colleagues[130] that evaluated more than 24,000 Taiwanese workers working evening or rotating shifts. No increased risk of gestational hypertension or preeclampsia above the risk for nonworking mothers was observed. However, it should be noted that the normal circadian variation of blood pressure is blunted in women with preeclampsia. This has led some investigators to postulate that there may be a link between the circadian clock gene and preeclampsia.[131]

Preliminary data on perinatal women with a major depressive disorder show variable shifts in the circadian rhythm that appear to correlate with depressive symptoms.[132]

Finally, there are some interesting data exploring the effect of circadian rhythms on labor. Spontaneous rupture of the membranes occurs most frequently in the middle of the night, with the onset of labor peaking in the early morning. In a randomized, controlled clinical trial comparing morning (8:00 AM) versus evening (8:00 PM) administration of prostaglandin, morning induction of labor was associated with a shorter induction to birth interval, and was less likely to result in instrumental vaginal births for women in their first pregnancies.[133] However, a recent meta-analysis[134] found no overall difference between morning and evening induction on either maternal or neonatal outcomes. Further work is needed to determine if timing of labor may play an important role, and if circadian disturbances are important.

In summary, there is some evidence in both animals and humans to suggest that disruption of circadian patterns may be detrimental. However, the mechanisms by which circadian misalignment leads to adverse perinatal consequences and the effect of treatment of circadian desynchrony on adverse outcomes need to be further investigated.

SUMMARY

Sleep disruption and poor sleep are quite common in pregnancy and peripartum; pregnancy physiology may predispose to the new-onset development of sleep disorders, as well as the worsening of others. Medication choices are more limited in the pregnant population because of concerns for fetal safety. However, poor sleep is associated with adverse pregnancy outcomes and possibly mediates the occurrence of some comorbid conditions. Hence, management of sleep disorders and poor sleep during pregnancy may prove to play an important part in the health and well-being of pregnancy.

REFERENCES

1. American Academy of Sleep Medicine. International classification of sleep disorders, revised: Diagnostic and coding manual. Chicago, Illinois: American Academy of Sleep Medicine; 2001.

2. Bourjeily G, Mohsenin V. Sleep physiology in pregnancy. In: Rosene-Montella K, Bourjeily G, editors. Pulmonary problems in pregnancy. New York: Humana Press; 2009. p. 37–55.

3. Habr F, Raker C, Lin CL, et al. Predictors of gastroesophageal reflux symptoms in pregnant women screened for sleep disordered breathing: A secondary analysis. Clin Res Hepatol Gastroenterol 2013;37(1):93–9.

4. Parboosingh J, Doig A. Studies of nocturia in normal pregnancy. J Obstet Gynaecol Br Commonw 1973;80(10):888–95.

5. Izci B, Riha RL, Martin SE, et al. The upper airway in pregnancy and pre-eclampsia. Am J Respir Crit Care Med 2003;167:137–40.

6. Pilkington S, Carli F, Dakin MJ, et al. Increase in Mallampati score during pregnancy. Br J Anaesth 1995;74:638–42.

7. Camann WR, Ostheimer GW. Physiological adaptations during pregnancy. Int Anesthesiol Clin 1990; 28:2–10.

8. Hegewald MJ, Crapo RO. Respiratory physiology in pregnancy. Clin Chest Med 2011;32:1–13.

9. Bourjeily G, Raker CA, Chalhoub M, et al. Pregnancy and fetal outcomes of symptoms of sleep-disordered breathing. Eur Respir J 2010;36:849–55.

10. Louis JM, Auckley D, Sokol RJ, et al. Maternal and neonatal morbidities associated with obstructive sleep apnea complicating pregnancy. Am J Obstet Gynecol 2010;202:261.e1–5.

11. Bourjeily G, El Sabbagh R, Sawan P, et al. Epworth Sleepiness Scale scores and adverse pregnancy outcomes. Sleep Breath 2013;17:1179–86.

12. Chen YH, Kang JH, Lin CC, et al. Obstructive sleep apnea and the risk of adverse pregnancy outcomes. Am J Obstet Gynecol 2012;206:136. e1–5.

13. Reutrakul S, Zaidi N, Wroblewski K, et al. Sleep disturbances and their relationship to glucose tolerance in pregnancy. Diabetes Care 2011;34:2454–7.

14. Reutrakul S, Zaidi N, Wroblewski K, et al. Interactions between pregnancy, obstructive sleep apnea, and gestational diabetes mellitus. J Clin Endocrinol Metab 2013;98:4195–202.

15. Franklin KA, Holmgren PA, Jonsson F, et al. Snoring, pregnancy-induced hypertension, and growth retardation of the fetus. Chest 2000;117:137–41.

16. Micheli K, Komninos I, Bagkeris E, et al. Sleep patterns in late pregnancy and risk of preterm birth and fetal growth restriction. Epidemiology 2011; 22:738–44.

17. Calaora-Tournadre D, Ragot S, Meurice JC, et al. Obstructive sleep apnea syndrome during pregnancy: prevalence of main symptoms and relationship with pregnancy-induced hypertension and intra-uterine growth retardation. Rev Med Interne 2006;27:291–5 [in French].

18. Leung PL, Hui DS, Leung TN, et al. Sleep disturbances in Chinese pregnant women. BJOG 2005; 112:1568–71.

19. Loube DI, Poceta JS, Morales MC, et al. Self-reported snoring in pregnancy. Association with fetal outcome. Chest 1996;109:885–9.

20. Tauman R, Many A, Deutsch V, et al. Maternal snoring during pregnancy is associated with enhanced fetal erythropoiesis—a preliminary study. Sleep Med 2011;12:518–22.

21. Charbonneau M, Falcone T, Cosio MG, et al. Obstructive sleep apnea during pregnancy. Therapy and implications for fetal health. Am Rev Respir Dis 1991;144:461–3.

22. Joel-Cohen SJ, Schoenfeld A. Fetal response to periodic sleep apnea: a new syndrome in obstetrics. Eur J Obstet Gynecol Reprod Biol 1978; 8:77–81.

23. Olivarez SA, Maheshwari B, McCarthy M, et al. Prospective trial on obstructive sleep apnea in pregnancy and fetal heart rate monitoring. Am J Obstet Gynecol 2010;202:552.e1–7.

24. Facco FL, Liu CS, Cabello AA, et al. Sleep-disordered breathing: a risk factor for adverse pregnancy outcomes? Am J Perinatol 2012;29:277–82.

25. Bourjeily G, Barbara N, Larson L, et al. Clinical manifestations of obstructive sleep apnoea in pregnancy: more than snoring and witnessed apnoeas. J Obstet Gynaecol 2012;32:434–8.

26. Guilleminault C, Kreutzer M, Chang JL. Pregnancy, sleep disordered breathing and treatment with nasal continuous positive airway pressure. Sleep Med 2004;5:43–51.

27. Bourjeily G, Habr F, Miller MA, et al. Symptoms of sleep-disordered breathing, BMI and pregnancy outcomes. Chest 2007;132(4):463a.

28. Coleman RM. Periodic movements in sleep (nocturnal myoclonus) and restless legs syndrome. In: Guilleminault C, editor. Sleeping and waking disorders: indications and techniques. Menlo Park (CA): Addison-Wesley; 1982. p. 265–95.

29. Ohayon MM, O'Hara R, Vitiello MV. Epidemiology of restless legs syndrome: a synthesis of the literature. Sleep Med Rev 2012;16:283–95.

30. Phillips B, Young T, Finn L, et al. Epidemiology of restless legs symptoms in adults. Arch Intern Med 2000;160:2137–41.

31. Chen PH, Liou KC, Chen CP, et al. Risk factors and prevalence rate of restless legs syndrome among pregnant women in Taiwan. Sleep Med 2012;13: 1153–7.

32. Manconi M, Govoni V, De Vito A, et al. Pregnancy as a risk factor for restless legs syndrome. Sleep Med 2004;5:305–8.

33. Harano S, Ohida T, Kaneita Y, et al. Prevalence of restless legs syndrome with pregnancy and the relationship with sleep disorders in the Japanese large population. Sleep Biol Rhythms 2008;6:102–9.

34. Suzuki K, Ohida T, Sone T, et al. The prevalence of restless legs syndrome among pregnant women in Japan and the relationship between restless legs syndrome and sleep problems. Sleep 2003;26: 673–7.

35. Manconi M, Govoni V, De Vito A, et al. Restless legs syndrome and pregnancy. Neurology 2004;63: 1065–9.

36. Sikandar R, Khealani BA, Wasay M. Predictors of restless legs syndrome in pregnancy: a hospital based cross sectional survey from Pakistan. Sleep Med 2009;10:676–8.

37. Tunc T, Karadag YS, Dogulu F, et al. Predisposing factors of restless legs syndrome in pregnancy. Mov Disord 2007;22:627–31.

38. Alves DA, Carvalho LB, Morais JF, et al. Restless legs syndrome during pregnancy in Brazilian women. Sleep Med 2010;11:1049–54.

39. Facco FL, Kramer J, Ho KH, et al. Sleep disturbances in pregnancy. Obstet Gynecol 2010;115: 77–83.

40. Uglane MT, Westad S, Backe B. Restless legs syndrome in pregnancy is a frequent disorder with a good prognosis. Acta Obstet Gynecol Scand 2011;90:1046–8.

41. Gambling L, Kennedy C, McArdle HJ. Iron and copper in fetal development. Semin Cell Dev Biol 2011;22:637–44.

42. Gambling L, Czopek A, Andersen HS, et al. Fetal iron status regulates maternal iron metabolism during pregnancy in the rat. Am J Physiol Regul Integr Comp Physiol 2009;296:R1063–70.

43. Fosset C, McGaw BA, Abramovich D, et al. Interrelations between ceruloplasmin and Fe status during human pregnancy. Biol Trace Elem Res 2004; 98:1–12.

44. Swensen AR, Harnack LJ, Ross JA. Nutritional assessment of pregnant women enrolled in the Special Supplemental Program for Women, Infants, and Children (WIC). J Am Diet Assoc 2001;101:903–8.

45. Aul EA, Davis BJ, Rodnitzky RL. The importance of formal serum iron studies in the assessment of restless legs syndrome. Neurology 1998;51:912.

46. Sun ER, Chen CA, Ho G, et al. Iron and the restless legs syndrome. Sleep 1998;21:371–7.

47. Botez MI, Lambert B. Folate deficiency and restless-legs syndrome in pregnancy. N Engl J Med 1977;297:670.

48. Lee KA, Zaffke ME, Baratte-Beebe K. Restless legs syndrome and sleep disturbance during pregnancy: the role of folate and iron. J Womens Health Gend Based Med 2001;10:335–41.

49. Kipp M, Karakaya S, Pawlak J, et al. Estrogen and the development and protection of nigrostriatal dopaminergic neurons: concerted action of a multitude of signals, protective molecules, and growth factors. Front Neuroendocrinol 2006;27:376–90.

50. Dzaja A, Wehrle R, Lancel M, et al. Elevated estradiol plasma levels in women with restless legs during pregnancy. Sleep 2009;32:169–74.

51. Hubner A, Krafft A, Gadient S, et al. Characteristics and determinants of restless legs syndrome in

pregnancy: a prospective study. Neurology 2013; 80:738–42.

52. Neau JP, Marion P, Mathis S, et al. Restless legs syndrome and pregnancy: follow-up of pregnant women before and after delivery. Eur Neurol 2010;64:361–6.

53. Batool-Anwar S, Malhotra A, Forman J, et al. Restless legs syndrome and hypertension in middle-aged women. Hypertension 2011;58:791–6.

54. Benediktsdottir B, Janson C, Lindberg E, et al. Prevalence of restless legs syndrome among adults in Iceland and Sweden: lung function, comorbidity, ferritin, biomarkers and quality of life. Sleep Med 2010;11:1043–8.

55. Ramirez JO, Cabrera SA, Hidalgo H, et al. Is pre-eclampsia associated with restless legs syndrome? Sleep Med 2013;14:894–6.

56. Baughman KR, Bourguet CC, Ober SK. Gender differences in the association between antidepressant use and restless legs syndrome. Mov Disord 2009;24:1054–9.

57. Kim SW, Shin IS, Kim JM, et al. Factors potentiating the risk of mirtazapine-associated restless legs syndrome. Hum Psychopharmacol 2008;23: 615–20.

58. Rottach KG, Schaner BM, Kirch MH, et al. Restless legs syndrome as side effect of second generation antidepressants. J Psychiatr Res 2008;43:70–5.

59. Brown LK, Dedrick DL, Doggett JW, et al. Antidepressant medication use and restless legs syndrome in patients presenting with insomnia. Sleep Med 2005;6:443–50.

60. Leutgeb U, Martus P. Regular intake of non-opioid analgesics is associated with an increased risk of restless legs syndrome in patients maintained on antidepressants. Eur J Med Res 2002;7:368–78.

61. Aurora RN, Kristo DA, Bista SR, et al. The treatment of restless legs syndrome and periodic limb movement disorder in adults—an update for 2012: practice parameters with an evidence-based systematic review and meta-analyses: an American Academy of Sleep Medicine Clinical Practice Guideline. Sleep 2012;35:1039–62.

62. Reproductive Toxicology Center. Reprotox. Available at: http://www.reprotox.org/. Accessed November 15, 2013.

63. Hale TW. Medications and mothers' milk. 2000. Available at: http://www.medsmilk.com/drugs/. 9th Retrieved November 22, 2013.

64. Schneider J, Krafft A, Bloch A, et al. Iron infusion in restless legs syndrome in the third trimester of pregnancy. Sleep Med 2011;12:S17–8.

65. National Sleep Foundation. "Sleep America Polls. 2007 Women and Sleep." 2007. Available at: http://ww.sleepfoundation.org/article/sleep-america-polls/2007-women-and-sleep. Retrieved November 21, 2013.

66. Lee KA, Zaffke ME, McEnany G. Parity and sleep patterns during and after pregnancy. Obstet Gynecol 2000;95:14–8.

67. Wilson DL, Barnes M, Ellett L, et al. Decreased sleep efficiency, increased wake after sleep onset and increased cortical arousals in late pregnancy. Aust N Z J Obstet Gynaecol 2011;51:38–46.

68. Hedman C, Pohjasvaara T, Tolonen U, et al. Effects of pregnancy on mothers' sleep. Sleep Med 2002; 3:37–42.

69. Mindell JA, Jacobson BJ. Sleep disturbances during pregnancy. J Obstet Gynecol Neonatal Nurs 2000;29:590–7.

70. Elek SM, Hudson DB, Fleck MO. Expectant parents' experience with fatigue and sleep during pregnancy. Birth 1997;24:49–54.

71. Hertz G, Fast A, Feinsilver SH, et al. Sleep in normal late pregnancy. Sleep 1992;15:246–51.

72. Lee KA, DeJoseph JF. Sleep disturbances, vitality, and fatigue among a select group of employed childbearing women. Birth 1992;19:208–13.

73. Lee KA. Sleep dysfunction in women and its management. Curr Treat Options Neurol 2006;8:376–86.

74. Dorheim SK, Bjorvatn B, Eberhard-Gran M. Insomnia and depressive symptoms in late pregnancy: a population-based study. Behav Sleep Med 2012;10:152–66.

75. Tsai SY, Kuo LT, Lee CN, et al. Reduced sleep duration and daytime naps in pregnant women in Taiwan. Nurs Res 2013;62:99–105.

76. Fernandez-Alonso AM, Trabalon-Pastor M, Chedraui P, et al. Factors related to insomnia and sleepiness in the late third trimester of pregnancy. Arch Gynecol Obstet 2012;286:55–61.

77. Ko H, Shin J, Kim MY, et al. Sleep disturbances in Korean pregnant and postpartum women. J Psychosom Obstet Gynaecol 2012;33:85–90.

78. Fung J, Messerlian G, Curran P, et al. Obstructive sleep apnea is associated with alterations in markers of feto-placental wellbeing. Accepted as oral presentation. European Respiratory Society Annual Congress. Barcelona, Spain, September 7–11, 2013.

79. Pien GW, Schwab RJ. Sleep disorders during pregnancy. Sleep 2004;27:1405–17.

80. Bourjeily G, Raker C, Chalhoub M, et al. Excessive daytime sleepiness in late pregnancy may not always be normal: results from a cross-sectional study. Sleep Breath 2013;17:735–40.

81. Bei B, Milgrom J, Ericksen J, et al. Subjective perception of sleep, but not its objective quality, is associated with immediate postpartum mood disturbances in healthy women. Sleep 2010;33: 531–8.

82. Dorheim SK, Bondevik GT, Eberhard-Gran M, et al. Sleep and depression in postpartum women: a population-based study. Sleep 2009;32:847–55.

83. Goyal D, Gay C, Lee K. Fragmented maternal sleep is more strongly correlated with depressive symptoms than infant temperament at three months postpartum. Arch Womens Ment Health 2009;12:229–37.

84. Marques M, Bos S, Soares MJ, et al. Is insomnia in late pregnancy a risk factor for postpartum depression/depressive symptomatology? Psychiatry Res 2011;186:272–80.

85. Swanson LM, Pickett SM, Flynn H, et al. Relationships among depression, anxiety, and insomnia symptoms in perinatal women seeking mental health treatment. J Womens Health (Larchmt) 2011;20:553–8.

86. Okun ML, Hanusa BH, Hall M, et al. Sleep complaints in late pregnancy and the recurrence of postpartum depression. Behav Sleep Med 2009; 7:106–17.

87. Khazaie H, Ghadami MR, Knight DC, et al. Insomnia treatment in the third trimester of pregnancy reduces postpartum depression symptoms: a randomized clinical trial. Psychiatry Res 2013; 210(3):901–5.

88. Swanson LM, Flynn H, Adams-Mundy JD, et al. An open pilot of cognitive-behavioral therapy for insomnia in women with postpartum depression. Behav Sleep Med 2013;11:297–307.

89. Lee KA, Gay CL. Sleep in late pregnancy predicts length of labor and type of delivery. Am J Obstet Gynecol 2004;191:2041–6.

90. Naghi I, Keypour F, Ahari SB, et al. Sleep disturbance in late pregnancy and type and duration of labour. J Obstet Gynaecol 2011;31:489–91.

91. Zafarghandi N, Hadavand S, Davati A, et al. The effects of sleep quality and duration in late pregnancy on labor and fetal outcome. J Matern Fetal Neonatal Med 2012;25:535–7.

92. Klebanoff MA, Shiono PH, Rhoads GG. Outcomes of pregnancy in a national sample of resident physicians. N Engl J Med 1990;323:1040–5.

93. Osborn LM, Harris DL, Reading JC, et al. Outcome of pregnancies experienced during residency. J Fam Pract 1990;31:618–22.

94. Okun ML, Schetter CD, Glynn LM. Poor sleep quality is associated with preterm birth. Sleep 2011;34: 1493–8.

95. Okun ML, Hall M, Coussons-Read ME. Sleep disturbances increase interleukin-6 production during pregnancy: implications for pregnancy complications. Reprod Sci 2007;14:560–7.

96. Okun ML, Coussons-Read ME. Sleep disruption during pregnancy: how does it influence serum cytokines? J Reprod Immunol 2007;73:158–65.

97. Okun ML, Luther JF, Wisniewski SR, et al. Disturbed sleep and inflammatory cytokines in depressed and nondepressed pregnant women: an exploratory analysis of pregnancy outcomes. Psychosom Med 2013;75:670–81.

98. Wikner BN, Kallen B. Are hypnotic benzodiazepine receptor agonists teratogenic in humans? J Clin Psychopharmacol 2011;31:356–9.

99. Longstreth WT Jr, Koepsell TD, Ton TG, et al. The epidemiology of narcolepsy. Sleep 2007;30:13–26.

100. Burgess CR, Scammell TE. Narcolepsy: neural mechanisms of sleepiness and cataplexy. J Neurosci 2012;32:12305–11.

101. Saper CB, Chou TC, Scammell TE. The sleep switch: hypothalamic control of sleep and wakefulness. Trends Neurosci 2001;24:726–31.

102. Scammell TE. The neurobiology, diagnosis, and treatment of narcolepsy. Ann Neurol 2003;53:154–66.

103. Chemelli RM, Willie JT, Sinton CM, et al. Narcolepsy in orexin knockout mice: molecular genetics of sleep regulation. Cell 1999;98:437–51.

104. Sakurai T, Amemiya A, Ishii M, et al. Orexins and orexin receptors: a family of hypothalamic neuropeptides and G protein-coupled receptors that regulate feeding behavior. Cell 1998;92:573–85.

105. Peyron C, Faraco J, Rogers W, et al. A mutation in a case of early onset narcolepsy and a generalized absence of hypocretin peptides in human narcoleptic brains. Nat Med 2000;6:991–7.

106. Dall'Aglio C, Pascucci L, Mercati F, et al. Immunohistochemical detection of the orexin system in the placenta of cats. Res Vet Sci 2012;92:362–5.

107. Maurovich-Horvat E, Kemlink D, Hogl B, et al. Narcolepsy and pregnancy: a retrospective European evaluation of 249 pregnancies. J Sleep Res 2013; 22:496–512.

108. Morgenthaler TI, Kapur VK, Brown T, et al. Practice parameters for the treatment of narcolepsy and other hypersomnias of central origin. Sleep 2007;30:1705–11.

109. Maurovich-Horvat E, Tormasiova M, Slonkova J, et al. Assessment of pregnancy outcomes in Czech and Slovak women with narcolepsy. Med Sci Monit 2010;16:SR35–40.

110. Ping LS, Yat FS, Kwok WY. Status cataplecticus leading to the obstetric complication of prolonged labor. J Clin Sleep Med 2007;3:56–7.

111. Thorpy M, Zhao CG, Dauvilliers Y. Management of narcolepsy during pregnancy. Sleep Med 2013;14: 367–76.

112. Shields N, Muza R, Kosky C, et al. An investigation into the use of stimulant therapy during pregnancy. Sleep Disord 2012;2012:308952.

113. Straif K, Baan R, Grosse Y, et al. Carcinogenicity of shift-work, painting, and fire-fighting. Lancet Oncol 2007;8:1065–6.

114. De Bacquer D, Van Risseghem M, Clays E, et al. Rotating shift work and the metabolic syndrome: a prospective study. Int J Epidemiol 2009;38:848–54.

115. Scheer FA, Hilton MF, Mantzoros CS, et al. Adverse metabolic and cardiovascular consequences of circadian misalignment. Proc Natl Acad Sci U S A 2009;106:4453–8.

116. Bisanti L, Olsen J, Basso O, et al. Shift work and subfecundity: a European multicenter study. European Study Group on Infertility and Subfecundity. J Occup Environ Med 1996;38:352–8.

117. Lauria L, Ballard TJ, Caldora M, et al. Reproductive disorders and pregnancy outcomes among female flight attendants. Aviat Space Environ Med 2006; 77:533–9.

118. Labyak S, Lava S, Turek F, et al. Effects of shiftwork on sleep and menstrual function in nurses. Health Care Women Int 2002;23:703–14.

119. Endo A, Watanabe T. Effects of non-24-hour days on reproductive efficacy and embryonic development in mice. Gamete Res 1989;22:435–41.

120. Varcoe TJ, Wight N, Voultsios A, et al. Chronic phase shifts of the photoperiod throughout pregnancy programs glucose intolerance and insulin resistance in the rat. PLoS One 2011;6:e18504.

121. Zhu JL, Hjollund NH, Andersen AM, et al. Shift work, job stress, and late fetal loss: the National Birth Cohort in Denmark. J Occup Environ Med 2004;46:1144–9.

122. Lin YC, Chen MH, Hsieh CJ, et al. Effect of rotating shift work on childbearing and birth weight: a study of women working in a semiconductor manufacturing factory. World J Pediatr 2011;7: 129–35.

123. Bonzini M, Palmer KT, Coggon D, et al. Shift work and pregnancy outcomes: a systematic review with meta-analysis of currently available epidemiological studies. BJOG 2011;118:1429–37.

124. Porkka-Heiskanen T, Zitting KM, Wigren HK. Sleep, its regulation and possible mechanisms of sleep disturbances. Acta Physiol (Oxf) 2013; 208:311–28.

125. van Amelsvoort LG, Schouten EG, Kok FJ. Duration of shiftwork related to body mass index and waist to hip ratio. Int J Obes Relat Metab Disord 1999; 23:973–8.

126. Lange T, Dimitrov S, Fehm HL, et al. Shift of monocyte function toward cellular immunity during sleep. Arch Intern Med 2006;166:1695–700.

127. Irwin M, McClintick J, Costlow C, et al. Partial night sleep deprivation reduces natural killer and cellular immune responses in humans. FASEB J 1996;10: 643–53.

128. Irwin MR, Wang M, Campomayor CO, et al. Sleep deprivation and activation of morning levels of cellular and genomic markers of inflammation. Arch Intern Med 2006;166:1756–62.

129. Haelterman E, Marcoux S, Croteau A, et al. Population-based study on occupational risk factors for preeclampsia and gestational hypertension. Scand J Work Environ Health 2007;33:304–17.

130. Chang PJ, Chu LC, Hsieh WS, et al. Working hours and risk of gestational hypertension and preeclampsia. Occup Med (Lond) 2010;60:66–71.

131. Ditisheim AJ, Dibner C, Philippe J, et al. Biological rhythms and preeclampsia. Front Endocrinol (Lausanne) 2013;4:47.

132. Sharkey KM, Pearlstein TB, Carskadon MA. Circadian phase shifts and mood across the perinatal period in women with a history of major depressive disorder: a preliminary communication. J Affect Disord 2013;150:1103–8.

133. Dodd JM, Crowther CA, Robinson JS. Morning compared with evening induction of labor: a nested randomized controlled trial. A nested randomized controlled trial. Obstet Gynecol 2006;108:350–60.

134. Bakker JJ, van der Goes BY, Pel M, et al. Morning versus evening induction of labour for improving outcomes. Cochrane Database Syst Rev 2013;(2):CD007707.

135. Dostal M, Felberg M, Weber-Schoendorfer C, et al. Treatment of restless legs syndrome during pregnancy. Reprod Toxicol 2010;30:236–7.

136. Tanase H, Hirose K, Shimada K, et al. The safety test of L-DOPA. II. Effect of L-DOPA on the development of pre- and post natal offsprings of experimental animals. Sankyo Kenyusho Nempo 1970; 22:165–86.

137. Staples RE, Mattis PA. Teratology of L-dopa [abstract]. Teratology 1973;8:238.

138. Samojlik E, Khing OJ, Chang MC. Effects of dopamine on reproductive processes and fetal development in rats. Am J Obstet Gynecol 1969;104:578–85.

139. Clark RB, Brunner JA 3rd. Dopamine for the treatment of spinal hypotension during cesarean section. Anesthesiology 1980;53:514–7.

140. Broussard CS, Rasmussen SA, Reefhuis J, et al. Maternal treatment with opioid analgesics and risk for birth defects. Am J Obstet Gynecol 2011; 204:314.e1–11.

141. Bracken MB, Holford TR. Exposure to prescribed drugs in pregnancy and association with congenital malformations. Obstet Gynecol 1981;58:336–44.

142. Heinonen OP, Slone D, Shapiro S. Birth defects and drugs in pregnancy. Littleton (MA): Pub. Sciences Group; 1977.

143. Schick B, Hom M, Tolosa G, et al. Preliminary analysis of first trimester exposure to oxycodone and hydrocodone. Reprod Toxicol 1996;10:162.

144. Huisjes HJ, Hadders-Algra M, Touwen BC. Is clonidine a behavioural teratogen in the human? Early Hum Dev 1986;14:43–8.

145. Fisher JB, Edgren BE, Mammel MC, et al. Neonatal apnea associated with maternal clonazepam therapy: a case report. Obstet Gynecol 1985;66:34S–5S.

146. Birnbaum CS, Cohen LS, Bailey JW, et al. Serum concentrations of antidepressants and benzodiazepines in nursing infants: a case series. Pediatrics 1999;104:e11.

147. Darwish M, Martin PT, Cevallos WH, et al. Rapid disappearance of zaleplon from breast milk after

oral administration to lactating women. J Clin Pharmacol 1999;39:670–4.

148. Wang LH, Lin HC, Lin CC, et al. Increased risk of adverse pregnancy outcomes in women receiving zolpidem during pregnancy. Clin Pharmacol Ther 2010;88:369–74.

149. Pons G, Francoual C, Guillet P, et al. Zolpidem excretion in breast milk. Eur J Clin Pharmacol 1989;37:245–8.

150. American Academy of Pediatrics Committee on Drugs. Transfer of drugs and other chemicals into human milk. Pediatrics 2001;108:776–89.

151. Diav-Citrin O, Okotore B, Lucarelli K, et al. Pregnancy outcome following first-trimester exposure to zopiclone: a prospective controlled cohort study. Am J Perinatol 1999;16:157–60.

152. Stephens S, Wilson G, Gilfillan C, et al. Preliminary data on therapeutic exposure to zopiclone during pregnancy. Reprod Toxicol 2008;26:73–4.

153. Mathieu OM, Thompson M, Leplaya M, et al. Case report: in utero exposure and safe breastfeeding in two premature twins of a chronically treated mother with high doses of zopiclone [abstract]. Fundam Clin Pharmacol 2010;24:424.

154. Takeda Pharmaceuticals America Inc. Micromedex Healthcare Series [intranet database] Version 5.1. Greenwood Village (CO): Thomson Healthcare. Available at: http://rxdrugsinfo.com/drug-info-label/rozerem. Retrieved July 1, 2014.

155. Greenberg G, Inman WH, Weatherall JA, et al. Maternal drug histories and congenital abnormalities. Br Med J 1977;2:853–6.

156. Winship KA, Cahal DA, Weber JC, et al. Maternal drug histories and central nervous system anomalies. Arch Dis Child 1984;59:1052–60.

157. Einarson A, Choi J, Einarson TR, et al. Incidence of major malformations in infants following antidepressant exposure in pregnancy: results of a large prospective cohort study. Can J Psychiatry 2009; 54:242–6.

158. Einarson A, Bonari L, Voyer-Lavigne S, et al. A multicentre prospective controlled study to determine the safety of trazodone and nefazodone use during pregnancy. Can J Psychiatry 2003;48: 106–10.

159. McElhatton PR, Garbis HM, Eléfant E, et al. The outcome of pregnancy in 689 women exposed to therapeutic doses of antidepressants. A collaborative study of the European Network of Teratology Information Services (ENTIS). Reprod Toxicol 1996;10:285–94.

160. Newport DJ, Ritchie JC, Knight BT, et al. Venlafaxine in human breast milk and nursing infant plasma: determination of exposure. J Clin Psychiatry 2009; 70:1304–10.

161. Bennett PN. Drugs and human lactation: a guide to the content and consequences of drugs, micronutrients, radiopharmaceuticals, and environmental and occupational chemicals in human milk. New York: Elsevier; 1988.

162. Anderka M, Mitchell AA, Louik C, et al. Medications used to treat nausea and vomiting of pregnancy and the risk of selected birth defects. Birth Defects Res A Clin Mol Teratol 2012;94:22–30.

163. Saxen I. Letter: Cleft palate and maternal diphenhydramine intake. Lancet 1974;1:407–8.

164. Gilboa SM, Strickland MJ, Olshan AF, et al. Use of antihistamine medications during early pregnancy and isolated major malformations. Birth Defects Res A Clin Mol Teratol 2009;85:137–50.

165. Kargas GA, Kargas SA, Bruyere HJ Jr, et al. Perinatal mortality due to interaction of diphenhydramine and temazepam. N Engl J Med 1985;313: 1417–8.

166. Little BB, Snell LM, Gilstrap LC 3rd. Methamphetamine abuse during pregnancy: outcome and fetal effects. Obstet Gynecol 1988;72:541–4.

167. Milkovich L, van der Berg BJ. Effects of antenatal exposure to anorectic drugs. Am J Obstet Gynecol 1977;129:637–42.

168. Nora JJ, Trasler DG, Fraser FC. Malformations in mice induced by dexamphetamine sulphate. Lancet 1965;2:1021–2.

169. American College of Obstetricians and Gynecologists Committee on Health Care for Underserved Women. Committee Opinion No. 479: methamphetamine abuse in women of reproductive age. Obstet Gynecol 2011;117:751–5.

170. Dideriksen D, Pottegard A, Hallas J, et al. First trimester in utero exposure to methylphenidate. Basic Clin Pharmacol Toxicol 2013;112:73–6.

171. Laget-Corsin L, Baroche J. Anesthesia with sodium gamma-hydroxybutyrate in cesarean section. Anesth Analg (Paris) 1972;29:43–9 [in French].

172. Lennestal R, Kallen B. Delivery outcome in relation to maternal use of some recently introduced antidepressants. J Clin Psychopharmacol 2007;27: 607–13.

173. Kallen B, Otterblad Olausson P. Antidepressant drugs during pregnancy and infant congenital heart defect. Reprod Toxicol 2006;21:221–2.

174. Berlin CM Jr. Advances in pediatric pharmacology and toxicology. Adv Pediatr 1995;42:593–629.

175. Webster PA. Withdrawal symptoms in neonates associated with maternal antidepressant therapy. Lancet 1973;2:318–9.

Environmental Factors That Can Affect Sleep and Breathing: Allergies

David T. Kent, MD[a], Ryan J. Soose, MD[b],*

KEYWORDS

- Allergic rhinitis • Nasal obstruction • Snoring • Sleep apnea • Sleep • Environment

KEY POINTS

- Sleep disorders, including insomnia and sleep-disordered breathing, are common in patients with allergic rhinitis and contribute greatly to the disease morbidity and effects on daytime function and quality of life.
- The degree of sleep disturbance is directly related to the severity of the allergic disease.
- The negative impact of allergic rhinitis on sleep is complex and multifactorial but is primarily mediated through nasal obstruction, which frequently has a diurnal variation and characteristic worsening in the overnight period and/or the supine position.
- Nasal obstruction increases the likelihood of snoring, obstructive sleep apnea, and intolerance to medical device therapies for sleep apnea.
- Although the impact of allergy and sinonasal treatment on polysomnography measures remains unclear and variable, medical and surgical therapy to lower nasal resistance has been shown to improve snoring, subjective sleep quality, daytime function, as well as disease-specific and general-health quality-of-life measures.

EPIDEMIOLOGIC CONSIDERATIONS

Environmental exposures have a significant role in sleep-disordered breathing. Sleep-related symptoms are common in patients with allergic rhinitis and have been observed for centuries. Hippocrates reported an association between poor sleep and nasal polyposis.[1] Almost 500 years ago, the Dutch physician Levinus Lemnius[2] reported that mouth breathing in the supine position causes restless sleep. Sleep impairment is likely a major contributor to the overall disease morbidity, direct and indirect health care costs, and the loss of work and academic productivity associated with allergic rhinitis. Allergic disease and sleep disturbance are linked via a complex constellation of pathophysiologic, environmental, and patient-related factors (**Fig. 1**).[3]

Epidemiologic studies have estimated that allergic rhinitis afflicts 9% to 42% of the US population, equating to approximately 58 million people as of 2007.[4] Its impact on disease-specific and general-health quality-of-life measures is well documented in large epidemiologic studies as well as controlled clinical trials.[5,6] In a survey of patients with allergies, 48% with seasonal allergic rhinitis (SAR) and 68% with perennial allergic rhinitis reported that their condition interfered

Disclosures: D.T. Kent, MD, none. R.J. Soose, MD, research support from Inspire Medical Systems, and consultant for Inspire Medical Systems, Philips-Respironics.
[a] Department of Otolaryngology, University of Pittsburgh School of Medicine, UPMC, Pittsburgh, PA, USA;
[b] Division of Sleep Surgery, Department of Otolaryngology, University of Pittsburgh School of Medicine, UPMC Mercy Building B, Suite 11500, 1400 Locust Street, Pittsburgh, PA 15219, USA
* Corresponding author.
E-mail address: sooserj@upmc.edu

Clin Chest Med 35 (2014) 589–601
http://dx.doi.org/10.1016/j.ccm.2014.06.013
0272-5231/14/$ – see front matter © 2014 Elsevier Inc. All rights reserved.

chestmed.theclinics.com

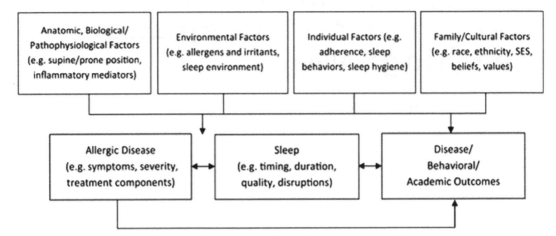

Fig. 1. Conceptual model of the association between allergic disease and sleep. SES, socioeconomic status. (*From* Koinis-Mitchell D, Craig T, Esteban CA. Sleep and allergic disease: a summary of the literature and future directions for research. J Allergy Clin Immunol 2012;130(6):1277; with permission from Elsevier Health Sciences.)

with their sleep.[7] In the Wisconsin Sleep Cohort (a prospective population study of almost 5000 patients), self-reported nocturnal congestion was associated with a 3-fold increased incidence of snoring and daytime sleepiness.[8] Craig and colleagues[9] surveyed more than 2000 patients with allergies and approximately half reported difficulty falling asleep or staying asleep as a result of their allergic condition (**Fig. 2**).

Leger and colleagues[5] showed that allergic rhinitis can affect multiple aspects of sleep with numerous consequences on daytime function. Sleep-related breathing disorders, insomnia, as well as daytime somnolence, morning headaches, and cognitive dysfunction, were all more common in patients with allergic rhinitis compared with controls. In the Wisconsin Sleep Cohort, patients with allergic rhinitis were 1.8 times more likely to have moderate to severe sleep-disordered breathing than those without allergic rhinitis.[8] Furthermore, patients with obstructive sleep apnea (OSA) with allergic rhinitis reported increased levels of general

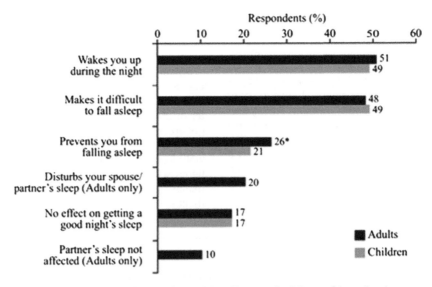

*Significant difference from adult sufferers at the 95% confidence level

Fig. 2. Results of a survey of 2355 patients with allergic rhinitis and the subjective impact of nasal congestion on sleep. Note that approximately half of the respondents reported that their allergy-related nasal congestion makes it difficult to both fall and stay asleep. (*From* Craig TJ, Ferguson BJ, Krouse JH. Sleep impairment in allergic rhinitis, rhinosinusitis, and nasal polyposis. Am J Otolaryngol 2008;29:211; with permission.)

stress and fatigue compared with matched patients with OSA without allergic rhinitis.[10]

In patients with SAR, seasonal variation in sleep-related symptoms has been shown with worsening of subjective sleep quality and daytime sleepiness during the allergy season.[5] Other research has found that subjective and objective sleep measures in patients with allergic rhinitis correlate with the severity of sinonasal disease.[6] As such, sleep disturbance is one of the key factors in the Allergic Rhinitis and its Impact on Asthma (ARIA) guidelines that distinguishes between mild and moderate-severe disease.[11] The degree of sleep impairment, the frequency and duration of respiratory events, and associated daytime dysfunction all seem to be directly related to the severity of the allergic rhinitis (**Figs. 3** and **4**).[6,12,13]

In addition to rhinitis caused by allergic disease, clinicians should recognize that symptomatic nasal obstruction and associated sleep disturbance may result from a multitude of other inflammatory and structural nasal disorders, often in combination. A recent study found that both patients with allergic rhinitis and patients with nonallergic have impaired sleep quality, with up to 83% of patients with nonallergic rhinitis reporting sleep disturbances.[14] McNicholas[15] noted that studies assessing sleep-disordered breathing were more likely to be associated with reversible nasal obstructive disease than chronic obstruction, implying that allergic rhinitis may have an even greater impact on sleep-disordered breathing than static structural problems such as a deviated septum. However, other large epidemiologic studies have confirmed that nasal obstruction of either type is an independent risk factor for both snoring and OSA.[16–18]

PATHOPHYSIOLOGY

The mechanisms by which allergic rhinitis affects sleep are likely multifactorial. Upper airway resistance, fraction of oral breathing, ventilatory effort, obstructive respiratory events, the confounding effects of allergy medication and sedative drugs, anxiety, depression, cytokine production, and other biochemical and hormonal effects all may play a role in the negative impact on sleep quality. Multiple inflammatory mediators have been linked to sleep dysregulation (including interferon gamma, tumor necrosis factor alpha, interleukin [IL]-1β, IL-4, and IL-10).[19,20] Some of these show a circadian rhythm with progressive worsening after midnight in patients with allergic rhinitis, peaking in the early morning hours (**Fig. 5**).[3,9] Proposed mechanisms for the observed diurnal variation in nasal congestion include the gravity effect of the dependent sleeping position, normal nocturnal decline in serum cortisol levels, and upregulation of inflammatory cytokines overnight. Simple elevation of the head of bed may counteract the gravity effect and significantly lower nasal resistance.[21] The increase in nasal congestion and inflammation in the second half of the night may be further compounded by the increased proportion of rapid eye movement (REM) sleep, which is already characterized by autonomic instability and reduced pharyngeal muscle activity.

Medical therapy for allergic rhinitis and/or sleep-disordered breathing may further contribute to the sleep disturbance. Oral antihistamines, frequently used to manage allergy symptoms, are also commonly used by the public as an over-the-counter insomnia treatment despite scant data on improvement in objective sleep measures.

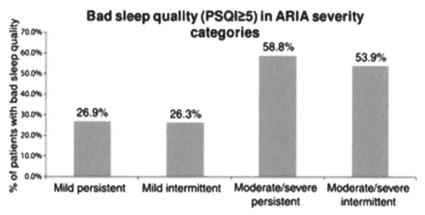

Fig. 3. Pittsburgh Sleep Quality Index (PSQI) scores in relation to ARIA severity categories in a survey of 2275 patients with allergic rhinitis. PSQI scores of greater than or equal to 5 define bad sleepers. (*From* Colás C, Galera H, Añibarro B, et al. Disease severity impairs sleep quality in allergic rhinitis (The SOMNIAAR study). Clin Exp Allergy 2012;42(7):1084; with permission.)

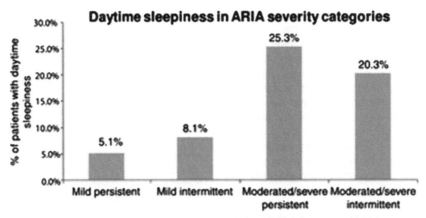

Fig. 4. Excessive daytime sleepiness in relation to ARIA severity categories in a survey of 2275 patients with allergic rhinitis. (*Reprinted from* Colás C, Galera H, Añibarro B, et al. Disease severity impairs sleep quality in allergic rhinitis (The SOMNIAAR study). Clin Exp Allergy 2012;42(7):1084; with permission.)

Oral antihistamines may cause side effects of drowsiness and fatigue as well as dryness of the mucous membranes caused by the anticholinergic effects. Decongestant medications and beta agonist inhalers may cause sleep-onset and sleep-maintenance insomnia. The impact of positive pressure therapy on the nose is still unclear and likely varies from patient to patient. In some

○ Female n = 435   ● Male n = 330

Blocked nose

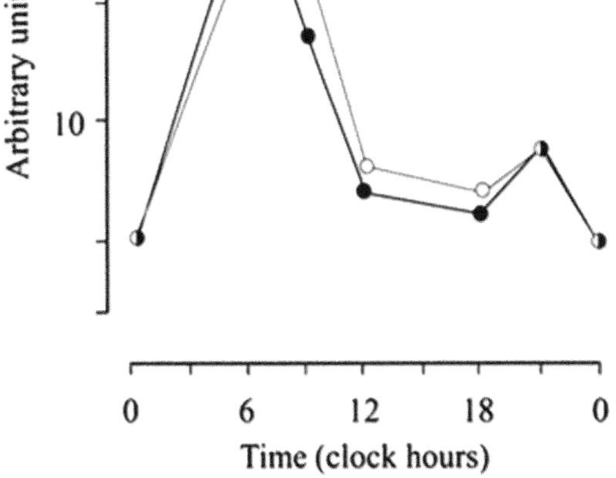

Fig. 5. Circadian variation of nasal congestion shows progressive worsening overnight with an average peak in nasal resistance at approximately 6 AM. (*From* Craig TJ, Ferguson BJ, Krouse JH. Sleep impairment in allergic rhinitis, rhinosinusitis, and nasal polyposis. Am J Otolaryngol 2008;29:211; with permission.)

patients with OSA, continuous positive airway pressure (CPAP) therapy with heated humidification lowers nasal resistance and improves symptoms. However, for other patients, CPAP causes or exacerbates sinonasal symptoms, which may be related to pressure requirements, mask type, and humidity level. A 2012 study by Alahmari and colleagues[22] found that CPAP therapy resulted in the dose-dependent upregulation of inflammatory markers associated with nasal and systemic inflammation as well as reduced mucociliary clearance.

Although the pathophysiology linking allergic rhinitis and sleep disturbance is complex and multifactorial, nasal obstruction seems to be the primary factor. Several airway models and experiments have suggested that nasal obstruction plays a role in sleep-disordered breathing through a variety of mechanisms, regardless of the cause of the nasal resistance (**Table 1**).[23]

Nasal breathing normally accounts for 92% and 96% of inhaled ventilation in awake and sleep states, respectively.[24] The Starling resistor model of the airway explains that increasing the resistance of airflow through the nose (which in normal individuals already accounts for 50% to 66% of total airway resistance[25]) may potentiate the risk of pharyngeal collapse because upstream nasal resistance of airflow generates greater negative intraluminal pressure within the oropharynx during inspiration.[26,27] Many individuals with inadequate nasal airflow also convert to maladaptive oral breathing, which may be associated with a 2.5-fold greater airway resistance[16] and subsequently a narrower and more collapsible pharyngeal airway.[28]

Multiple studies have shown that experimentally induced nasal obstruction leads to abnormal sleep

Table 1
Proposed pathophysiologic mechanisms linking nasal obstruction and sleep-disordered breathing

Starling resistor model	Increased nasal resistance upstream results in increased negative intraluminal pressure (suction force) in the oropharyngeal airway downstream
Unstable oral breathing	Increased nasal resistance results in compensatory increase in oral breathing fraction and shift to breathing through an unstable oral airway, resulting in an increase in total airway resistance
Nasal ventilatory reflex	Decreased nasal airflow results in decreased activation of nasal neurologic receptors with subsequent reduction in pharyngeal muscle activity and central control of breathing
Nitric oxide	Decreased nasal airflow causes reduced lung nitric oxide with resultant potential perfusion ventilation mismatch as well as other central and pharyngeal effects

Adapted from Georgalas C. The role of the nose in snoring and obstructive sleep apnoea: an update. Eur Arch Otorhinolaryngol 2011;268(9):1366; with permission.

continuity, abnormal sleep architecture, and increased obstructive respiratory events in normal patients.[29–34] In contrast, the nasal route of breathing additionally has been shown to improve minute ventilation and increase pharyngeal muscle activity.[35,36] In a randomized, single-blind, placebo-controlled, and sham-controlled crossover study, McLean and colleagues[37] compared the impact of the fraction of oral breathing on objective sleep measures. With polysomnography, they showed that patients with lower nasal resistance and a normal nasal route of breathing had decreased light sleep (stage 1), increased deep sleep (slow wave), increased REM sleep, and improved sleep efficiency. However, nasal obstruction, caused by postoperative nasal packing for example, significantly worsens the apnea-hypopnea index (AHI) in patients with and without OSA.[38]

In addition to physical nasal obstruction, sensorineural feedback from the nose also seems to play a key role in control of breathing during sleep. Even in the absence of anatomic obstruction, abolishment of nasal receptor reflexes with topical lidocaine seems to increase the frequency of obstructive events and depress central respiratory drive.[39] In a controlled crossover study, patients treated with nasal lidocaine (4%) with decongestant had a mean AHI increase from 6.4 to 25.8, compared with the same patients treated with nasal saline with decongestant. An increase in both central and obstructive respiratory events was observed, leading the investigators to conclude that nasal receptor stimulation is critical for central respiratory control and maintenance of pharyngeal muscle activity. Decreased stimulation of these receptors has been found to increase the frequency of apneic episodes as well as their severity.[39,40] In contrast, their activation during normal breathing increases resting respiratory rate and minute ventilation.[41] This pathway may be mediated in part by nitric oxide, which is produced in large quantities in the nose.[42] Nitric oxide acts as a pulmonary vasculature vasodilator, affects pharyngeal muscle activity, and also has central effects on breathing and sleep regulation that are not yet well understood.[42,43]

EVALUATION OF ALLERGIC RHINITIS AND NASAL OBSTRUCTION

A thorough sinonasal history and an upper airway examination are integral components of successful management of patients with sleep-disordered breathing. Symptomatic nasal obstruction and associated sleep disturbance may be caused by a wide variety of medical and structural disorders (**Table 2**). Although considerable overlap exists, in general terms, the inflammatory/mucosal conditions are commonly treated with medical therapy, whereas the structural problems are often modifiable with surgical therapy.

Initial evaluation should focus on a detailed clinical history of allergic and nasal obstructive symptoms as well as a thorough examination to evaluate for both inflammatory and anatomic abnormalities. A thorough nasal evaluation can be brief and inexpensive in the routine patient, and does not necessarily require sophisticated rhinomanometry, imaging, or endoscopic techniques. In-office examination of the external nasal dorsum and anterior rhinoscopy with a nasal speculum and light source is often adequate and informative for most patients and can distinguish between structural and inflammatory causes of nasal obstruction.

History is critical in the evaluation of environmental factors contributing to nasal obstruction. A history of SAR is easy to elicit because most

Table 2
Examples of causes of symptomatic nasal obstruction and associated sleep disturbance

Medical	Structural
Allergic rhinitis	Deviated nasal septum
Vasomotor rhinitis	Inferior turbinate
Atrophic rhinitis	hypertrophy
Rhinitis	Acquired nasal
medicamentosa	deformity
NARES	Nasal valve collapse
Medications (eg,	Concha bullosa
antihypertensives,	Nasal polyps
aspirin, oral	Adenoid hypertrophy
contraceptives)	Tonsillar hypertrophy
Infection (eg, common	Narrow pyriform
cold, chronic	aperture/hard
rhinosinusitis)	palate
Hormonal (eg,	Inverting papilloma
pregnancy,	Neoplasm
hypothyroidism)	Foreign body
Autoimmune (eg,	Synechiae
lupus, Wegener,	Meningocele
rheumatoid	Granulomatous
arthritis)	disease
Occupational (eg,	
chemicals, paint	
fumes, chalk dust,	
sawdust, perfumes)	
Smoking	

Abbreviation: NARES, nonallergic rhinitis with eosinophilia syndrome.

patients can recall the recurrent onset of symptoms in relation to changing seasons or locations. A history of perennial allergic rhinitis may be more difficult to assess, because patients may not recall a clear association between exposure and onset of symptoms. Questions targeting symptoms during a change in environment (such as recent travel) may be helpful in identifying these exposures. Patients may also recall acute exposure events, such as a moldy basement, or work-related exposures, such as sawdust or coal dust. A sinonasal history should also include home or occupational exposures as well as previously attempted successful and unsuccessful medical therapies. Patients may have acclimated to a lifetime of chronic nasal obstruction and may not initially realize the significance of their symptoms. It is also important to assess the temporality of nasal obstruction, because many patients with allergic rhinitis and sleep-disordered breathing primarily experience nasal symptoms when supine and/or overnight. A clinician may miss or underestimate sinonasal disorders if relying only on daytime questioning and examination.

Reliable, validated questionnaires such as the Nasal Obstruction Symptom Evaluation (NOSE) scale or the Sinonasal Questionnaire are quick and easy to administer and may be useful for further quantifying nasal obstruction (**Fig. 6**, **Table 3**).[44,45] Inhalant and food allergy testing, either via skin prick sensitivity or immunoglobulin E–specific blood work, can also provide useful information to implement environmental controls and avoidance strategies. Allergy testing results can also serve as the basis for subcutaneous or sublingual immunotherapy treatment options.

EVIDENCE FOR MEDICAL THERAPY

Treatment of nasal obstruction may be classified broadly into either medical or surgical management strategies, although in practice many patients undertake individualized therapy tailored to their specific symptoms and anatomy. Many allergy exposures can be modulated with behavioral changes including allergen avoidance, dietary modification, and smoking cessation. Medical therapy may be approached through symptomatic management using decongestants, antihistamines, and topical steroid therapy. In patients with more severe allergic rhinitis or persistent symptoms despite environmental and medical treatment options, subcutaneous or sublingual immunotherapy may be beneficial.

Nasal steroids are the most extensively studied medical treatment of allergic rhinitis as it relates to sleep disturbance, and several randomized controlled trials have evaluated their efficacy along with other pharmacologic therapy (**Table 4**).

The largest trial examining the use of intranasal corticosteroids in patients with OSA was recently published by Lavigne and colleagues,[46] who reported statistically significant improvement in supine AHI as well as baseline O_2 saturation in 34 patients with OSA and allergic rhinitis compared with 21 patients without allergic rhinitis. However, the patient group with allergic rhinitis had statistically significant worse AHI at enrollment. Another study, completed by Craig and colleagues[47–50] in 2005, examined the results of 3 previously completed double-blind, placebo-controlled crossover studies on patients with non-OSA allergic rhinitis with sleep-related symptoms. All 3 trials excluded patients with OSA, and varied only in the nasal steroid applied in each trial (budesonide, flunisolide, or fluticasone). Pooled results described a significant decrease in nasal congestion and daytime somnolence, as well as a significant negative correlation between nasal congestion and improved sleep quality as measured using a nonvalidated, self-reported measurement scale.

Over the last 3 months how often, on average, did you have the following symptoms?

	Never	1 - 4 times per month	2 - 6 times per week	Daily
Runny Nose	☐	☐	☐	☐
Post nasal drip	☐	☐	☐	☐
Need to blow your nose	☐	☐	☐	☐
Facial pain/pressure	☐	☐	☐	☐
Nasal obstruction	☐	☐	☐	☐

Scoring: Never (0), 1-4 times per month (1), 2- 6 times per week (2), and daily (3).

Score reported as average of 5 items: range of possible scores 0 - 3.

Fig. 6. The Sinonasal Questionnaire. (*From* Dixon AE, Sugar EA, Zinreich SJ, et al. Criteria to screen for chronic sinonasal disease. Chest 2009;136(5):1330; with permission.)

Keily and colleagues[51] reported on the use of fluticasone in 24 consecutive snoring patients with associated rhinitis using a randomized, placebo-controlled crossover design in 2004. Patients were divided into apneic and nonapneic groups based on an AHI cutoff of 10. The investigators reported a decrease in AHI from 30.3 to 23.3 in the apneic group despite no subjective symptom improvements. Daytime alertness was improved in nonapneic patients without any significant improvement in AHI.

A double-blind parallel study of mometasone versus saline published by Meltzer and colleagues[52] in 2010 found an improvement in sleep quality and quality of life as measured using the Rhinoconjunctivitis Quality of Life Questionnaire–Standardized score (RQLQ), Epworth Sleepiness Scale score (ESS), and Work Productivity and Activities Impairment–Allergy Specific (WPAI-AS) questionnaire score. None of the 30 patients had an AHI greater than 20, and no significant change in AHI or snoring was noted.

The benefit of topical antihistamine therapy on sleep is less clear. In a randomized, double-blinded crossover trial by Golden and colleagues,[53] subjective outcome measures were assessed in patients with allergic rhinitis with sleep-disordered breathing. Twenty-four patients

Table 3
The NOSE scale

	Not a Problem	Very Mild Problem	Moderate Problem	Fairly Bad Problem	Severe Problem
Nasal congestion or stuffiness	0	1	2	3	4
Nasal blockage or obstruction	0	1	2	3	4
Trouble breathing through my nose	0	1	2	3	4
Trouble sleeping	0	1	2	3	4
Unable to get enough air through my nose during exercise or exertion	0	1	2	3	4

From Stewart MG, Witsell DL, Smith TL, et al. Development and validation of the Nasal Obstruction Symptom Evaluation (NOSE) scale. Otolaryngol Head Neck Surg 2004;130:162; with permission.

Table 4
Randomized controlled trials of pharmacologic therapy for nasal obstruction and sleep-disordered breathing

Investigators	Study Design	Patient Population	Objective Outcomes	Subjective Outcomes
Lavigne et al,[46] 2013	Prospective cohort study	21 patients with OSA and AR vs 34 patients with OSA and no AR	Improved O_2 nadir and supine AHI in AR group	Significant improvement in daytime somnolence in AR group
Craig et al,[47] 2005	Pooled data from 3 randomized, double-blind, placebo-controlled crossover studies	69 patients with AR but no OSA	No significant change in AHI (only measured in 1 study)	Decreased daytime somnolence and nasal congestion
Meltzer et al,[52] 2010	Double-blind evaluation of mometasone vs saline	30 patients with AR	No significant change in AHI	Improved QOL; decreased nasal congestion and daytime somnolence
Kiely et al,[51] 2004	Double-blind crossover study of fluticasone vs saline	10 patients without OSA (AHI<10); 13 patients with OSA (AHI>10)	AHI decrease from 30.3 to 23.3 in patients with OSA treated with fluticasone	Improved daytime somnolence in patients without OSA
Golden et al,[53] 2000	Randomized, double-blind crossover trial of azelastine vs saline	24 patients with perennial AR (seasonal AR excluded)	Not measured	Improved rhinorrhea and sleep quality; no improvement in congestion or daytime somnolence
Santos et al,[54] 2008	Randomized, double-blind crossover trial of montelukast vs placebo	31 patients with perennial AR (seasonal AR excluded)	Not measured	Significant improvement in daytime somnolence and fatigue
Kerr et al,[57] 1992	Single-blind crossover study of oxymetazoline and nasal dilator vs placebo	10 patients with OSA	No change in AHI	Improved sleep quality
McLean et al,[37] 2005	Single-blind crossover study of oxymetazoline and nasal dilator vs placebo	10 patients with OSA	Improved AHI, nasal resistance, and sleep architecture	No change in daytime somnolence
Clarenbach et al,[58] 2008	Double-blind crossover study of oxymetazoline vs placebo	12 patients with OSA	No change in AHI	No change in daytime somnolence or sleep quality

Abbreviations: AHI, apnea-hypopnea index; AR, allergic rhinitis; QOL, quality of life.

were randomized to either treatment with azelastine or saline spray. Subjects reported that sleep was subjectively improved with azelastine; however, neither daytime sleepiness nor congestion was significantly improved.

Subjective response to montelukast therapy was examined in a randomized, double-blinded controlled trial by Santos and colleagues[54] in patients with allergic rhinitis. Significant improvement in daytime somnolence and daytime fatigue were noted with montelukast use compared with the placebo group.

Two studies have examined the role of nasal dilators in patients with nasal obstruction.[55,56] A double-blind, crossover study by Pevernagie and colleagues[55] examining an external nasal valve dilator found a decrease in snoring frequency but otherwise no significant improvements in AHI or sleep architecture. Djupesland and colleagues[56] reported worsened AHI with an external valve dilator and no improvement in subjective or objective symptoms. Other available studies examined the use of sympathomimetic decongestant agents that are not likely to be suitable for long-term therapy because of concern for rebound effects, limiting their usefulness for treatment.[37,57,58]

Summarizing the available literature, in patients with sleep-disordered breathing and rhinitis, intranasal steroids may improve both subjective and objective outcome measures, are associated with minimal risk/morbidity, and may provide a useful adjunct to CPAP and other more definitive forms of OSA therapy. Nevertheless, the consistency of the results remains unclear and adherence to intranasal steroids may be suboptimal and difficult to monitor. Further research is needed to determine the role of intranasal steroids, as well as nasal decongestants and other nasal medical therapy, in patients with sleep-disordered breathing and allergic rhinitis.

SURGICAL THERAPY FOR NASAL OBSTRUCTION

In many patients with allergic rhinitis, the symptomatic nasal obstruction and sleep-disordered breathing may be attributable to a combination of both inflammatory and structural disorders. A recent study by de Aguiar Vidigal and colleagues[59] found that patients with moderate to severe sleep apnea were significantly more likely to have significant nasal septal deviation or inferior turbinate hypertrophy.

The management approach to these patients generally involves first identifying and medically treating any underlying inflammatory process that may be present. For structural anatomic problems, surgical therapy can be effective but the specific procedures indicated vary from patient to patient based on the specific anatomic and clinical problem. Surgical therapy also has a role in improving adherence to CPAP.

Structural causes of increased nasal resistance may not be confined to the nasal cavity alone. For example, Benninger and colleagues[60] reported that subjective sleep quality improved significantly following endoscopic sinus surgery in patients with chronic rhinosinusitis. It is well known, particularly in pediatric patients, that adenoid hypertrophy contributes significantly to nasal obstruction and sleep-disordered breathing, and that adenoidectomy can dramatically improve sleep and breathing. However, the impact of tonsillar hypertrophy on nasal resistance may be greatly underestimated. In 2007, Nakata and colleagues[61] showed that patients with OSA with 3 to 4+ tonsils had significantly higher nasal resistance. Furthermore, simple tonsillectomy alone not only improved subjective and objective sleep measures but also greatly lowered nasal resistance.

Although adenotonsillectomy alone often successfully treats most children with OSA, many pediatric patients with allergic rhinitis require concurrent treatment of turbinate hypertrophy. In a large retrospective study, Sullivan and colleagues[62] showed that pediatric patients with enlarged inferior turbinates often had both subjective and polysomnographic evidence of persistent sleep-disordered breathing after adenotonsillectomy alone. These residual symptoms and AHI increase were subsequently improved further with the addition of radiofrequency inferior turbinate reduction. Thus, overlooking treatment of nasal obstruction in children may lead to inadequate sleep apnea management.

Several recent studies have reported on the effect of surgically lowering nasal resistance on both subjective and objective measures of sleep-disordered breathing, although cautious interpretation is needed because of the heterogeneity of the reports and variable outcome measures. A meta-analysis of 13 studies completed by Li and colleagues[63] in 2011 found multiple reports of improved nasal resistance and subjective sinonasal and sleep-related symptoms, despite a lack of significant change in the overall AHI (35.3–33.5; $P = .69$). Reports of improvement in other objective measures of success such as oxygen saturation nadir and improved sleep architecture were more variable. Two additional case series published in 2011 and 2012 additionally failed to show an improvement in AHI, although both reported improved sleep architecture.[64,65]

These reports are consistent with a recent publication by Victores and Takashima,[66] which showed that nasal surgery did not significantly alter patterns of pharyngeal collapse after surgery as assessed by drug-induced sleep endoscopy, nor did it significantly improve the AHI in 24 patients.

It is again important to note that consistent improvement in objective measures of sleep and snoring may be difficult to identify in previous studies because of heterogeneous patient populations and definitions of surgical success. Despite these difficulties, there are significant data regarding subjective outcomes with regard to treatment of nasal obstruction and sleep symptoms. Significant improvement in subjective symptoms were reported in 9 of the 11 aforementioned studies that examined them, with large gains being made in measures of sleepiness and quality of life using tools such as the Epworth Sleepiness Scale and the Short Form Health Survey.[64,67–74] Although AHI provides an important gauge of OSA severity in many patients, it remains only 1 metric of the complex relationship between sleep and breathing. A critical opportunity to improve patients' sleep may be lost by focusing only on the AHI rather than evaluating and managing the patients' subjective symptoms.

Although the current literature suggests that, across a heterogeneous population, lowering nasal resistance has little overall effect on the AHI, select patients, with otherwise good pharyngeal and craniofacial anatomy, in whom the nasal obstruction is a primary contributor to the OSA pathophysiology, may achieve meaningful improvement in AHI with nasal surgery. Findings that have been attributable to successful lowering of the AHI with nasal surgery alone include small tonsils, low modified Mallampati score, and a normal mandibular plane to hyoid distance on cephalometry. In contrast, large tonsils, modified Mallampati III/IV, and/or a low hyoid position suggest an unfavorable improvement in the AHI with nasal surgery alone.[37,67,75]

In addition, treatment of nasal obstruction in patients with OSA can significantly improve adherence and effectiveness of CPAP and oral appliance therapy. Mounting evidence suggests that increased nasal resistance negatively affects success rates and tolerance of medical therapy devices for OSA, which critically depends on regular usage to be effective. High nasal resistance was one of only 2 independent predictors (in addition to body mass index) of inadequate treatment response to oral appliance therapy.[76] Suguira and colleagues[77] concluded that increased nasal resistance was also associated with nonacceptance of CPAP. Further, in patients with poor CPAP compliance and nasal obstruction, lowering nasal resistance with surgical therapy has been shown to lower mean CPAP pressures and improve adherence.[69] Poirier and colleagues[78] recently showed that with careful selection of patients intolerant of CPAP therapy because of nasal obstruction, corrective nasal surgery could dramatically decrease obstructive nasal symptoms, increase CPAP adherence (0.5 hours per night before surgery to 5 hours per night after surgery; $P<.05$), and convert CPAP failures into successes.

SUMMARY

Nasal obstruction is common in both allergic rhinitis and sleep-disordered breathing patient populations. Allergic rhinitis and associated symptomatic nasal obstruction negatively affect sleep through a variety of mechanisms and may contribute to persistent symptoms and poor adherence with medical device therapy for sleep apnea. A history of sinonasal symptoms, particularly those that occur at night or in the supine position, is the cornerstone of the medical evaluation. Validated questionnaires are available to facilitate this process. A brief nasal examination with anterior rhinoscopy provides important information on the inflammatory and structural contributions to the nasal obstruction and helps to guide treatment. More advanced or refractory cases may benefit from otolaryngology consultation and additional radiographic or endoscopic evaluation.

Of the available medical therapy options, intranasal steroids currently have the most data supporting improvement in both sinonasal and sleep-related symptoms, although further investigation is needed. In patients with allergic rhinitis with anatomic contributions to nasal obstruction (particularly those who have failed medical therapy), surgical therapy to lower nasal resistance may improve snoring, subjective sleep quality, daytime alertness, disease-specific and general quality-of-life measures, as well as objective measures of sleep continuity and sleep architecture. Further research efforts would benefit from standardized measurement and outcomes variables as well as the power to carefully elucidate small subgroups of patients who would derive benefit from targeted therapies.

REFERENCES

1. Freind J. Hippocrates, De morbis popularibus. 1717.
2. Lemnius L. Occulta natura miracula. Antwerp (Belgium): Willem Simon; 1559.

3. Koinis-Mitchell D, Craig T, Esteban CA, et al. Sleep and allergic disease: a summary of the literature and future directions for research. J Allergy Clin Immunol 2012;130:1275–81.

4. Charnock DR, Settipane RA. Epidemiology of rhinitis: allergic and nonallergic. Clin Allergy Immunol 2007;19:23–34.

5. Leger D, Annesi-Maesano I, Carat F, et al. Allergic rhinitis and its consequences on quality of sleep: an unexplored area. Arch Intern Med 2006;16: 1744–8.

6. Stuck BA, Czajkowski J, Hagner AE, et al. Changes in daytime sleepiness, quality of life, and objective sleep patterns in seasonal allergic rhinitis: a controlled clinical trial. J Allergy Clin Immunol 2004;113:663–8.

7. Reigel T, Philpot E, Blaiss M, et al. A study to determine the impact of rhinitis on sufferers' sleep and daily routine. J Allergy Clin Immunol 2005;115:S197.

8. Young T, Finn L, Kim H. Nasal obstruction as a risk factor for sleep-disordered breathing. The University of Wisconsin Sleep and Respiratory Research Group. J Allergy Clin Immunol 1997;99:S757–62.

9. Craig TJ, Ferguson BJ, Krouse JH. Sleep impairment in allergic rhinitis, rhinosinusitis, and nasal polyposis. Am J Otolaryngol 2008;29:209–17.

10. Park CE, Shin SY, Lee KH, et al. The effect of allergic rhinitis on the degree of stress, fatigue and quality of life in OSA patients. Eur Arch Otorhinolaryngol 2012;269:2061–4.

11. Mullol J, Maurer M, Bousquet J. Sleep and allergic rhinitis. J Investig Allergol Clin Immunol 2008;18: 415–9.

12. McNicholas WT, Tarlo S, Cole P, et al. Obstructive apneas during sleep in patients with seasonal allergic rhinitis. Am Rev Respir Dis 1982;126:625–8.

13. Colas C, Galera H, Añibarro B, et al. Disease severity impairs sleep quality in allergic rhinitis (The SOMNIAAR study). Clin Exp Allergy 2012; 42:1080–7.

14. Kalpaklioğlu AF, Kavut AB, Ekici M. Allergic and nonallergic rhinitis: the threat for obstructive sleep apnea. Ann Allergy Asthma Immunol 2009;103:20–5.

15. McNicholas WT. The nose and OSA: variable nasal obstruction may be more important in pathophysiology than fixed obstruction. Eur Respir J 2008; 32:3–8.

16. Young T, Finn L, Palta M. Chronic nasal congestion at night is a risk factor for snoring in a population-based cohort study. Arch Intern Med 2001;161: 1514–9.

17. Stradling JR, Crosby JH. Predictors and prevalence of obstructive sleep apnea in 1001 middle-aged men. Thorax 1991;46:85–90.

18. Lofaso F, Coste A, d'Ortho MP, et al. Nasal obstruction as a risk factor for sleep apnoea syndrome. Eur Respir J 2000;16:639–43.

19. Ferguson BJ. Influences of allergic rhinitis on sleep. Otolaryngol Head Neck Surg 2004;130: 617–29.

20. Krouse HJ, Davis JE, Krouse JH. Immune mediators in allergic rhinitis and sleep. Otolaryngol Head Neck Surg 2002;126:607–13.

21. Toh ST, Lin CH, Guilleminault C. Usage of four-phase high-resolution rhinomanometry and measurement of nasal resistance in sleep-disordered breathing. Laryngoscope 2012;122:2343–9.

22. Alahmari MD, Sapsford RJ, Wedzicha JA, et al. Dose response of continuous positive airway pressure on nasal symptoms, obstruction and inflammation in vivo and in vitro. Eur Respir J 2012;40: 1180–90.

23. Georgalas C. The role of the nose in snoring and obstructive sleep apnoea: an update. Eur Arch Otorhinolaryngol 2011;268:1365–73.

24. Fitzpatrick M, Driver H, Chatha N. Partitioning of inhaled ventilation between the nasal and oral routes during sleep in normal subjects. J Appl Physiol (1985) 2003;94:883–90.

25. Ferris BG, Mead J, Opie L. Partitioning of respiratory flow resistance in man. J Appl Physiol 1964; 19:653–8.

26. Smith PL, Wise RA, Gold AR, et al. Upper airway pressure-flow relationships in obstructive sleep apnea. J Appl Physiol 1988;64:789–95.

27. Park SS. Flow-regulatory function of upper airway in health and disease: a unified pathogenetic view of sleep-disordered breathing. Lung 1993; 171:311–33.

28. Meurice J, Marc I, Carrier G. Effects of mouth opening on upper airway collapsibility in normal sleeping subjects. Am J Respir Crit Care Med 1996;153:255–9.

29. Millman RP, Acebo C, Rosenberg C, et al. Sleep, breathing, and cephalometrics in older children and young adults. Chest 1996;109:673–9.

30. Carskadon MA, Bearpark HM, Sharkey KM. Effects of menopause and nasal occlusion on breathing during sleep. Am J Respir Crit Care Med 1997; 155:205–10.

31. Fitzpatrick MF, McLean H, Urton AM. Effect of nasal or oral breathing route on upper airway resistance during sleep. Eur Respir J 2003;22:827–32.

32. Suratt PM, Turner BL, Wilhoit SC. Effect of intranasal obstruction on breathing during sleep. Chest 1986;90:324–9.

33. Lavie P, Fischel N, Zomer J, et al. The effects of partial and complete mechanical occlusion of the nasal passages on sleep structure and breathing in sleep. Acta Otolaryngol 1983;95:161–3.

34. Zwillich C, Pickett C, Hanson F, et al. Disturbed sleep and prolonged apnea during nasal obstruction in normal men. Am Rev Respir Dis 1981;124: 158–60.

35. McNicholas W, Coffey M, Boyle T. Effects of nasal airflow on breathing during sleep in normal humans. Am Rev Respir Dis 1993;147:620–3.

36. Basner R, Simon P, Schwartzstein R, et al. Breathing route influences upper airway muscle activity in awake normal adults. J Appl Physiol 1989;66:1766–71.

37. McLean HA, Urton AM, Driver HS, et al. Effect of treating severe nasal obstruction on the severity of obstructive sleep apnoea. Eur Resp J 2005;25:521–7.

38. Regli A, von Ungern-Sternberg B, Strobel W, et al. The impact of postoperative nasal packing on sleep-disordered breathing and nocturnal oxygen saturation in patients with obstructive sleep apnea syndrome. Anesth Analg 2006;102:615–20.

39. White D, Cadieux R, Lomard R, et al. The effects of nasal anesthesia on breathing during sleep. Am Rev Respir Dis 1985;132:972–5.

40. Berry RB, Kouchi KG, Bower JL, et al. Effect of upper airway anesthesia on obstructive sleep apnea. Am J Respir Crit Care Med 1995;151(6):1857–61.

41. Douglas NJ, White DP, Weil JV, et al. Effect of breathing route on ventilation and ventilatory drive. Respir Physiol 1983;51(2):209–18.

42. Blitzer ML, Loh E, Roddy MA, et al. Endothelium-derived nitric oxide regulates systemic and pulmonary vascular resistance during acute hypoxia in humans. J Am Coll Cardiol 1996;28(3):591–6.

43. Haight JS, Djupesland PG. Nitric oxide (NO) and obstructive sleep apnea (OSA). Sleep Breath 2003;7(2):53–62.

44. Stewart MG, Witsell DL, Smith TL, et al. Development and validation of the Nasal Obstruction Symptom Evaluation (NOSE) scale. Otolaryngol Head Neck Surg 2004;130:157–63.

45. Dixon AE, Sugar EA, Zinreich SJ, et al. Criteria to screen for chronic sinonasal disease. Chest 2009;136(5):1324–32.

46. Lavigne F, Petrof BJ, Johnson JR, et al. Effect of topical corticosteroids on allergic airway inflammation and disease severity in obstructive sleep apnoea. Clin Exp Allergy 2013;43(10):1124–33.

47. Craig T, Hanks C, Fisher L. How do topical nasal corticosteroids improve sleep and daytime somnolence in allergic rhinitis? J Allergy Clin Immunol 2005;116:1264–6.

48. Craig T, Mende C, Hughes K, et al. The effect of topical nasal fluticasone on objective sleep testing and the symptoms of rhinitis, sleep, and daytime somnolence in perennial allergic rhinitis. Allergy Asthma Proc 2003;24:53–8.

49. Craig T, Teets S, Lehman E, et al. Nasal congestion secondary to allergic rhinitis as a cause of sleep disturbance and daytime fatigue and the response to topical nasal corticosteroids. J Allergy Clin Immunol 1998;101:633–7.

50. Hughes K, Glass C, Ripchinski M, et al. Efficacy of the topical nasal steroid budesonide on improving sleep and daytime somnolence in patients with perennial allergic rhinitis. Allergy 2003;58:380–5.

51. Kiely J, Nolan P, McNicholas W. Intranasal corticosteroid therapy for obstructive sleep apnoea in patients with co-existing rhinitis. Thorax 2004;59:50–5.

52. Meltzer E, Munafo D, Chung W, et al. Intranasal mometasone furoate therapy for allergic rhinitis symptoms and rhinitis-disturbed sleep. Ann Allergy Asthma Immunol 2010;105:65–74.

53. Golden S, Teets SJ, Lehman EB, et al. Effect of topical nasal azelastine on the symptoms of rhinitis, sleep, and daytime somnolence in perennial allergic rhinitis. Ann Allergy Asthma Immunol 2000;85(1):53–7.

54. Santos CB, Hanks C, McCann J, et al. The role of montelukast on perennial allergic rhinitis and associated sleep disturbances and daytime somnolence. Allergy Asthma Proc 2008;29(2):140–5.

55. Pevernagie D, Hamans E, Van Cauwenberge P, et al. External nasal dilation reduces snoring in chronic rhinitis patients: a randomized controlled trial. Eur Respir J 2000;15:996–1000.

56. Djupesland P, Skatvedt O, Borgersen A. Dichotomous physiological effects of nocturnal external nasal dilation in heavy snorers: the answer to a rhinologic controversy? Am J Rhinol 2001;15:95–103.

57. Kerr P, Millar T, Buckle P, et al. The importance of nasal resistance in obstructive sleep apnea syndrome. J Otolaryngol 1992;21:189–95.

58. Clarenbach C, Kohler M, Senn O, et al. Does nasal decongestion improve obstructive sleep apnea? J Sleep Res 2008;17:444–9.

59. de Aguiar Vidigal T, Martinho Haddad FL, Gregório LC, et al. Subjective, anatomical, and functional nasal evaluation of patients with obstructive sleep apnea syndrome. Sleep Breath 2013;17(1):427–33.

60. Benninger MS, Khalid AN, Benninger RM, et al. Surgery for chronic rhinosinusitis may improve sleep and sexual function. Laryngoscope 2010;120:1696–700.

61. Nakata S, Miyazaki S, Ohki M, et al. Reduced nasal resistance after simple tonsillectomy in patients with OSA. Am J Rhinol 2007;21:192–5.

62. Sullivan S, Kasey Li, Guilleminault C. Nasal obstruction in children with sleep-disordered breathing. Ann Acad Med Singapore 2008;37:645–8.

63. Li H, Wang P, Chen Y, et al. Critical appraisal and meta-analysis of nasal surgery for obstructive sleep apnea. Am J Rhinol Allergy 2011;25:45–9.

64. Sufioğlu M, Ozmen OA, Kasapoglu F, et al. The efficacy of nasal surgery in obstructive sleep apnea syndrome: a prospective clinical study. Eur Arch Otorhinolaryngol 2012;269(2):487–94.

65. Choi J, Kim E, Kim Y, et al. Effectiveness of nasal surgery alone on sleep quality, architecture, position, and sleep-disordered breathing in obstructive sleep apnea syndrome with nasal obstruction. Am J Rhinol Allergy 2011;25:338–41.

66. Victores AJ, Takashima M. Effects of nasal surgery on the upper airway: a drug-induced sleep endoscopy study. Laryngoscope 2012;122(11):2606–10.

67. Li H, Lee L, Wang P, et al. Can nasal surgery improve obstructive sleep apnea: subjective or objective? Am J Rhinol Allergy 2009;23:e51–5.

68. Koutsourelakis I, Georgoulopoulos G, Perraki E, et al. Randomized trial of nasal surgery for fixed nasal obstruction in obstructive sleep apnoea. Eur Respir J 2008;31:110–7.

69. Nakata S, Noda A, Yagi H, et al. Nasal resistance for determinant factor of nasal surgery in CPAP failure patients with obstructive sleep apnea syndrome. Rhinology 2005;44:296–9.

70. Nakata S, Noda A, Yasuma F, et al. Effects of nasal surgery on sleep quality in obstructive sleep apnea syndrome with nasal obstruction. Am J Rhinol 2008;22:59–63.

71. Verse T, Maurer J, Pirsig W. Effect of nasal surgery on sleep-related breathing disorders. Laryngoscope 2002;112:64–8.

72. Friedman M, Tanyeri H, Lim J, et al. Effect of improved nasal breathing on obstructive sleep apnea. Otolaryngol Head Neck Surg 2000;122:71–4.

73. Tosun F, Kemikli K, Yetkin S, et al. Impact of endoscopic sinus surgery on sleep quality in patients with chronic nasal obstruction due to nasal polyposis. J Craniofac Surg 2009;20:446–9.

74. Li H, Lin Y, Chen N, et al. Improvement in quality of life after nasal surgery alone for patients with obstructive sleep apnea and nasal obstruction. Arch Otolaryngol Head Neck Surg 2008;134: 429–33.

75. Series F, St Pierre S, Carrier G. Surgical correction of nasal obstruction in the treatment of mild sleep apnea: importance of cephalometry in predicting outcome. Thorax 1993;48:360–3.

76. Zeng B, Ng AT, Qian J, et al. Influence of nasal resistance on oral appliance treatment outcome in obstructive sleep apnea. Sleep 2008;31(4):543–7.

77. Suguira T, Noda A, Nakata S, et al. Influence of nasal resistance on initial acceptance of CPAP in treatment of OSAS. Respiration 2007;74:56–60.

78. Poirier J, George C, Rotenberg B. The effect of nasal surgery on nasal continuous positive airway pressure compliance. Laryngoscope 2014;124(1): 317–9.

Index

Note: Page numbers of article titles are in **boldface** type.

A

Abuse
  alcohol- and drug-related
    CCHS and, 542–543
Acetazolamide
  sleep and breathing effects of, 562
Acquired central alveolar hypoventilation
  SDB and, 554
Adaptive servo-ventilation
  for sleep apnea related to heart failure, 530
Air temperature
  in nocturnal asthma, 488–489
Airway resistance
  breathing during sleep effects of, 452–453
  in nocturnal asthma, 483–484
Airway secretions
  in nocturnal asthma, 489
Alcohol
  sleep and breathing effects of, 564
Alcohol abuse
  CCHS and, 542–543
Allergen exposure
  in nocturnal asthma, 489
Allergic rhinitis
  evaluation of, 593–594
ALS. *See* Amyotrophic lateral sclerosis (ALS)
Alzheimer disease
  sleep disruption in, 552
Amyotrophic lateral sclerosis (ALS)
  sleep in, 509–510
    breathing effects on, 547–548
ANSD. *See* Autonomic nervous system dysregulation (ANSD)
Anticholinergic agents
  in nocturnal asthma management, 490
Antidepressants
  sleep and breathing effects of, 561
Antihistamines
  sleep and breathing effects of, 560
Antipsychotics
  atypical
    sleep and breathing effects of, 561–562
Apnea(s)
  central sleep. *See* Central sleep apnea (CSA)
  in children, 460–461
    type, duration, and frequency of, 460–461
  in full-term infants, 460–461
  nocturnal asthma and, 489

in preterm infants, 461
Apnea threshold/CO_2 reserve and changes with sleep
  onset, 475
Arousal responses
  in nocturnal asthma, 487–488
  ventilatory control and, 475–476
Asthma
  nocturnal, **483–493**
    allergen exposure in, 489
    arousal and ventilatory responses in, 487–488
    body and air temperature effects on, 488–489
    bronchial hyper-responsiveness in, 484
    epidemiology of, 483
    flow rates and airway resistance in, 483–484
    GERD and, 489
    hormonal changes in, 485
    inflammatory changes in, 485–486
    lung volume changes in, 486–487
    management of, 490
    mucociliary transport and airway secretions
      in, 489
    parasympathetic system in, 484–486
    pathophysiology of, 483–487
    precipitating factors for, 484–489
    sleep apnea and, 489
    sleep architecture in, 488
  sleep in, **483–493**. *See also* Asthma, nocturnal
Autonomic nervous system dysregulation (ANSD)
  in CCHS, 538

B

β-agonist bronchodilators
  long-acting
    in nocturnal asthma management, 490
Becker muscular dystrophy
  breathing during sleep effects of, 549
Benzodiazepines
  sleep and breathing effects of, 558
Bilevel positive airway pressure (BPAP)
  for sleep apnea related to heart failure, 529–530
Body temperature
  in nocturnal asthma, 488–489
BPAP. *See* Bilevel positive airway pressure (BPAP)
Breathing
  in CHF, **521–534**
  environmental factors affecting, **589–601**.
    See also Environmental factors, sleep and
    breathing effects of

Clin Chest Med 35 (2014) 603–608
http://dx.doi.org/10.1016/S0272-5231(14)00061-6
0272-5231/14/$ – see front matter © 2014 Elsevier Inc. All rights reserved.

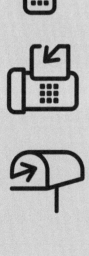
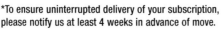

Printed and bound by CPI Group (UK) Ltd, Croydon, CR0 4YY

03/10/2024

01040375-0015